SO-EDI-998

# A·N·N·U·A·L E·D·I·T·I·O·N·S

# Nutrition

*Eleventh Edition*

# 99/00

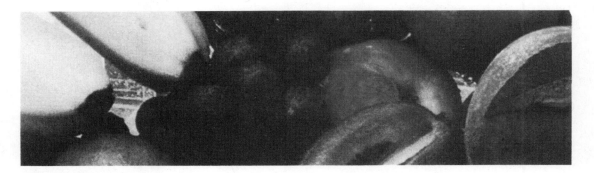

## EDITOR

### Charlotte C. Cook-Fuller
*Towson University*

Charlotte Cook-Fuller has a Ph.D. in community health education and graduate and undergraduate degrees in nutrition. She has worked for several years in public health services and has also been involved with the federally funded WIC (Women, Infants, and Children) program. Now as a professor, she teaches nutrition within both professional and consumer contexts, as well as courses for health education students. She has coauthored a nutrition curriculum for grades K–12 and is currently involved in a multidisciplinary effort to provide strategies to public school teachers for teaching about global issues such as hunger.

## Editorial Consultant

### Stephen Barrett, M.D.
**Editor, *Nutrition Forum***

*Dushkin/McGraw-Hill*
Sluice Dock, Guilford, Connecticut 06437

## Visit us on the Internet
*http://www.dushkin.com/annualeditions/*

## Credits

**1. Trends Today and Tomorrow**
Facing overview—Dushkin/McGraw-Hill illustration by Mike Eagle.
**2. Nutrients**
Facing overview—Photo courtesy of the American Egg Board.
**3. Through the Life Span: Diet and Disease**
Facing overview—© 1999 by Cleo Freelance Photography.
**4. Fat and Weight Control**
Facing overview—© 1999 by PhotoDisc, Inc.
**5. Food Safety**
Facing overview—Dushkin/McGraw-Hill photo by Frank Tarsitano.
**6. Health Claims**
Facing overview—Dushkin/McGraw-Hill photo by Nick Zavalishin.
**7. World Hunger and Malnutrition**
Facing overview—United Nations photo.

## Copyright

Cataloging in Publication Data
Main entry under title: Annual editions: Nutrition. 1999/2000.
1. Nutrition—Periodicals. 2. Diet—Periodicals. I. Cook-Fuller, Charlotte C., *comp.* II. Title: Nutrition.
ISBN 0–07–040354–6        613.2'.05        91–641611        ISSN 1055–6990

© 1999 by Dushkin/McGraw-Hill, Guilford, CT 06437, A Division of The McGraw-Hill Companies.

Copyright law prohibits the reproduction, storage, or transmission in any form by any means of any portion of this publication without the express written permission of Dushkin/McGraw-Hill, and of the copyright holder (if different) of the part of the publication to be reproduced. The Guidelines for Classroom Copying endorsed by Congress explicitly state that unauthorized copying may not be used to create, to replace, or to substitute for anthologies, compilations, or collective works.

Annual Editions® is a Registered Trademark of Dushkin/McGraw-Hill, A Division of The McGraw-Hill Companies.

Eleventh Edition

Cover image © 1999 PhotoDisc, Inc.

Printed in the United States of America        1234567890BAHBAH5432109        Printed on Recycled Paper

Members of the Advisory Board are instrumental in the final selection of articles for each edition of ANNUAL EDITIONS. Their review of articles for content, level, currentness, and appropriateness provides critical direction to the editor and staff. We think that you will find their careful consideration well reflected in this volume.

**Editors/Advisory Board**

## EDITORS

**Charlotte C. Cook-Fuller**
*Towson University*

**with Stephen Barrett, M.D.**
*Editor, Nutrition Forum*

## ADVISORY BOARD

**Becky Alejandre**
*American River College*

**John S. Braubitz**
*Cayuga Community College*

**Valencia Browning**
*Eastern Illinois University*

**Georgia W. Crews**
*South Dakota State University*

**Patricia Erickson**
*Skyline College*

**Sarah T. Hawkins**
*Indiana State University*

**Suzanne Hendrich**
*Iowa State University*

**David H. Hyde**
*University of Maryland
College Park*

**Dorothea J. Klimis**
*University of Maine
Orono*

**Manfred Kroger**
*Pennsylvania State University
University Park*

**Rebecca M. Mullis**
*Georgia State University*

**Gretchen Myers-Hill**
*Michigan State University*

**M. Zafar Nomani**
*West Virginia University*

**Thomas M. Richard**
*Keene State College*

**Karen J. Schmitz**
*Madonna University*

**Donna R. Seibels**
*Samford University*

**Diana M. Spillman**
*Miami University*

**Danielle Torisky**
*James Madison University*

**Linda Elaine Wendt**
*University of Wisconsin
Eau Claire*

**Royal E. Wohl**
*Washburn University*

## EDITORIAL STAFF

**Ian A. Nielsen,** Publisher
**Roberta Monaco,** Senior Developmental Editor
**Dorothy Fink,** Associate Developmental Editor
**Addie Raucci,** Senior Administrative Editor
**Cheryl Greenleaf,** Permissions Editor
**Joseph Offredi,** Permissions/Editorial Assistant
**Diane Barker,** Proofreader
**Lisa Holmes-Doebrick,** Program Coordinator

## PRODUCTION STAFF

**Brenda S. Filley,** Production Manager
**Charles Vitelli,** Designer
**Lara M. Johnson,** Design/
Advertising Coordinator
**Laura Levine,** Graphics
**Mike Campbell,** Graphics
**Tom Goddard,** Graphics
**Juliana Arbo,** Typesetting Supervisor
**Jane Jaegersen,** Typesetter
**Marie Lazauskas,** Word Processor
**Kathleen D'Amico,** Word Processor
**Larry Killian,** Copier Coordinator

**Staff**

# To the Reader

In publishing ANNUAL EDITIONS we recognize the enormous role played by the magazines, newspapers, and journals of the public press in providing current, first-rate educational information in a broad spectrum of interest areas. Many of these articles are appropriate for students, researchers, and professionals seeking accurate, current material to help bridge the gap between principles and theories and the real world. These articles, however, become more useful for study when those of lasting value are carefully collected, organized, indexed, and reproduced in a low-cost format, which provides easy and permanent access when the material is needed. That is the role played by ANNUAL EDITIONS.

New to ANNUAL EDITIONS is the inclusion of related World Wide Web sites. These sites have been selected by our editorial staff to represent some of the best resources found on the World Wide Web today. Through our carefully developed topic guide, we have linked these Web resources to the articles covered in this ANNUAL EDITIONS reader. We think that you will find this volume useful, and we hope that you will take a moment to visit us on the Web at **http://www.dushkin.com** to tell us what you think.

You may agree with Pudd'nhead Wilson (a character created by Mark Twain) who said, "The only way to keep your health is to eat what you don't want, drink what you don't like, and do what you'd rather not." Nutritionists would argue that you can't achieve or maintain good health on a diet of soft drinks and vending machine foods. But you might be surprised to learn that many of your favorite foods can fit into a good diet. In making food choices, remember that variety and moderation are two key words that will assist you in achieving positive health outcomes and avoiding the negative results of excesses or deficiencies.

An array of resources is available to help you make decisions, including popular publications, the news media, scientific journals, and people from many educational backgrounds. Your dilemma is to select reliable sources that will supply factual information based on science rather than exaggerations based on bias. It is important to avoid overreacting to nutrition- and food-related news items or promotional materials, especially if they sound sensational or have shock value. The exaggeration and the myth are what much of the public grasps and, in large measure, reacts to. My challenge to you is to use *Annual Editions: Nutrition 99/00*, preferably with a standard nutrition text, as an invitation to learning. Become a discriminating learner. Compare what you hear and read to the accepted body of knowledge. If this volume provides you with useful information, challenges your thinking, broadens your understanding, or motivates you to take some useful action, it will have fulfilled its purpose.

While this entire volume is essentially one of current events and current thinking, the first unit focuses on trends that give a preview of the future and that relate to characteristics of today's food consumer, the food industry, and views of foods and food components. The next three units are devoted to nutrients, diet and disease, and weight control. All are topics that directly relate to our health, and the dynamic state of knowledge on these subjects requires each of us to be con-

stantly learning and adjusting. Units on food safety and health claims follow, areas in which consumers are especially vulnerable to media and promotional hype and misinformation. The last unit addresses hunger and malnutrition as social and political issues. This unit is intended primarily as a forum for global concerns, but it has become abundantly clear that hunger is also a national issue.

Although the units in this book are distinct, many of the articles have broader significance. The *topic guide* will help you to find other articles on a given subject. Also, World Wide Web sites can be used to further explore topics. These sites are cross-referenced by number in the topic guide. You also will find that many of the articles contain at least some element of controversy, the origin of which may be incomplete knowledge, questionable policy, pseudoscience, or competing needs. Sometimes these are difficult issues to resolve, and frequently any resolution creates further dilemmas. But creatively solving problems is our challenge. We take the world as it is and use it as the foundation for tomorrow's discoveries and solutions.

*Annual Editions: Nutrition 99/00* is an anthology, and any anthology can be improved, including this one. You can influence the content of future editions by returning the postage-paid article rating form on the last page of this book with your comments and suggestions.

*Charlotte C. Cook-Fuller*

Charlotte C. Cook-Fuller
*Editor*

# Contents

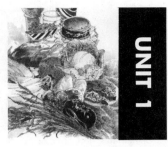

**UNIT 1**

## Trends Today and Tomorrow

Ten articles examine the eating patterns of people today. Some of the topics considered include nutrients in our diet, eating trends, food labeling, and self-service outlets.

---

The concepts in bold italics are developed in the article. For further expansion please refer to the Topic Guide, the Glossary, and the Index. v

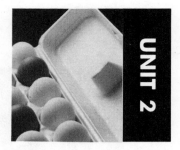

## UNIT 2

## Nutrients

Nine articles discuss the importance of nutrients and fiber in our diet. Topics include dietary standards, carbohydrates, fiber, vitamins, supplements, and minerals.

The concepts in bold italics are developed in the article. For further expansion please refer to the Topic Guide, the Glossary, and the Index.

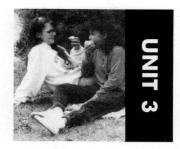

**UNIT 3**

# Through the Life Span: Diet and Disease

Eleven articles examine our health
as it is affected by diet throughout
our lives. Some topics include the
links between diet and disease,
cholesterol, and eating habits.

The concepts in bold italics are developed in the article. For further expansion please refer to the Topic Guide, the Glossary, and the Index.

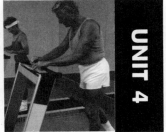

UNIT 4

# Fat and Weight Control

Twelve articles examine weight management. Topics include the relationship between dieting and exercise, the effects of various diet plans, and the relationship between being overweight and fit.

**UNIT 5**

# Food Safety

Seven articles discuss the safety of
food. Topics include foodborne
illness, pesticide residues, naturally
occurring toxins, and food preservatives.

The concepts in bold italics are developed in the article. For further expansion please refer to the Topic Guide, the Glossary, and the Index.

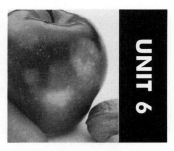

UNIT 6

# Health Claims

Twelve articles examine some of the health claims made by today's "specialists." Topics include quacks, fad diets, and nutrition myths and misinformation.

The concepts in bold italics are developed in the article. For further expansion please refer to the Topic Guide, the Glossary, and the Index.

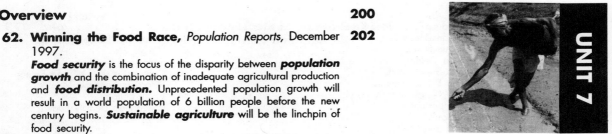

UNIT 7

# World Hunger and Malnutrition

Four articles discuss the world's
food supply. Topics include
global malnutritioin, water
quality, agriculture, and famine.

# Topic Guide

This topic guide suggests how the selections and World Wide Web sites found in the next section of this book relate to topics of traditional concern to students and professionals involved with the study of nutrition. It is useful for locating interrelated articles and Web sites for reading and research. The guide is arranged alphabetically according to topic.

The relevant Web sites, which are numbered and annotated on pages 4 and 5, are easily identified by the Web icon ( ☺ ) under the topic articles. By linking the articles and the Web sites by topic, this ANNUAL EDITIONS reader becomes a powerful learning and research tool.

| TOPIC AREA | TREATED IN | TOPIC AREA | TREATED IN |
|---|---|---|---|
| **Alcohol** | 30. Alcohol and Health<br>☺ ***1, 2, 4, 12, 16, 23*** | | 22. Heart Association Dietary Guidelines<br>23. Answering Nine of Your Cholesterol Questions<br>24. Evidence Mounts for Heart Disease Marker<br>25. New Blood Pressure Guidelines<br>☺ ***1, 2, 3, 4, 5, 8, 10, 11, 12, 13, 14, 15, 16, 18, 21, 23, 24*** |
| **Athletes** | 60. Don't Buy Phony 'Ergogenic Aids'<br>☺ ***31*** | | |
| **Attitudes/ Knowledge** | 1. "What We Eat in America"<br>7. Clearing Up Common Misconceptions<br>61. Unethical Behavior of Pharmacists<br>☺ ***4, 5, 6, 7, 10, 11, 21*** | **Dieting** | 2. Are Reduced-Fat Foods Keeping Americans Healthier?<br>21. Most Frequently Asked Questions<br>34. What It Takes to Take Off Weight<br>35. Skinny on Weight Loss<br>37. Winnowing Weight-Loss Programs<br>38. "Natural" Therapeutics for Weight Loss<br>39. History of Dieting<br>40. Congress Asked to Take Eating Disorders Seriously<br>41. Binge Eating<br>57. Ephedrine's Deadly Edge<br>☺ ***2, 3, 4, 5, 20, 21, 22, 23, 24*** |
| **Cancer** | 11. Are You Getting Enough Fat?<br>20. Fighting Cancer with Food<br>29. Physical Activity and Nutrition<br>☺ ***2, 4, 7, 13*** | | |
| **Controversies** | 2. Are Reduced-Fat Foods Keeping Americans Healthier?<br>5. Freshness Fallacy<br>11. Are You Getting Enough Fat?<br>15. Vitamin Supplements<br>16. Vitamin E Supplements<br>17. Do You Need More Minerals?<br>19. How Important Is Salt Restriction?<br>30. Alcohol and Health<br>32. Body Mass Index and Mortality<br>38. "Natural" Therapeutics for Weight Loss<br>39. History of Dieting<br>54. Alternative Medicine<br>55. 'Dietary Supplement' Mess<br>62. Winning the Food Race<br>☺ ***2, 3, 4, 7, 9, 10, 11, 12, 21, 22, 23, 24, 25, 30*** | | |
| | | **Eating Disorders** | 27. When Eating Goes Awry<br>39. History of Dieting<br>40. Congress Asked to Take Eating Disorders Seriously<br>41. Binge Eating<br>42. Dysfunctional Eating<br>☺ ***2, 16, 22, 23, 24*** |
| | | **Elderly** | 18. Making the Most of Calcium<br>29. Physical Activity and Nutrition<br>32. Body Mass Index and Mortality<br>56. Minding Your Memory<br>☺ ***10, 18, 19*** |
| **Coronary Heart Disease** | 11. Are You Getting Enough Fat?<br>12. Trans Fat<br>21. Most Frequently Asked Questions<br>22. Heart Association Dietary Guidelines<br>23. Answering Nine of Your Cholesterol Questions<br>24. Evidence Mounts for Heart Disease Marker<br>29. Physical Activity and Nutrition<br>☺ ***2, 3, 4, 14, 16, 21, 23, 24*** | **Fats/Substitutes** | 2. Are Reduced-Fat Foods Keeping Americans Healthier?<br>11. Are You Getting Enough Fat?<br>12. Trans Fat<br>23. Answering Nine of Your Cholesterol Questions<br>☺ ***20, 21, 23, 24*** |
| | | **Fiber** | 13. 'Bran-New' Look<br>☺ ***10, 11, 21, 23, 24*** |
| **Diet/Disease** | 8. Doing the DRIs<br>10. Fruits and Vegetables<br>11. Are You Getting Enough Fat?<br>12. Trans Fat<br>13. 'Bran-New' Look<br>17. Do You Need More Minerals?<br>18. Making the Most of Calcium<br>19. How Important Is Salt Restriction?<br>20. Fighting Cancer with Food<br>21. Most Frequently Asked Questions | **Food Allergies** | 28. Food Allergy Myths<br>☺ ***15*** |
| | | **Food Safety** | 44. New Risks in Ground Beef<br>45. Why You Need a Kitchen Thermometer<br>46. For Safety's Sake<br>47. Mad Cows and Americans<br>48. Irradiation<br>49. Codex<br>☺ ***25, 26, 27, 28*** |

2

# World Wide Web Sites

DUSHKIN ONLINE

# ◉ AE: Nutrition

The following World Wide Web sites have been carefully researched and selected to support the articles found in this reader. If you are interested in learning more about specific topics found in this book, these Web sites are a good place to start. The sites are cross-referenced by number and appear in the topic guide on the previous two pages. Also, you can link to these Web sites through our DUSHKIN ONLINE support site at *http://www.dushkin.com/online/*.

**The following sites were available at the time of publication. Visit our Web site—we update DUSHKIN ONLINE regularly to reflect any changes.**

## General Sources

### 1. American Medical Association
*http://www.ama-assn.org*
The venerable AMA offers this site for consumers and health practitioners to find up-to-date nutritional and medical information, discussions of such topics as women's health, and important publications such as the *AMA's journal*.

### 2. Hardin MD
*http://www.lib.uiowa.edu/hardin/md/nutr.html*
This site lists "the *best* sites" that list nutrition, diet, and food sites on the Web. It assigns a "clean bill of health" by placing an asterisk after each site description, and offers instant links to these good sites.

### 3. Health Links
*http://www.hslib.washington.edu*
Open this site to find links to sites of interest to people with knowledge of nutrition and other health sciences. There are links to international health statistics, journals, public health topics, library services, and so on.

### 4. U.S. National Institutes of Health
*http://www.nih.gov*
Consult this site for links to extensive health information and scientific resources. Comprised of 24 separate institutes, centers, and divisions—including the Institute of Mental Health—the NIH is one of eight health agencies of the Public Health Service, which, in turn, is part of the U.S. Department of Health and Human Services.

## Trends Today and Tomorrow

### 5. Food Science and Human Nutrition Extension
*http://www.exnet.iastate.edu/Pages/families/fshn/*
This extensive Iowa State University site links to latest news and reports, consumer publications, food safety information, and many other useful nutrition-related sites.

### 6. U.S. Department of Agriculture
*http://www.usda.gov/news/news.htm*
Visit this site of the USDA to keep up with nutritional news and information. The site provides links to publications, educational resources, and related congressional news.

### 7. U.S. Food and Drug Administration
*http://www.fda.gov/default.htm*
This is the home page of the FDA, which describes itself as the United States' "foremost consumer protection agency." Visit this site and its links to learn about food safety, food and nutrition labeling, and other topics of importance.

### 8. Vegetarian Pages
*http://www.veg.org/veg/*
The Vegetarian Pages are intended to be an independent, definitive Internet guide for vegetarians, vegans, and others. The index and listings will lead you to information about all things vegetarian.

## Nutrients

### 9. Encyclopedia Britannica
*http://www.ebig.com*
This huge Internet guide leads to many informational sites and references and is a good starting point for research into vitamins and other nutrients.

### 10. Food and Nutrition Information Center
*http://www.nal.usda.gov/fnic/*
Use this site to find dietary and nutrition information provided by various USDA agencies, to find links to food and nutrition resources on the Internet, and to access FNIC publications and databases.

### 11. Nutrient Data Laboratory
*http://www.nal.usda.gov/fnic/foodcomp/*
This USDA Agricultural Research Service site provides information about the USDA Nutrient Database. Search here for answers to FAQs, a glossary of terms, facts about food composition, and useful links.

### 12. U.S. National Library of Medicine
*http://www.nlm.nih.gov*
This huge site permits you to search a number of databases and electronic information sources such as MEDLINE, learn about research projects, keep up on nutrition-related news, and peruse the national network of medical libraries.

## Through the Life Span: Diet and Disease

### 13. American Cancer Society
*http://www.cancer.org/frames.html*
Open this site and its various links to learn the concerns—and lifestyle advice—of the American Cancer Society. It provides information on tobacco, alternative therapies, other Web resources, and more.

### 14. American Heart Association
*http://www.amhrt.org*
The AMA offers this site to provide the most comprehensive information on heart disease and stroke as well as late-breaking news. The site presents facts on warning signs, a reference guide, and explanations of diseases and treatments.

### 15. The Food Allergy Network
*http://www.foodallergy.org*
This site, which welcomes consumers, health professionals, and reporters, includes product alerts and updates, information about food allergy, daily tips, and links to other sites.

### 16. Go Ask Alice! from Columbia University Health Services
*http://www.goaskalice.columbia.edu*
This interactive site provides discussion and insight into a number of issues of interest to college-age people—and those younger and older. Many questions about physical and emotional well-being, fitness and nutrition, and alcohol, nicotine, and other drugs are answered.

**17. LaLeche League International**
*http://www.lalecheleague.org*
This site provides important information to mothers who are contemplating breastfeeding. There are links to other sites.

**18. National Osteoporosis Foundation**
*http://www.nof.org*
The NOF has a mission of reducing the widespread prevalence of osteoporosis. It contains information about causes, prevention, detection, and treatment.

**19. National Institute on Aging**
*http://www.nih.gov/nia/*
The NIA, one of the institutes of the U.S. National Institutes of Health, presents this home page to lead you to a variety of resources on health and lifestyle issues that are of interest to people as they grow older.

## Fat and Weight Control

**20. American Society of Exercise Physiologists**
*http://www.css.edu/users/tboone2/asep/toc.htm*
ASEP is devoted to promoting people's health and physical fitness. This extensive site provides links to publications related to exercise, career opportunities in exercise physiology, and the process of professionalization of the field.

**21. The Blonz Guide to Nutrition**
*http://www.wenet.net/blonz/*
The categories in this valuable site report news in the fields of nutrition, food science, foods, fitness, and health. There is also a selection of search engines and links.

**22. Cath's Links to Eating Disorders Resources on the Net**
*http://www.stud.ntnu.no/studorg/ikstrh/ed/*
This collection of links leads to much information on compulsive eating, bulimia, anorexia, and other eating disorders.

**23. Healthfinder**
*http://www.healthfinder.gov*
This U.S. Department of Health and Human Services consumer site has extensive links to information on such topics as the health benefits of exercise, weight control, and prudent lifestyle choices.

**24. MedWeb Plus**
*http://www.medwebplus.com/subject/*
This massive site has links to information and resources on all topics in nutritional health, from dietary supplements to eating disorders. It is useful for research into other topics in health science, such as weight control.

## Food Safety

**25. Centers for Disease Control and Prevention**
*http://www.cdc.gov*
The CDC offers this home page, from which you can learn information about travelers' health, data and statistics related to disease control and prevention, general nutritional and health information, publications, and more.

**26. Center for Food Safety and Applied Nutrition**
*http://vm.cfsan.fda.gov*
This informative site leads you to other sites that will tell you everything you might want to know about food safety and what government agencies are doing to ensure it.

**27. Food Safety and Inspection Service**
*http://www.fsis.usda.gov*
The FSIS, part of the U.S. Department of Agriculture, is the government agency "responsible for ensuring that the nation's commercial supply of meat, poultry, and egg products is safe, wholesome, and correctly labeled and packaged." This is its home page.

**28. Food Safety Project**
*http://www.exnet.iastate.edu/Pages/ families/fs/*
The goal of this project is to develop educational materials that help the public to minimize the risk of foodborne illness. The site contains food safety lessons, 10 steps to a safe kitchen, consumer control points, and food law and food irradiation facts.

## Health Claims

**29. Alt-MEDMarket**
*http://alt.medmarket.com/indexes/indexmfr.html*
This commercial site bills itself as "the Internet guide to alternative therapies and products." Click on the "Alternative Health E-Mall" for an alternative medicine directory and herbal information center; alternative medicine providers, listed by geographic area and specialty; a listing of articles; herbs with their corresponding treatments; and other information.

**30. National Center for Complementary Alternative Medicine (NCCAM)**
*http://altmed.od.nih.gov/nccam/*
Established by Congress in 1998, NCCAM sponsors this Web site, which provides helpful information on alternative medicine therapies and treatments.

**31. QuackWatch**
*http://www.quackwatch.com*
Quackwatch Inc., a nonprofit corporation, provides this consumer guide to examine health fraud and quackery. Data for intelligent decision making on traditional and alternative health topics are also presented.

## World Hunger and Malnutrition

**32. Population Reference Bureau**
*http://www.prb.org*
This is a key source for global population information—a good place to pursue data on nutrition problems worldwide.

**33. World Health Organization**
*http://www.who.ch/Welcome.html*
This home page of the World Health Organization will provide you with links to a wealth of statistical and analytical information about health and nutrition around the world.

**34. World Hunger Year**
*http://www.iglou.com/why/ria.htm*
WHY offers this site as part of its program called Reinvesting in America, its effort to help people fight hunger and poverty in their communities. Various resources and models for grassroots action are included here.

**35. WWW Virtual Library: Demography & Population Studies**
*http://coombs.anu.edu.au/ResFacilities/DemographyPage.html*
This is a definitive guide to demography and population studies. A multitude of important links to information about global poverty and hunger can be found here.

**We highly recommend that you review our Web site for expanded information and our other product lines. We are continually updating and adding links to our Web site in order to offer you the most usable and useful information that will support and expand the value of your Annual Editions. You can reach us at:**
*http://www.dushkin.com/annualeditions/.*

www.dushkin.com/online/

## Unit Selections

1. **"What We Eat in America" Survey,** *Nutrition Today*
2. **Are Reduced-Fat Foods Keeping Americans Healthier?** *Tufts University Health & Nutrition Letter*
3. **Low-Calorie Sweeteners: Adding Reduced-Calorie Delights to a Healthful Diet,** *Food Insight*
4. **Are Fruits and Vegetables Less Nutritious Today?** *University of California at Berkeley Wellness Letter*
5. **The Freshness Fallacy,** Minna Morse
6. **The Truth about Organic 'Certification,'** Stephen Barrett
7. **Clearing up Common Misconceptions about Vegetarianism,** *Tufts University Health & Nutrition Letter*
8. **Doing the DRIs,** Stephen Barrett
9. **An FDA Guide to Dietary Supplements,** Paula Kurtzweil
10. **Fruits and Vegetables: Nature's Best Protection,** *Consumer Reports on Health*

## Key Points to Consider

❖ What current consumer trends and food industry trends will and will not support healthier lifestyles?

❖ Find several reduced-fat foods in the grocery store. Compare them to their regular counterparts and explain what you find.

❖ What demands do you think your generation will place on the food industry two or three decades from now?

❖ What do you see as the issues related to the use of organic foods? How would you decide whether or not to buy them?

❖ Does change always equal progress? Why or why not? Give examples from the nutrition field.

❖ Is the philosophical change that has occurred with the change from RDAs to DRIs a good one? Defend your answer.

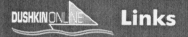 **Links** **www.dushkin.com/online/**

5. **Food Science and Human Nutrition Extension**
   *http://www.exnet.iastate.edu/Pages/families/fshn/*
6. **U.S. Department of Agriculture**
   *http://www.usda.gov/news/news.htm*
7. **U.S. Food and Drug Administration**
   *http://www.fda.gov/default.htm*
8. **Vegetarian Pages**
   *http://www.veg.org/veg/*

These sites are annotated on pages 4 and 5.

# Trends Today and Tomorrow

*It is change, continuing change, inevitable change, that is the dominant factor in society today. No sensible decision can be made any longer without taking into account not only the world as it is, but the world as it will be.*

*—Isaac Asimov, 1981*

The average consumer is a phantom, constantly reshaping and reemerging under the influences of the food industry, the media, activist organizations, and whatever health headlines are currently most persuasive. For the sake of heart health, we have been persuaded first to switch from animal fats to vegetable oils and margarine, then to avoid tropical oils, and now to beware of trans-fatty acids produced in the manufacture of solid margarine. Americans are constantly bombarded by health and nutrition messages and admonitions, many of which are misleading and contradictory. It is no wonder that consumers are confused and disenchanted with conventional sources of advice. As more and more people access the Internet, this problem may be exacerbated rather than lessened.

American consumers appear to understand the link between nutrition and good health; yet many admit they don't always act on their knowledge. Most still believe in good and bad foods, unaware that it is the total diet and not single foods that counts. The first article in this book provides data showing the correlation between people's attitudes and knowledge about nutrition and their nutrient intakes and food choices. Market trends indicate that consumers increasingly are less likely to prepare food and more willing to spend for ready-to-eat, great-tasting, and easily accessible meals. They also are more likely to find these meals at supermarkets rather than restaurants and fast food outlets. Today nearly half of all current culinary school graduates are employed in supermarkets, where the increasing diversity of gourmet, ethnic, and organic options is evident.

Consumers' beliefs and behaviors are not always consistent. On the one hand, shoppers agree that a plethora of reduced- and no-fat products are one of the most important recent developments in the market, yet taste has become the most important factor when choosing food. Consumption of a spartan meal followed by an exceptionally rich dessert is not uncommon, and food companies are promoting this indulgence with language designed to leave the consumer guilt-free. The Food Marketing Institute says consumers find that their cravings are not satisfied with fat-free foods. Perhaps that is why the McLeans Deluxe burger, Sara Lee's low-fat desserts, Taco Bell's light tacos, and Kentucky Fried Chicken's skinless chicken options all bombed. One can, of course, inquire whether the reduced-fat foods have resulted in greater consumer health. The answers found in the second article may surprise you.

With a renewed focus on calories rather than on fat, interest in low-calorie sweeteners may increase as well. The third article describes the sweeteners that are in use and those that are awaiting approval from the FDA. One of these, sucralose, has since been approved. Information about the approval process is also informative.

The next three articles discuss plant products and may dispel common misinformation. In recognition of strong supporting evidence, the FDA has recently agreed to allow canned fruits and vegetables, as well as fresh and frozen ones, to be sold as "healthy." In fact, nutritionally speaking, fresh equals frozen equals canned. Furthermore, and contrary to common belief, it is not the vitamin content of a crop that suffers from being grown on depleted soil but rather the size of the crop produced. Common sense tells us that farmers can't afford this lack of productivity and must replenish their soil. The nutrient value of plants will vary by climate, handling, and the genetic potential of different varieties. Then there is the issue of organic foods, a huge industry that is growing about 20 percent yearly. But what makes foods "organic"? Currently 33 private and 11 state certifying bodies make these decisions, and each has its own seal and set of criteria. The USDA has been trying to reach consensus with farmers and food processors about a common set of standards. It is hoped that they will be successful by the time this book is in print.

Although more people report being vegetarians than appear to be totally dedicated to the concept, there is still a great deal of interest in this lifestyle. Much confusion about it remains, however, including how healthy it is and what desirable effects this lifestyle may have on the environment. Straightforward answers are provided in the article on vegetarianism, which should clarify some of the issues.

Since 1941 the familiar RDAs, or Recommended Dietary Allowances, have provided us with recommendations for amounts of nutrients to be consumed daily. These guidelines are revised every few years, and changes are based on new knowledge of human dietary needs and physiology. The newest version, now called DRIs for Dietary Reference Intakes, is being released in a series of reports. The first set to be published relates to bone health, and—as expected—there are changes in calcium recommendations. The new guidelines mirror a shift in philosophical emphasis, from that of preventing deficiencies to that of preventing chronic diseases, which is based on our expanded knowledge of diet/disease relationships.

A continuing trend worthy of note is reliance on the supposed health benefits of herbal and other dietary supplements, the topic of another article in this unit. Yet many questions of both safety and efficacy remain. Consumers often mistakenly believe that the government protects them against all such products if harmful, but this is not the case. The 1994 Dietary Supplement Health and Education Act allows consumers greater access to more supplements and limits the power of the FDA to regulate them. Once on the market, a dietary supplement must be proved unsafe before the FDA can act to restrict its use. Some members of the supplement industry are working to regulate themselves by establishing good manufacturing practices and voluntarily alerting consumers to the potentially negative effects of some supplements.

The final article in this unit reminds us that the best current wisdom dictates eating a wide variety of foods with emphasis on fruits, vegetables, and whole grains. The benefits of such a diet are considerable, for fruits and vegetables contain not only large amounts of valuable nutrients, but many other chemicals which act as antioxidants to protect the body against chronic and degenerative diseases. If followed, this diet negates the need to consider supplements or manufactured foods.

7

# "What We Eat in America" Survey

### Highlights from USDA's 1994 Continuing Survey of Food Intakes by Individuals and 1994 Diet and Health Knowledge Survey[a]

Results of the first year of the USDA's 10th Nationwide Food Consumption Survey has been released in a set of 14 tables. Information from the table recording the mean nutrient intake per individual by age and sex for 1 day in 1994 is presented in Table 1. The complete set of data tables can be accessed on the Internet at http://www.barc.usda.gov/bhnrc/foodsurvey/csfii94.htm.

These surveys are being conducted by the Agricultural Research Service (ARS) of the US Department of Agriculture (USDA). The CSFII 1994–96, popularly known as "What we Eat in America", is the third in a series of continuing surveys conducted since 1985. The Diet and Health Knowledge Survey (DHKS), which is a telephone follow-up to CSFII, was initiated in 1989. Both surveys were uniquely designed so that individuals' attitudes and knowledge about healthy eating could be linked with their food choices and nutrient intakes.

## OBJECTIVES AND SCOPE

The objectives of the surveys are to:

- **Measure the kinds and amounts of food eaten by Americans.** This objective addresses the requirements of the National Nutrition Monitoring and Related Research Act of 1990 (P.L. 101-445) for continuous monitoring of the nutritional status of the American population, including the low-income population.
- **Measure attitudes and knowledge about diet and health among Americans.**

Following a pilot study of the data collection methods, data collection for the full survey began in January 1994. In each of the 3 survey years, a nationally representative sample of approximately 5000 individuals is asked to provide, through in-person interviews, food intake for 2 nonconsecutive days and socioeconomic and health-related information. About 2 weeks after the CSFII, 2000 selected individuals from the survey households are asked to answer a series of questions in a telephone about knowledge and attitudes toward dietary guidance and health. The number of CSFII respondents is anticipated to be between 15,000 and 16,000 over 3 years. The number of DHKS respondents is expected to be between 4,000 and 5,000 over 3 years. The results of the 2nd and 3rd years will be released in subsequent reports.

## CHANGES

The CSFII/DHKS 1994–96 differs from the 1989–91 surveys in several important ways. Compared with earlier surveys, the 1994–96 surveys include:

[a]Highlights presented were based on information provided by L. E. Cleveland, J. D. Goldman, and L. G. Borrund. Data tables: Results from USDA's Continuing Survey of Food Intakes by Individuals and 1994 Diet and Health Knowledge Survey. Agricultural Research Service, US Department of Agriculture, Riverdale, MD 20737.

From *Nutrition Today*, January/February 1997, pp. 37-40. © 1997 by Williams & Wilkins. Reprinted by permission.

## Table 1
## Mean Nutrient Intake per Individual by Age and Sex for 1 Day[a]

| Sex and Age (yr) | Percentage of population | Food energy (kcal) | Protein (g) | Total fat (g) | Saturated fatty acids (g) | Mono-unsaturated fatty acids (g) | Poly-unsaturated fatty acids (g) | Cholesterol (mg) | Carbohydrate (g) | Dietary fiber (g) | Vitamin A[b] (µg) | Carotenes[b] (µg) | Vitamin E[c] (mg) | Vitamin C (mg) | Thiamin (mg) | Riboflavin (mg) | Niacin (mg) | Vitamin B-6 (mg) | Folate (µg) | Vitamin B-12 (µg) | Calcium (mg) | Phosphorus (mg) | Magnesium (mg) | Iron (mg) | Zinc (mg) | Copper (mg) | Sodium (mg) | Potassium (mg) |
|---|---|---|---|---|---|---|---|---|---|---|---|---|---|---|---|---|---|---|---|---|---|---|---|---|---|---|---|---|
| **Males and females:** | | | | | | | | | | | | | | | | | | | | | | | | | | | | |
| >1 | 1.0 | 840 | 22.8 | 37.4 | 15.8 | 10.5 | 82 | 66 | 104.3 | 3.1 | 993 | 194 | 13.6 | 96 | .90 | 1.40 | 10.9 | 0.63 | 113 | 3.72 | 671 | 536 | 94 | 16.0 | 5.7 | .8 | 507 | 1084 |
| 1–2 | 3.2 | 1322 | 50.0 | 48.0 | 19.6 | 17.6 | 72 | 185 | 177.4 | 8.8 | 741 | 273 | 4.6 | 98 | 1.11 | 1.67 | 13.0 | 1.31 | 176 | 3.34 | 823 | 952 | 185 | 10.9 | 7.2 | .7 | 1988 | 2000 |
| 3–5 | 4.7 | 1552 | 55.0 | 58.0 | 219 | 222 | 9.8 | 183 | 208.8 | 10.2 | 758 | 244 | 5.6 | 93 | 1.29 | 1.75 | 15.6 | 1.40 | 206 | 3.49 | 796 | 1010 | 196 | 11.9 | 7.9 | .8 | 2419 | 1999 |
| ≥5 | 8.9 | 1392 | 49.7 | 52.1 | 20.3 | 19.3 | 8.7 | 171 | 186.1 | 8.9 | 776 | 249 | 6.1 | 95 | 1.18 | 1.68 | 14.2 | 1.29 | 185 | 3.46 | 792 | 938 | 181 | 12.0 | 7.4 | .8 | 2056 | 1900 |
| **Males** | | | | | | | | | | | | | | | | | | | | | | | | | | | | |
| 6–11 | 4.6 | 1980 | 70.4 | 73.8 | 27.4 | 28S | 12.5 | 234 | 266.1 | 13.3 | 1061 | 354 | 6.9 | 96 | 1.76 | 2.29 | 21.3 | 1.86 | 288 | 4.83 | 972 | 1251 | 243 | 15.9 | 10.5 | 1.0 | 3067 | 2409 |
| 12–19 | 5.7 | 2760 | 97.4 | 00.6 | 35.4 | 39.2 | 18.4 | 327 | 372.1 | 17.4 | 1010 | 297 | 9.7 | 122 | 2.10 | 2.57 | 28.0 | 2.21 | 328 | 5.86 | 1,125 | 1619 | 311 | 19.2 | 14.2 | 1.4 | 4223 | 3023 |
| 20–29 | 7.0 | 2943 | 110.8 | 108.9 | 37.6 | 42.2 | 20.6 | 375 | 344.9 | 18.6 | 953 | 428 | 10.1 | 121 | 2.06 | 2.50 | 32.9 | 2.47 | 321 | 5.97 | 1,025 | 1691 | 350 | 19.3 | 15.1 | 1.6 | 4574 | 3337 |
| 30–39 | 8.8 | 2614 | 100.3 | 100.8 | 33.9 | 39.0 | 20.2 | 351 | 316.8 | 19.2 | 1087 | 482 | 12.2 | 113 | 2.07 | 2.36 | 29.6 | 2.37 | 325 | 6.14 | 943 | 1546 | 341 | 19.4 | 15.0 | 1.6 | 4317 | 3326 |
| 40–49 | 6.7 | 2448 | 100.1 | 93.6 | 31.2 | 36.2 | 18.7 | 343 | 288.7 | 18.6 | 1161 | 543 | 10.0 | 104 | 1.96 | 2.23 | 28.7 | 2.16 | 297 | 5.98 | 895 | 1527 | 344 | 17.9 | 13.4 | 15 | 4197 | 3346 |
| 50–59 | 4.7 | 2160 | 85.0 | 82.2 | 26.1 | 31.9 | 17.8 | 295 | 262.7 | 17.5 | 1038 | 528 | 9.3 | 102 | 1.78 | 1.99 | 26.3 | 2.04 | 281 | 5.48 | 728 | 1300 | 302 | 16.0 | 12.6 | 1.4 | 3746 | 2987 |
| 60–69 | 3.5 | 2079 | 83.7 | 80.5 | 26.4 | 31.0 | 16.6 | 302 | 250.1 | 18.6 | 1244 | 641 | 9.2 | 100 | 1.70 | 2.03 | 25.1 | 2.01 | 279 | 6.04 | 766 | 1308 | 310 | 17.5 | 12.6 | 1.4 | 3549 | 3054 |
| ≥70 | 3.3 | 1873 | 74.0 | 71.1 | 24.0 | 27.4 | 14.0 | 275 | 234.8 | 18.2 | 1560 | 641 | 9.6 | 100 | 1.69 | 2.10 | 22.5 | 1.98 | 297 | 7.42 | 750 | 1217 | 288 | 17.1 | 12.3 | 1.4 | 3234 | 2799 |
| ≥20 | 34.0 | 2460 | 96.1 | 93.6 | 31.4 | 36.2 | 18.7 | 334 | 294.9 | 18.6 | 1129 | 521 | 10.4 | 109 | 1.93 | 2.25 | 28.5 | 2.23 | 305 | 6.10 | 884 | 1482 | 330 | 18.2 | 13.9 | 1.5 | 4048 | 3207 |
| **Females** | | | | | | | | | | | | | | | | | | | | | | | | | | | | |
| 6–11 | 4.4 | 1747 | 61.1 | 64.8 | 23.8 | 24.8 | 11.4 | 195 | 237.2 | 11.6 | 792 | 246 | 6.4 | 98 | 1.45 | 1.92 | 17.7 | 1.48 | 237 | 3.74 | 859 | 1121 | 217 | 13.0 | 9.0 | .9 | 2724 | 2113 |
| 12–19 | 5.5 | 1898 | 67.5 | 69.4 | 24.8 | 26.6 | 12.7 | 220 | 257.7 | 13.1 | 884 | 373 | 6.8 | 96 | 1.47 | 1.82 | 18.8 | 1.54 | 236 | 4.12 | 809 | 1148 | 225 | 13.8 | 10.2 | 1.0 | 3081 | 2279 |
| 20–29 | 7.1 | 1791 | 65.9 | 66.1 | 22.8 | 25.0 | 13.3 | 225 | 228.5 | 12.4 | 764 | 340 | 7.2 | 89 | 1.34 | 1.65 | 19.0 | 1.52 | 224 | 3.94 | 725 | 1098 | 223 | 12.7 | 9.5 | 1.1 | 2917 | 2208 |
| 30–39 | 8.9 | 1648 | 64.0 | 60.4 | 19.9 | 23.1 | 12.6 | 209 | 210.7 | 13.4 | 982 | 521 | 7.0 | 79 | 1.33 | 1.60 | 19.0 | 1.54 | 228 | 4.19 | 638 | 1031 | 231 | 12.8 | 9.6 | 1.0 | 2850 | 2253 |
| 40–49 | 6.7 | 1663 | 65.3 | 61.6 | 20.2 | 23.5 | 13.1 | 213 | 214.0 | 14.4 | 952 | 570 | 8.2 | 94 | 1.34 | 1.58 | 19.5 | 1.49 | 227 | 3.85 | 663 | 1029 | 244 | 13.2 | 9.5 | 1.1 | 2833 | 2477 |
| 50–59 | 52 | 1559 | 629 | 59.4 | 19.3 | 22. | 13.2 | 217 | 192.5 | 14.0 | 943 | 513 | 7.2 | 93 | 1.27 | 1.50 | 18.7 | 1.51 | 218 | 4.40 | 607 | 1001 | 237 | 12.8 | 8.4 | 1.0 | 2702 | 2399 |
| 60–69 | 4.3 | 1507 | 61.0 | 56.4 | 18.6 | 212 | 12.0 | 215 | 191.8 | 15.3 | 1115 | 586 | 6.8 | 103 | 1.29 | 1.55 | 18.0 | 1.48 | 224 | 5.25 | 602 | 968 | 236 | 12.8 | 8.7 | 1.1 | 2718 | 2415 |
| ≥70 | 4.7 | 1363 | 56.4 | 47.9 | 15.7 | 18.0 | 10.3 | 188 | 182.1 | 14.0 | 1049 | 509 | 6.0 | 87 | 1.24 | 1.50 | 17.6 | 1.48 | 229 | 4.62 | 547 | 893 | 217 | 12.0 | 8.3 | 1.0 | 2413 | 2177 |
| ≥20 | 36.9 | 1613 | 63.2 | 59.5 | 19.8 | 22.5 | 12.6 | 212 | 206.4 | 13.8 | 953 | 500 | 7.0 | 89 | 1.31 | 1.57 | 18.8 | 1.15 | 225 | 4.29 | 639 | 1015 | 231 | 12.6 | 9.1 | 1.1 | 2768 | 2315 |
| All individuals | 100.0 | 1985 | 75.6 | 74.2 | 25.4 | 28.4 | 14.6 | 257 | 251.0 | 15.0 | 994 | 448 | 8.2 | 99 | 1.59 | 1.93 | 22.3 | 1.79 | 259 | 4.91 | 798 | 1224 | 264 | 15.1 | 11.0 | 1.2 | 3264 | 2615 |

[a] Excludes breast-fed children.
[b] Retinol equivalents.
[c] Tocopherol equivalents.

- A target population of noninstitutionalized individuals in all 50 states rather than the 48 coterminous states.
- The collection of 2 nonconsecutive days of food intake through in-person interviews rather than 3 consecutive days of food intake using a 1-day recall and a 2-day record.
- Oversampling of the low-income population, rather than a separate low-income survey.
- A larger sample in selected age-sex categories, specifically young children and elderly.
- Subsampling within households, rather than the collection of information from all members of a household.
- Collection of DHKS data from adults 20 years of age and older, rather from only main meal-planners/-preparers.
- Additional questions on attitudes and knowledge about using food labels, and
- Tighter management controls to minimize nonresponse.

The tables provide national probability estimates for the US population. The results are weighted to adjust for differential rates of selection and nonresponse and to calibrate the sample to match population characteristics that are correlated with eating behavior. Sample sizes on which estimates are based are provided in an Appendix. In general, the sample sizes for each sex-age group provide a sufficient level of precision to ensure statistical reliability of the estimates. The one exception is the sample size for children less than 1 year of age. Estimates for that group should be used with caution. Statistical issues are discussed in another Appendix.

### SELECTED HIGHLIGHTS FROM TABLE 1: NUTRIENT INTAKE OF INDIVIDUALS

Among adults 20 years of age and older:

- Men consume an average of about 2500 calories per day. Women consume an average of about 1600 calories/day.
- The average cholesterol intake by men (334 mg/day) exceeds

the recommendation to consume no more than 300 mg/day. Women's average intake (212 mg/day) meets the recommendation.

- Average daily sodium intakes from foods alone are over 4000 mg for men and almost 3000 mg for women. Total intakes of sodium are even higher, because these values do not include sodium from salt added to foods at the table. These intakes exceed the recommendation to consume no more than 2400 mg/day.
- Men consume an average of 19 g of dietary fiber/day, and women consume an average of 14 g. The National Cancer Institute recommends that people consume 20 to 30 g of dietary fiber daily.
- Although Americans have a wide variety of nutritious foods from which to choose, some people choose diets that put them at risk for nutrient shortfalls. Average intakes of women 20 years of age and older are below Recommended Dietary Allowances (RDAs) for six nutrients—vitamin E, vitamin B-6, calcium, magnesium, iron, and zinc. Average intakes of men are below RDAs for zinc and magnesium. The farther that average intakes fall below the RDAs, the greater the likelihood that some people have inadequate intakes.

**Highlights from Data on Percentage of Individuals Meeting 100% of the 1989 RDAs by Sex and Age, 2-Day Average, 1994.** Interpreting the data in this table: "The RDAs provide a safety factor appropriate to each nutrient, and exceed the actual requirements of most individuals." Thus, individuals with intakes below the RDA do not necessarily have inadequate intakes. However, as the percentage of the population with intakes below 100% of a given RDA increases, so does the likelihood that some individuals in the population are at nutritional risk.

*Selected Highlights.*

- Less than one fourth of women 20 years of age and older have

diets that provide 100% of the RDAs for calcium (21%), magnesium (22%), and zinc (17%).

- Less than one half the men of the same age, 45%, 37%, and 35%, have diets providing 100% of the RDA for these nutrients, respectively.

**Intakes for Total Fat, Saturated Fat, and Cholesterol, 2-Day Average, 1994.** *Selected Highlights.* The 1995 Dietary Guidelines for Americans recommend that people 2 years of age and older choose a diet with no more than 30% of calories from total fat, less than 10% of calories from saturated fat, and no more than 300 mg/day from cholesterol. Among individuals 20 years of age and older:

- 35% of women and 29% of men meet the recommendation for total fat of 30% or less of calories
- 41% of women and 34% of men meet the recommendation for saturated fat of less than 10% of calories.
- 78% of women and 56% of men meet the recommendation for cholesterol of 300 mg or less.

On the basis of 1-day intake:

- Women consume 32% of calories from fat and 11% from saturated fat
- Men consume 34% of calories from fat and 11% from saturated fat
- Intake of alcohol for men and women 20 years of age and older represented 2.8% and 1.3%, respectively, of total calories.
- Male and female respondents 20 to 29 years of age consumed 4.3% and 1.9% of calories from alcohol, respectively, for men and women.

**Food eaten away from home:**

- About one fourth of calories consumed by both men and women 20 years of age and older are from foods obtained and eaten away from home.
- Among adults, calories from foods obtained and eaten away from home are highest among those 20 to 29 years of age and

lowest among those 70 years of age and older.

- Nutrients contributed by foods eaten at breakfast:

- Men consume an average of 17% of calories, 16% of total fat, and 18% of cholesterol at breakfast.
- Women have similar percentages.
- Percentage of calories and total fat contributed by foods eaten at breakfast increase with age for men.
- Women consume only 18% of their calories at breakfast, but about 23% to 24% of their calcium, iron, and magnesium and 22% to 26% of riboflavin, folate, vitamins A and C, and thiamin, nutrients often low in the diets of women.

**Highlights of Nutrient Intakes Contributed by Foods Eaten as Snacks.** In this table, "snack" refers to any eating occasion designated by the respondent as a food and/or beverage break, including the snack, alcoholic beverage, and other beverage categories.

- Americans consume an average of 17% of their calories and 15% of their total fat intake as snacks.
- Adolescents consume about 21% of their calories and about 20% of both total fat and saturated fat from snacks.
- Girls obtain over 20% of their intake of vitamins A and E and calcium from snacks.

**Selected Highlights about Quantities of Food Consumed by Individuals.** The 1995 Dietary Guidelines for Americans advise people to choose a diet with most of the calories from grain products, vegetables, fruits, low-fat milk products, lean meats, fish, poultry, and dry beans and choose fewer calories from fats and sweets. They place special emphasis on grain products, vegetables, and fruits as key parts of a varied diet.

- Americans consume an average of 300 g of grain products each day. More than one third (112 g) is consumed as grain mixtures—such as lasagna and pizza. Yeast

breads and rolls and cereals, rice, and pasta are also substantial contributors.

- Americans consume low levels of nutrient-packed dark green and deep yellow vegetables, despite guidance to do otherwise. Men 20 years of age and older consume an average of 21 g of dark green and deep yellow vegetables/day, and women consume an average of 24 g.
- More than half of the white potatoes eaten by children 6 to 19 years old are in the form of fried potatoes.
- Adolescent boys consume about 1¼ cups (305 g) of fluid milk/day; adolescent girls consume less than 1 cup. For both, about one third is whole milk and about two thirds is low-fat or skim milk. By contrast, adolescent boys consumed about 2⅔ (658 g) of carbonated soft drinks; adolescent girls, about 1½ cups (381 g).
- On any given day, only about half (54%) of Americans eat fruit, and only about three fourths (79%) consume milk or milk products.
- One fourth of all Americans eat fried potatoes on any given day.
- One half of all Americans drink carbonated soft drinks on any given day.

**Perceived Diet Quality by Self-Assessment.** Respondents were asked: *Compared with what is healthy, do you think your diet is too low, too high, or about right in* (NUTRIENT/FOOD COMPONENT)?

The question covers the following nutrients and food components: calories, calcium, iron, vitamin C, protein, fat, saturated fat, cholesterol, salt or sodium, fiber, and sugar and sweets.

*Selected Highlights.* Among adults 20 years of age and older:

- 36% of men and 43% of women think their diets are *too high* in calories.
- 48% of men and women think their diets are *too high* in fat.
- 29% of men and 24% of women think their diets are *too high* in salt or sodium.
- 42% of women think their diets

are *too low* in calcium.
- 36% of women think their diets are *too low* in iron.

Respondents were asked the following question: *To you, personally, is it very important, somewhat important, not too important, or not at all important to* (statement)?

Each statement covers one of the Dietary Guidelines for Americans.

Guidelines published in 1995 advise Americans to:

- Eat a variety of foods
- Balance the food you eat with physical activity—maintain or improve your weight
- Choose a diet with plenty of grain products, vegetables, and fruits
- Choose a diet low in fat, saturated fat, and cholesterol
- Choose a diet moderate in sugars
- Choose a diet moderate in salt and sodium
- If you drink alcoholic beverages, do so in moderation

**Selected Highlights of Respondents Perception of the Importance of Dietary Guidance.**

Among adults 20 years of age and older:

- Most say it is important to them to maintain a healthy weight. In fact, 70% of men and 79% of women say it is very important.
- Many also say it is very important to them to choose a diet with plenty of fruits and vegetables—61% of men and 73% of women.
- However, only 30% of men and 37% of women say choosing a diet with plenty of breads, cereals, rice, and pasta is very important despite the emphasis on these foods in the Dietary Guidelines

Individuals who wish to conduct their own analyses can order the macro data on CD-ROM ($50) or magnetic tape ($240) from National Technical Information Service at 5285, Port Royal Road, Springfield, VA 22161 (703-487-4650).

# Are Reduced-Fat Foods Keeping Americans Healthier?

I N 1990, THE U.S. Public Health Service asked the food industry to create 5,000 reduced-fat, processed products by the year 2000. Industry met the goal in 1992, eight years ahead of schedule. And thousands more reduced-fat products have since been introduced.

But has the proliferation of lower-fat cookies, crackers, soups, salad dressings and the like led to lower-fat diets—and a healthier America? At least one set of data from the U.S. Department of Agriculture suggests that people who make high use of reduced-fat foods are more likely to end up taking in less fat—and fewer calories—than others.

Still, Americans are getting heavier overall, even though lower-fat is generally expected to mean lower in calories. And our incidence of chronic, weight-related conditions such as diabetes appears to be on the rise.

The irony in all of this is that the number of grams of fat that Americans eat dropped between 1965 and 1989— before reduced-fat foods hit the market in a big way. But **throughout the 1990s, as reduced-fat foods have been appearing in supermarkets with increasing frequency, there have been indications that fat consumption has actually started to drift upward once again.**

Clearly, the way in which reduced-fat foods might be integrated into the U.S. diet to make it more healthful has not yet become evident. "We are involved in a grand experiment," says Bruce Bistrian, MD, a professor of medicine at Harvard Medical School.

How the experiment will ultimately turn out no one knows for sure. In the meantime, researchers, industry representatives, consumer advocates, government health trackers, and public health educators convened recently at a Tufts University conference to try to get a handle on the potential role of reduced-fat foods in constructing healthful diets.* And they had some very definite ideas about why the increasing availability of lower-fat foods hasn't led to a corresponding rise in lower-fat people.

### Message has overshot the mark

Most health care professionals agree that the message to reduce fat has been overemphasized to the point that other health messages which are just as important have been excluded. And that may have fostered unrealistic expectations that eating reduced-fat products has a magic-bullet effect in improving health.

Many people may have come to feel that as long as they toss reduced-fat foods into their shopping carts, they're doing everything they need to do for themselves. It doesn't matter, for instance, whether those foods are high in sugar, even though the *U.S. Dietary Guidelines* say that consuming a diet moderate in sugars is an important component of healthful eating. The result: reduced-fat cakes and

*The Tufts Dialogue Conference on the Role of Fat-Modified Foods in Dietary Change was underwritten by a grant from Procter & Gamble, makers of Olestra.*

*Did you know...* Even low-intensity exercise like walking can add years to your life. In a 12-year study of 700 retired men in their 60s, 70s, and 80s, those who logged two miles a day cut their risk of dying almost in half, compared with those who walked less than one mile. The more the men walked, the greater the benefit.

From *Tufts University Diet & Nutrition Letter*, March 1998, pp. 4-5. © 1998 by Tufts University Diet & Nutrition Letter. Reprinted by permission.

cookies, which are often high in sugar, are mistakenly seen as nutritionally equivalent to other reduced- or low-fat foods like skim and low-fat milk, meat trimmed of excess fat, and vegetables and fruits—all of which tend to be much lower in sugar and much higher in vitamins and minerals.

Balancing food intake with physical activity, another of the government's guidelines, gets short shrift, too—even though physical activity, not eating less fat, is the lifestyle factor most consistently linked to long-term weight loss and weight maintenance.

In light of the fact that the term "reduced-fat" has come to be viewed as *the* answer for living more healthfully, Alice Lichtenstein, DSc, a heart disease researcher at Tufts, goes so far as to say that the array of reduced-fat foods we have to choose from may have actually proven counterproductive—at least when it comes to the snack and dessert aisles. "The good thing is that we are living in a land of extraordinary abundance, and food is extraordinarily cheap," she comments. "But it's also the bad thing. It tempts people with a false safety net by making them feel that just because they've chosen something reduced in fat, they've improved their health. But I think there are a lot of people who, if they just had the choice between high-fat cake and nothing else, would choose to eat nothing else, or they might choose to have an apple, pear, or grapes."

Linda Sandefur, a vice president at Procter & Gamble, doesn't go that far. She believes reduced-fat desserts and snacks simply provide different kinds of options for people who are trying to eat more healthfully. She does say, however, that it would be useful for people to recognize that reduced-fat cakes, cookies, potato chips and other foods that are not particularly high in nutrients are not healthful per se. Rather, they are simply less *un*healthful than their full-fat versions.

It would also be useful for consumers to recognize that the term "reduced-fat" on a label should not be seen as carte blanche to eat without regard for the number of calories consumed. As the chart shows, low-fat versions of foods often have as many—

## The calories in reduced-fat foods: a double take—literally

ACCORDING TO ONE SURVEY, more than 50 percent of consumers look at the fat content of foods on nutrition labels. But only 10 percent look at calories—and therein may lie some of this country's growing problem with weight control. People often assume that less fat means fewer calories, but many reduced-fat and low-fat processed foods have as many—or more—calories than their full-fat counterparts. Check out the examples we found while browsing through the supermarket.

| | calories |
|---|---|
| Campbell's Vegetable Soup Made with Beef Stock, 1/2 cup | 80 |
| Campbell's 98% Fat Free Healthy Request Vegetable Soup [with beef stock], 1/2 cup | 90 |
| Drake's Yodels, 2 | 280 |
| Drake's Reduced-Fat Yodels, 2 | 290 |
| Franco-American Slow Roast Turkey Gravy, 1/4 cup | 30 |
| Franco-American Fat Free Slow Roast Turkey Gravy, 1/4 cup | 30 |
| Jif Peanut Butter, 2 tablespoons | 190 |
| Reduced-Fat Jif, 2 tablespoons | 190 |
| Nabisco Saltine Crackers, 5 | 60 |
| Nabisco Fat-Free Saltine Crackers, 5 | 60 |
| Ore Ida Country Style Steak Fries, 3 oz | 110 |
| Ore Ida Low Fat Steak Fries, 3 oz | 110 |
| Quaker Peanut Butter & Chocolate Chunk Chewy Granola Bar, 1 | 120 |
| Quaker Reduced Fat Peanut Butter & Chocolate Chunk Chewy Granola Bar, 1 | 120 |
| Smucker's Special Recipe Butterscotch Caramel Topping, 2 tablespoons | 130 |
| Smucker's Fat Free Caramel Topping, 2 tablespoons | 130 |

or more—calories than their traditional counterparts. And that may have something to do with the fact that as Americans' consumption of reduced-fat foods has been rising, so has their calorie consumption.

## Time to downshift expectations

Perhaps it seems as if the government's call for more low-fat foods was well-intended but ill-conceived. After all, these items are not making the population thinner; they often aren't particularly nutritious; and they appear to make some people eat even more than they would otherwise.

Indeed, according to a group of participants at the Tufts conference, "it seems unlikely that even widespread use of low-fat...diets will have a major impact on pre-existing obesity." Susan Roberts, PhD, chief of the Energy Metabolism Laboratory at Tufts, backs up that assertion by pointing to research which shows that even in studies where people reduced their fat consumption from 40 percent of their calories to 25 percent, weight loss ranged

only from about two to seven pounds.

Even so, a number of experts, including Dr. Roberts herself, believes maybe the answer isn't to eschew lower-fat processed foods completely but, rather, to lower our expectations of what they can do for us. "They're not completely useless," she says. "They're just not as important as people used to think."

How might reduced-fat products help? Consider that while a seven-pound weight loss may not sound like much, it's known that even losing five to 10 pounds can result in a significant drop in blood pressure in some people with hypertension. Similarly, small reductions in weight can reduce blood sugar in people with diabetes.

Furthermore, **maybe eating less fat, particularly less saturated fat, even with minimal to no weight loss, can reduce the risk for heart disease.** In fact, that's in part why the U.S. Public Health Service charged industry with creating more reduced-fat products in the first place. And the argument can be made that the strategy may very well be working. Although Americans have been getting heavier, heart disease has declined. Less fat in the diet may even help reduce the risk for certain types of cancer (although the evidence on that has been inconsistent).

In the same vein, it might be that while eating reduced-fat products doesn't "cure" obesity, it may help prevent it in people who are not yet overweight. As Dr. Roberts puts it, "these foods may not help us lose weight, but they may help us not gain weight."

Unfortunately, that possibility has not been addressed by the scientific community. And the food industry, whose job is to make money rather than improve consumers' health, has not used its advertising dollars to focus on maintaining weight or losing small amounts of weight. Rather, it uses "reduced-fat" and "low-fat" as marketing tools to sell the promise of slimness.

And that's what consumers are buying. "People are looking for significant weight loss for cosmetic reasons," says Priscilla Clarkson, PhD, associate dean for the School of Public Health and Health Sciences at the University of Massachusetts. They equate small losses with a failure to look good rather than with a possible improvement in their health. But if people could change their focus from looking for big results on the scale to looking for meaningful results on blood tests and so forth, they might view even a modest loss of weight as successful.

It's a point worth considering, especially for those who are not ready to engage in a multi-pronged approach to better eating and increased physical activity. In other words, they might want to try starting with just the single step of substituting some reduced-fat, lower-calorie foods for their full-fat counterparts. If they also made sure that the foods they chose were reduced in saturated fat, and, as Tufts's Dr. Lichtenstein notes, if they managed to make the changes without overcompensating by eating as many or more calories altogether, there very likely would be some benefits—even if they didn't show up in the mirror.

# Low-Calorie Sweeteners:

*Adding Reduced-Calorie Delights to a Healthful Diet*

This is a likely scenario: A person is shopping in a grocery store, picks a packaged food from the shelf, immediately skips the first line of the nutrition facts panel, information on "Calories Per Serving," and scans to "Total Fat." With the neglect of calories in the past few years, this is not surprising.

The calorie is back—not that it ever left, it just got lost in the shadow of Americans' focus on fat. We are seeing more reminders that being conscious of calories is just as important as being attentive to other nutrients.

Among our many choices, there are a lot of options for reduced-calorie foods and beverages to help balance our overall energy intake. Because no one sweetener meets all consumer and food preparation needs, a variety of reduced-calorie sweeteners (commonly referred to as low-calorie sweeteners), has been developed and is available. *Food Insight* presents an update on these ingredients that give the satisfyingly sweet taste to many reduced-calorie products.

## More Than Just a Sweet Taste

Low-calorie sweeteners taste very similar to sucrose (table sugar) but are much sweeter. Most do not contain any calories. Even though some sweeteners, such as aspartame, contain calories, they are used in such small amounts that they add essentially no calories to foods and beverages. As a result, these sweeteners practically eliminate or substantially reduce calories in some foods and beverages such as carbonated soft drinks, light yogurt and sugar-free pudding.

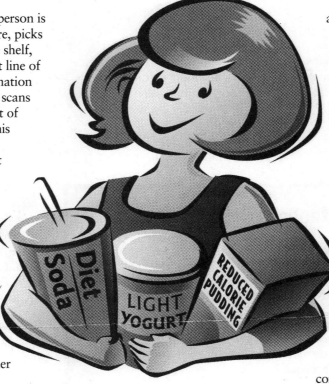

## Low-calorie Sweeteners in the United States

The Food and Drug Administration (FDA) has to date approved three low-calorie sweeteners for use in the United States: aspartame, acesulfame-K and saccharin.

*Aspartame* tastes very similar to sucrose but is 200-times sweeter. It is broken down to compounds normally found in the foods we eat everyday: aspartic acid, phenylalanine and a small amount of methanol. Aspartic acid and phenylalanine are essential amino acids (the building blocks of protein) and methanol is found naturally in many foods, such as fruit and vegetable juices. In fact, a glass of tomato juice provides six times as much methanol as a similar amount of diet soda. Many prepared foods contain aspartame which is also available as a tabletop sweetener.

Aspartame underwent extensive safety testing for more than a decade before the FDA concluded in 1981 that aspartame is safe for use by consumers and thus approved its use. Products made with aspartame, however, must carry a statement on the label that they contain phenylalanine. The statement is important for people with phenylketonuria, a rare hereditary disease, because they cannot properly metabolize phenylalanine.

*Acesulfame-K,* or acesulfame potassium, is produced by using derivatives of acetoncetic acid (a derivative of acetic acid or vinegar). It also is 200-times sweeter than sucrose. Over 90 studies were conducted to test its safety before the FDA approved its use in 1988.

Available as a tabletop sweetener, acesulfame-K also is used in many prepared foods. When eaten alone in high concentrations, acesulfame-K may produce a slight aftertaste. However, blending acesulfame-K with other low-calorie sweeteners helps improve the taste of low-calorie products as well as their sweetness, shelf-life and stability. Also, with blended sweeteners, a synergy often occurs that makes it possible to produce the desired sweetness using a lower total amount of sweeteners.

*Saccharin* is the oldest of low-calorie sweeteners and has been used to sweeten foods and beverages since the turn of the century. It has a taste 300-times sweeter than sucrose. Saccharin is highly stable, but has a slightly bitter aftertaste.

The FDA proposed a ban on saccharin in 1977 based on animal research

Reprinted with permission from *Food Insight*, January/February 1998, pp. 2-3. © 1998 by the International Food Information Council Foundation (IFIC).

that suggested it was a weak bladder carcinogen. However, a congressional moratorium was placed on the ban to allow for more research on saccharin's safety. The moratorium on the ban has been extended seven times based on the need for further scientific study and continued consumer demand. The FDA withdrew the ban in 1991, but the moratorium is still in effect until the year 2002. While numerous studies since 1977 have clearly shown that saccharin does not cause cancer in humans, labels on products with saccharin must continue to have a statement that it has caused cancer in laboratory animals.

No final decision has been made regarding delisting saccharin from Health and Human Services' Public Health Services' National Toxicology Program's (NTP) Report on Carcinogens. Three separate committees have reviewed saccharin: Two internal NTP committees voted to delist saccharin, and a third, external advisory group in a close vote recommended keeping it on the list. A final decision will be made at a later date.

### Waiting in the Wings

The FDA is currently considering petitions to approve other low-calorie sweeteners, including sucralose, alitame and cyclamate, all of which are already approved for use in numerous other countries.

*Sucralose* is the only low-calorie sweetener that is made from sugar. It is approximately 600-times sweeter and does not contain calories. Sucralose is highly stable under a wide variety of processing conditions. Thus, it can be used virtually anywhere sugar can, including cooking and baking, without losing any of its sugar-like sweetness.

Today, sucralose is approved in over 25 countries around the world for use in food and beverages. In the United States, sucralose has been petitioned to the FDA for use in 15 different food and beverage categories.

*Alitame* is formed from amino acids (L-aspartic acid, L-alanine, and a novel amide). It offers a taste that is 2,000-times sweeter than sucrose, and can be used in cooking and baking. If approved, alitame would be suitable for use in a wide variety of products, including beverages, tabletop sweeteners, frozen desserts and baked goods.

*Cyclamate* is approved for use in Canada and more than 50 countries in Europe, Asia, South America and Africa. Cyclamate is 30-times sweeter than sucrose and is heat-stable. Since 1970, however, its use has been banned in the United States, based on a study suggesting cyclamates may be related to development of bladder tumors in rats. While 75 subsequent studies have failed to show cyclamate is carcinogenic, the sweetener has yet to be reapproved for use in this country.

### Low-Calorie Delights

Low-calorie sweeteners help satisfy desires for a sweet taste, and allow people to follow a healthful eating plan that includes their favorite foods. According to Adam Drewnowski, Ph.D., professor at the University of Michigan, "Low-calorie sweeteners offer the best method to date of reducing calories while maintaining the palatability of the diet."

Low-calorie sweeteners are an option for reducing the number of calories in our diet. Although calorie reduction goes hand-in-hand with weight loss, it must be recognized that low-calorie sweeteners in and of themselves will not magically solve our struggles with weight. Successful weight management requires habits that include a balanced diet and regular physical activity.

## Anatomy of a Sweetener Approval

How does a new sweetener get approved for use in foods and beverages in the United States? The most common way taken is the food additive petition route. If the information and data provided to the Food and Drug Administration (FDA) is satisfactory, the agency will indicate that the petition has been "accepted for filing."

In the course of what is usually a lengthy (in some instances 10 years) and intensive review, the FDA requires substantial supporting data for their scientists to analyze. Additional external peer review may also be required. At a minimum, the following data are needed:

■ How will the product be consumed and how much?

■ Who, including children, adults, men and women, will consume the ingredient, and how much will each group consume?

■ What does the ingredient do as an additive to food?

■ Is the ingredient toxic and what levels are safe?

■ Does the product have the potential to: cause cancer; affect reproduction; be stored in the body; be metabolized into other, potentially unsafe products; or cause allergic reaction?

■ How and where is the ingredient made, who makes it, how pure is it?

■ Is the ingredient suitable to food processing and consumer use?

During approval, the FDA also sets an acceptable daily intake (ADI) for the ingredient, which is the amount that can be safely consumed on a daily basis over a person's lifetime. The ADI for aspartame, for example, is 50 milligrams per kilogram per day. For a 150-pound adult, this translates to 20 12-ounce containers of carbonated soft drink or 97 packets of tabletop sweetener per day over a lifetime.

The process does not stop with approval. The FDA usually requires an ingredient to be monitored for consumer complaints in addition to dietary surveys to determine consumption. ■

# Are fruits and vegetables less nutritious today?

Our readers often tell us they are concerned that the soil is mineral-depleted and that the produce they buy is not nutritious—understandable concerns, given the compost heap of misinformation that's out there. So we decided to dig into the subject.

As has been known for centuries, agriculture tends to wear out the soil. Erosion, as well as planting, depletes top soil. Replenishing the soil is what agriculture is all about, and always has been. Fertilizers, in some form, have been used by farmers since the beginnings of agriculture. The main goal is to replace minerals, especially trace minerals. Another goal is not to add too much fertilizer. There are many, many methods that improve and maintain soil quality: water management, erosion control, planting legumes to replace nitrogen in the soil, crop rotation, adding compost, manure, and chemical fertilizers, and otherwise boosting organic matter. Enormous expertise is brought to bear on these problems—they do not go unnoticed.

Indeed, the fertility of the soil here and in the rest of the world is a matter of intense concern to farmers, governments, international investors, and thousands of scientists. The amount of nutrients in the soil controls crop development and agricultural yield. Will the soil of planet Earth produce enough food to keep up with population growth, particularly if people who now go hungry are also fed? Will there be enough to nourish everybody in the year 2010? 2050? The Food and Agriculture Organization of the United Nations and the World Bank study such questions, along with the USDA and our land-grant colleges, to name only a few of the interested parties. Predicting the future, even from solid scientific data, is always difficult. So far, however, predictions are optimistic, assuming that sound agricultural policies will

be followed. Each year, around the world, there are international conferences to discuss these issues.

### The one essential fact

"Fruits, vegetables, and grains will not grow, cannot be sold, and will not be bought if they contain insufficient nutrition. If there's an inadequate amount of nutrients in the soil, plants may die because of insect infestation or disease, or cannot be sold because of poor appearance." These are the words of Dr. Gary Banuelos, a soil scientist with the USDA Research Service in Fresno, California, and they echo the conclusions of other experts. As any gardener knows, plants just won't grow properly in depleted soil. Vitamins in plants are created by the plants themselves. Minerals—such as phosphorus, potassium, iodine, calcium, copper, iron, selenium, fluoride, molybdenum, and zinc—must come from the soil. If the elements aren't there, the plant droops, fails to flower, and may die. *If the fruits and vegetables you buy look healthy, you can be certain they contain the nutrients they should.*

According to Joanne Ikeda, a cooperative extension nutrition-education specialist at UC Berkeley, "The idea that the soil is being depleted of nutrients and thus our food doesn't contain nutrients is one of those myths we can't seem to eradicate, though I have certainly spent years trying."

**Bottom line:** *People who tell you that the soil is depleted and our food is no longer nutritious are unacquainted with the truth, or not telling it. They're usually trying to get you to take some sort of mineral supplements. Certainly, nutrients will vary from one batch of produce to another, depending on climate, handling, and other factors. But a varied, balanced diet will make up for this over the long term.*

Reprinted with permission from *University of California at Berkeley Wellness Letter,* May 1998, p. 1. © 1998 by Health Letter Associates. For information, call (800) 829-9170.

# The Freshness Fallacy

## Who says the veggies in the produce bin are better for you than the ones in the freezer?

I am, I confess, a frozen-vegetable devotee. From chopped spinach to green beans, asparagus to broccoli, veggies that have spent most of their lives in a freezer

### By MINNA MORSE

compartment are the mainstay of my diet. When company is coming I seek out fresh, but when I'm on my own, dinner is often a plate of frozen brussels sprouts, cooked in the microwave and topped with melted cheddar cheese.

For one thing, it's so easy. There's no chopping involved, no stringing or peeling, and thanks to the microwave, I've got only one dish to wash at the end of the meal. Besides, when I do buy fresh produce, much of it ends up going to waste.

The vast majority of Americans would probably think I'm crazy—or at least nutritionally deprived. According to a study by the Opinion Research Corporation in Princeton, New Jersey, 92 percent believe that fresh vegetables pack more vitamins and minerals than frozen. At the same time, however, they say they're too busy to prepare fresh vegetables, so they don't bother to eat many at all. Only 5 percent meet the daily recommended amount of five or more servings a day.

Fortunately, they're wrong (and I'm vindicated). In a recent study at the University of Illinois at Urbana, researchers compared the nutritional profiles of four fresh vegetables with their frozen counterparts. After almost one year of storage, the frozen samples had roughly the same amount of vitamin C—one of the least stable vitamins—as fresh green beans and corn at eight days, broccoli at 14 days, and carrots at 21 days.

This isn't the first time research has touted the nutritional benefit of frozen foods. But Barbara Klein, the food scientist who led the study, says most other analyses compared the results of separate studies—one on fresh, say, and another on frozen. In this one, however, researchers divided a large batch of vegetables into groups, then left some of each variety sitting on the shelf and sent some to the freezer. (A third group was canned, and it scored nearly as high as the frozen—even without the liquid that the vegetables had been canned in.)

"We pretty much knew what we were going to find," says Klein. "But we also knew about people's distrust of frozen vegetables. So we figured this would be a definitive way to prove the point and hopefully get folks to eat more veggies."

Why exactly aren't fresh carrots and corn much more nutritious than frozen? Because fresh isn't always what it seems. It turns out there are two primary ways to sap nutrients from a vegetable: by letting it sit around after it's been harvested and by cooking it.

From *Health*, March 1998, pp. 38, 41. © 1998 by Time Inc. Health, a division of Time Publishing Ventures, Inc. Reprinted by permission.

Fresh vegetables suffer the most from the first part of this rule. From the time they're picked in the field to the moment you serve them for dinner, a good two weeks may have passed. During that stretch they can lose anywhere from 10 to 50 percent of some of their nutrients.

Case in point: Most of the green beans you buy in winter are grown in the Culiacán region on the west coast of Mexico. After those beans are harvested, they may be in transit for five or more days before they arrive at a grocery near you. There they might sit for another few days, and who knows what'll happen once you get them home? Sure, you planned on making three-bean salad the next night, but you worked late and didn't feel like cooking, and the night after that you're invited out for dinner. Before you know it, three more days have gone by.

Frozen vegetables, on the other hand, end up on ice within hours of being picked. By this count, in fact, they'd seem to be doing *better* than their fresh brothers and sisters. But before a vegetable is sent to the freezer, it's plunged into hot water for a minute or two. This process stabilizes the vegetable and helps preserve its color and texture, but for certain nutrients it can be just as bad as sitting around. The rate of vitamin loss varies depending on the vegetable, but in general, says Klein, fresh and frozen come out pretty even down the line.

And not just on vitamin C. Happily, most of the health goodies contained in a vegetable are a lot more stable than you might think. Fiber, beta-carotene, and all of its minerals are locked into the vegetable whatever treatment it receives.

The reason C is so vulnerable is that it oxidizes easily. When a plant is on the vine, its vitamins are protected. But as soon as it's picked, the cell walls start to break down, allowing oxygen to enter and come into contact with the vitamins. And oxygen alters the chemical structure of vitamin C, rendering it inactive. (Vitamin C also dissolves in water, but that's mainly a problem in cooking, not storage.) Folic acid is another easily oxidized vitamin, though according to Klein, it's a little less vulnerable than C because it binds to the plant's proteins, which help keep it intact.

Of course, no matter how vitamin-rich a frozen vegetable may be, there's still the issue of taste. How can a frozen stalk of broccoli possibly compare to fresh?

## Protecting Your Frozen Assets

Not all frozen vegetables get the star treatment provided in commercial facilities: namely, airtight packaging and ultracold temperatures. But you can spot some signs of poor handling when shopping for frozen foods. And when freezing at home, you can take steps to ensure a professional outcome.

**Check packages** for signs of water migration. At some point during their lifetime—in transit, perhaps, or waiting around at the grocery before its shelves are restocked—the vegetables may have partially thawed. The result: When they refreeze, the vegetables form ice crystals and can clump together, both of which lead to greater nutrient loss and softening in texture. (The same thing happens on a small scale every time your freezer goes through its self-defrosting cycle.) If you're looking at a bag of frozen peas, the vegetables should be loose or break apart easily; if it's a solid box of spinach, the greens should fill the package rather than bunching to one side.

**Set your refrigerator** at zero, the temperature used in commercial facilities. (Your ice cream will come out too hard to serve, however, so remember to let it sit awhile after you take it out.) Vegetables can last up to six months at this temperature. If your freezer does not have a separate temperature control, it may be as much as ten degrees warmer than that, in which case your veggies will be good only for about three months.

**When freezing** your own produce, make sure you pack it in an airtight container or a plastic bag. To squeeze air out of a filled bag, try this trick: Fill a bowl or basin with water. Dunk the loaded bag into the water almost up to the top, then seal. When you pull the bag out, the plastic will cling tightly to the contents. If you do a lot of freezing at home, consider buying a gadget that vacuum-seals plastic bags.

Well, it may not if you're talking about one that's freshly picked and steamed to perfection. And there's no doubt that the texture won't be quite up to snuff. But even a food professional like Arthur Schwartz, cookbook author and former restaurant critic for the *New York Daily News,* says that many frozen vegetables taste just fine, particularly when mixed into a casserole or stew. Carrots and onions are two exceptions: "Their taste begins to die as soon as you cut them."

Having had my frozen-veggie habit validated by a nutritionist *and* a restaurant critic, I decided it was time to see how much freshness really mattered to my foodie friends. I would throw a dinner party using almost exclusively frozen ingredients, but I wouldn't tell any of the guests about the menu.

I went all out. First, a vegetarian pâté made of pureed green beans and walnuts. Next, individual puff pastries filled with spinach and feta cheese. I even used corn kernels and broccoli florets in a pasta salad, where they couldn't hide beneath a sauce or a buttery crust. Finally, the pièce de résistance: angel food cake smothered with a scarlet sauce of pureed raspberries.

The forks clanked, the conversation bubbled, the chairs slid back. And I heard nothing but raves.

# The Truth about Organic 'Certification'

*Does it help ensure safer foods— or just costlier ones?*

## by Stephen Barrett, MD

"If you as a consumer have a desire to purchase a fake or a fraud of one kind or another, should your government guarantee your right to do so? More than that, is your government obligated to prosecute one who, knowing of your propensity for fraud, tricks you into buying the genuine in place of buying the fake? Remembering that 'your government' is all the rest of us, is it right for you to take our time and money to underwrite such ridiculous exercises as making sure you are cheated when you want to be cheated? And must we penalize the man who breaks his promise to cheat you?"

These astute questions were raised in 1972 by Dick Beeler, editor of *Animal Health and Nutrition,* who was concerned about laws being adopted in California and Oregon to certify "organic" foods. Those laws signaled the beginning of efforts that culminated in 1990 with passage of the U.S. Organic Foods Production Act, which ordered the U.S. Department of Agriculture (USDA) to set certification standards. Although the USDA had opposed passage of the act, the Alar scare plus a campaign by environmental, consumer, and farm groups persuaded Congress to include it in the 1990 Farm Bill (*NF* 8:25–29, 1991).

As directed by the law, the secretary of agriculture established a National Organic Standards Board to help develop a list of substances permissible in organic production and handling and to advise the secretary on other aspects of implementing a National Organic Program. In 1992, the secretary appointed 15 people, 8 of whom were industry members. The board held 12 full-board meetings and 5 joint committee meetings and received additional input through public hearings and written submissions from interested persons. It presented its recommendations to the secretary in 1994 and issued 30 subsequent addenda.

*Studies have found that the pesticide levels in foods designated organic were similar to those that were not.*

## The Current Marketplace

Total retail sales of the organic industry have reportedly risen from $1 billion in 1990 to $3.5 billion in 1996. "Certified" organic cropland production expanded from 473,000 acres to 667,000 acres between 1992 and 1994 and is expected to reach two million acres by the year 2000. Despite this rapid growth, the organic industry represents a very small percentage of total agricultural production and sales.

The most common concept of "organically grown" food was articulated in 1972 by Robert Rodale, editor of *Organic Gardening and Farming* magazine, at a public hearing: "Food grown without pesticides; grown without artificial fertilizers; grown in soil whose humus content is increased by the additions of organic matter; grown in soil whose mineral content is increased by the application of natural mineral fertilizers; has not been treated with preservatives, hormones, antibiotics, etc."

However, in 1980, a team of scientists appointed by the USDA concluded that there was no universally accepted definition of "organic farming." Their report stated:

The organic movement represents a spectrum of practices, attitudes, and philosophies. On the one hand are those organic practitioners who would not use chemical fertilizers or pesticides under any circumstances. These producers hold rigidly to their purist philosophy. At the other end of the spectrum, organic farmers espouse a more flexible approach. While striving to avoid the use of chemical fertilizers and pesticides, these practitioners do not rule them out entirely. Instead, when absolutely necessary, some fertilizers and also herbicides are very selectively and sparingly used as a second line of defense. Nevertheless, these farmers, too, consider themselves to be organic farmers.

Today, approximately 4,000 farmers and 600 handlers are certified by 33 private or 11 state agencies. Each certifying agency has its own standards and identifying marks. No industrywide agreement exists about which substances should be permitted or prohibited for organic production and handling.

## The Proposed Rule

On December 16, 1997, the USDA Agricultural Marketing Service proposed rules for a National Organic Program (Federal Register 62:65850–65967, 1997). The proposal includes: (1) national standards for production and handling, (2) a National List of approved synthetic sub-

From *Nutrition Forum,* March/April 1998, pp. 9-13. © 1998 by Prometheus Books, 59 John Glenn Drive, Amherst, NY 14228. Reprinted by permission of the publisher.

stances, (3) a certification program, (4) a program for accrediting certifiers, (5) labeling requirements, (6) enforcement provisions, and (7) rules for importing equivalent products. A new USDA seal will be the only permissible marker.

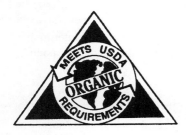

The proposed rule defines organic farming and handling as:

A system that is designed and managed to produce agricultural products by the use of methods and substances that maintain the integrity of organic agricultural products until they reach the consumer. This is accomplished by using, where possible, cultural, biological and mechanical methods, as opposed to using substances, to fulfill any specific function within the system so as to: maintain long-term soil fertility; increase soil biological activity; ensure effective pest management; recycle wastes to return nutrients to the land; provide attentive care for farm animals; and handle the agricultural products without the use of extraneous synthetic additives or processing in accordance with the Act and the regulations in this part.

The weed and pest-control methods to which this refers include crop rotation, hand cultivation, mulching, soil enrichment, and encouraging beneficial predators and microorganisms. If these methods are not sufficient, various listed chemicals can be used. (The list does not include cytotoxic chemicals that are carbon-based.) The proposal does not call for monitoring specific indicators of soil and water quality, but leaves the selection of monitoring activities to the producer in consultation with the certifying agent.

For raising animals, antibiotics are not permitted as growth stimulants but are

permitted to counter infections. The rules permit up to 20% of animal feed to be obtained from nonorganic sources. This was done because some nutrients (such as trace minerals) are not always available organically. Irradiation, which can reduce or eliminate certain pests, kill disease-causing bacteria, and prolong food shelf-life, is permitted during processing. Genetic engineering is also permissible.

In an accompanying news release, USDA Secretary Dan Glickman stated:

What is organic? Generally, it is agriculture produced through a natural as opposed to synthetic process. The natural portion of the definition is fairly obvious, but process is an equally critical distinction. When we certify organic, we are certifying not just a product but the farming and handling practices that yield it. When you buy a certified organic tomato, for instance, you are buying the product of an organic farm. And, consumers are willing to fork over a little more for that tomato. They've shown that they will pay a premium for organic food. National standards are our way of ensuring that consumers get what they pay for.

## More Nutritious?

The USDA proposal applies to all types of agricultural products and all aspects of their production and handling, ranging from soil fertility management to the packaging and labeling of the final product. The document is intended to address production methods rather than the physical qualities of the products themselves. In fact, it states: "No distinctions should be made between organically and non-organically produced products in terms of quality, appearance, or safety." In other words, no claim should be made that the foods themselves are better—or even different!

Organic foods are certainly not more nutritious. The nutrient content of plants is determined primarily by heredity. Mineral content may be affected by the mineral content of the soil, but this has no significance in the overall diet. If essential nutrients are missing from the soil, the plant will not

grow. If plants grow, that means the essential nutrients are present. Experiments conducted for many years have found no difference in the nutrient content of organically grown crops and those grown under standard agricultural conditions.

## Safer?

"Organic" proponents suggest that their foods are safer because they have lower levels of pesticide residues. However, the pesticide levels in our food supply are not high. To protect consumers, the FDA sets tolerance levels in foods and conducts frequent "market basket" studies wherein foods from regions throughout the United States are purchased and analyzed. The agency has found that about two-thirds of the fruits and vegetables have no detectable pesticides and only about 1% of domestic and 3% of imported foods had violative levels. Its annual Total Diet Study has found that dietary intakes of pesticides for all population groups are well within international and EPA standards.

Studies conducted since the early 1970s have found that the pesticide levels in foods designated organic were similar to those that were not. In 1997, *Consumer Reports* purchased about a thousand pounds of tomatoes, peaches, green bell peppers, and apples in five cities and tested them for more than 300 synthetic pesticides. Traces were detected in 77% of conventional foods and 25% of organically labeled foods, but only one sample of each exceeded the federal limit (*Consumer Reports* 63[1]:12–18, 1998).

Pesticides can locate on the surface of foods as well as beneath the surface. The amounts that washing can remove depends on their location, the amount and temperature of the rinse water, and whether detergent is used. Most people rinse their fruits and vegetables with plain water before eating them. *Consumer Reports* stated that it did not do so because the FDA tests unwashed products. The amount of pesticide removed by simple rinsing has not been scientifically studied but is probably small. *Consumer Reports* missed a golden opportunity to assess this.

Do pesticides found in conventional foods pose a health threat? Does the difference in pesticide content warrant buying "organic" foods? *Consumer Reports* equivocates: "For consumers in general, the unsettling truth is that no one really knows what a lifetime of consuming the tiny quantities in foods might do to a person. The effect, if any, is likely to be small for most individuals—but may be significant for the population at large." But the editors also advise, "No one should avoid fruits and vegetables for fear of pesticides; the health benefits of these foods overwhelm any possible risk."

*NF* Senior Associate Editor Manfred Kroger, Ph.D., Professor of Food Science at Pennsylvania State University, puts the matter more bluntly: "Scientific agriculture has provided Americans with the safest and most abundant food supply in the world. Agricultural chemicals are needed to maintain this supply. The risk from pesticide residue, if any, is minuscule, is not worth worrying about, and does not warrant paying higher prices."

## Tastier?

Taste is determined primarily by freshness. In the early 1990s, Israeli researchers made 460 assessments of 9 different fruits and vegetables and found no significant difference in quality between "organic" and conventionally grown samples (*American Journal of Alternative Agriculture* 7:129–136, 1992). The *Consumer Reports* study found no consistent differences in appearance, flavor, or texture.

Organically produced ("free-range") poultry are said to be raised in an environment where they are free to roam. To use this term, handlers must sign an affidavit saying that the chickens are provided with access to the outdoors. A recent taste test conducted by *Consumer Reports* rated two brands of free-range chicken as average among nine brands tested. Its March 1998 issue stated that few chickens choose to roam and that one manager said that free-ranging probably detracts from taste because it decreases the quality of the bird's food intake (*Consumer Reports* 63[3]:12–18, 1998).

## Organic Proponents Object

Health-food-industry trade and consumer publications indicate widespread dissatisfaction with the proposed rules. The Organic Farmers Marketing Association (**http://www.ota.com**) states:

> The definition of organic as written in the proposed national organic standards lacks the holistic approach central to organic practices. The proposed rules take a reductionist approach to organic food production that eliminates key concepts such as the health of the agro-ecosystem and biodiversity on the farm.

Industry sources state that the USDA has received more than 4,000 comments on the proposed rules. One distributors association official wrote that if the rules are implemented, his members would seek to buy its agricultural products from foreign sources. Others have complained that the proposed fees are too high.

Most objections pertain to the provisions that permit irradiation, genetic engineering, and the use of sewage sludge as fertilizer. Other objections include permitted use of amino acids as growth promoters, antibiotics (when necessary to save the animal's life), synthetic animal drugs, food additives, and animal feed from nonorganic sources.

Certification agencies with "higher standards" have objected that they are prohibited from stating this on their labels. Some poultry farmers have objected to provisions enabling intermingling of free-range poultry and other poultry.

## The Bottom Line

Organic certification, no matter what the rules, will not protect consumers. Foods certified as "organic" will neither be safer nor more nutritious than "regular" foods. They will just cost more and may lessen consumer confidence in the safety of "ordinary" foods.

(Copies of the proposed rule can be purchased for $8 from the Federal Register by calling [202] 512–1800. Additional information can be accessed through the National Organic Program Web page at **http://www. ams.usda. gov/nop**. Comments on the proposed rule can be sent from the Web site or mailed to: Eileen S. Stommes, Deputy Administrator, USDA-AMS-TM-NOP, Room 4007-So., Ag Stop 0275, P.O. Box 96456, Washington, DC 20090. Comments will eventually be posted on the Web page.)

*Stephen Barrett, MD, a retired psychiatrist who resides in Allentown, Pennsylvania, is a board member of the National Council Against Health Fraud and board chairman of Quackwatch, Inc.*

# Clearing Up Common Misconceptions about *Vegetarianism*

YOU KNOW vegetarianism has gone mainstream when you can buy a meatless burger at a Subway shop. But while the image of who might be a vegetarian has gone from a granola-munching hippie to your average Joe grabbing a meal at a fast-food outlet, myths about vegetarianism persist. Herewith, five of the most common ones—and the truths behind them.

**Myth number 1:** *Vegetarian diets are automatically more healthful than diets that include animal foods.*

**Fact:** Vegetarian diets are often much lower in saturated fat and cholesterol and higher in fiber than non-vegetarian diets. And studies suggest that in general, vegetarians are less likely to suffer from chronic degenerative conditions that plague the American population: diabetes, high blood pressure, heart disease, and obesity.

But just leaving out animal foods does not undo all the "wrongs" of the typical American diet. Consider that a lacto-ovo vegetarian, meaning one who eats dairy products and eggs, can pile on the saturated fat with full-fat dairy products like butter, cream, and cheese. Candy, chips, and other foods that fall under the vegetarian heading also tend to have a lot of fat—and calories—and relatively little in the way of nutrients.

By the same token, healthful vegetarian diets have to be planned (just like the diets of meat eaters) according to the rules of nutrition science. Without sufficient knowledge of nutrient needs, going on a vegetarian diet because it seems "cool" or like the right thing to do could lead to serious vitamin and mineral deficiencies.

**Myth number 2:** *Vegetarians eat weird foods.*

**Fact:** Vegetarians often do eat items that are not part of traditional American meals: soybean-based products like tofu and tempeh and different types of beans, nuts, and seeds. Such foods are particularly important for vegetarians known as vegans, who eat no animal products whatsoever, dairy foods and eggs included. The soy items, beans, and nuts provide them with the calcium that others get from milk, yogurt, and cheese. Many of these items also contain iron—a good thing for all vegetarians because anyone who foregoes beef and poultry foregoes the major sources of iron in the American diet.

Still, in no way does eating a vegetarian diet have to mean giving up familiar fare, especially for lacto-ovo vegetarians. Eggplant parmesan; vegetable lasagna; split pea or lentil soup with a hunk of bread and a garden salad; meatless chili; stuffed peppers; pizza—all these fit into a vegetarian menu.

**Myth number 3:** *Vegetarians don't get enough protein.*

**Fact:** Even vegans, who go without all the protein in dairy foods and eggs, tend not to be deficient in protein. A 160-pound man needs about 60 grams of protein a day; a 125-pound woman, about 45 grams. But a cup and a half of pasta alone contains 11 grams. Add in a cup of broccoli and a half cup of tomato sauce, and the protein tally jumps to 19 grams. And that's just at dinner.

Related to the not-enough-protein myth is the myth that vegetarians have to eat certain foods at the same time to make their proteins "complete." Granted, unlike a meat or dairy product, any one plant food is "incomplete" on its own because it does not contain all the amino acids (protein building blocks) that the body is unable to synthesize by itself. Therefore, vegan diets must include various combinations of plant foods to ensure that the amino acids absent from one are provided by another.

But researchers now have some evidence that those combinations—beans with grains or cereals; cereals with leafy vegetables; peanuts with wheat, oats, corn or rice; soy with corn,

---

## Vegetarian for a Day

THE FOLLOWING MENU is for a vegan, who would eat no dairy foods or eggs. Lacto-ovo vegetarians, who include milk, yogurt, cheese, and eggs in their diets, would have an even easier time meeting nutrient requirements.

The one-day example here provides 1,850 calories. It also supplies 66 grams of protein, 29 grams of iron, 870 milligrams of calcium, and 10 milligrams of zinc—meeting or exceeding current recommendations for most of those minerals, which are traditionally thought of as animal-food nutrients. In addition, it contributes just 10 grams of saturated fat—a mere 5 percent of total calories.

**Breakfast**
1 cup Kellogg's Raisin Bran
1 cup soymilk
1 cup calcium-fortified orange juice
**Midmorning snack**
1 banana
1 tablespoon peanut butter

**Lunch**
1 cup split pea soup
2 slices whole wheat bread
Salad tossed with 1 tablespoon slivered
    almonds
**Midafternoon snack**
2 tablespoons sunflower seeds

**Dinner**
1½ cups pasta
½ cup tomato sauce
1 cup broccoli mixed with ¼ cup tofu
**Evening snack**
1 cup cut-up cantaloupe

---

*Did you know...* Americans average 24 gallons of milk each year, down from 29 gallons in 1975. That comes to an annual per-capita drop in calcium consumption of 24,000 milligrams—almost a month's worth of the recommended allowance for that bone-building mineral.

From *Tufts University Health & Nutrition Letter*, April 1998, pp. 4-5. © 1998 by Tufts University Diet & Nutrition Letter. Reprinted by permission.

wheat, or rye—do not have to be eaten at the same time. An over-the-course-of-the day approach appears fine.

From a practical standpoint, it doesn't matter either way. Rice and beans, peanut butter and jelly sandwiches, bread dipped into a bean-based soup—these and many other meals that people eat without thinking about protein needs meet the requirement.

**Myth number 4:** *Vegetarians are seriously deficient in iron, calcium, and other essential nutrients.*

**Fact:** There are five nutrients that present special concerns for vegetarians: iron, calcium, vitamin D, vitamin $B_{12}$, and zinc. But that said, the rate of iron-deficiency anemia is similar in vegetarians and meat eaters. And calcium consumption, at least among lacto-ovo vegetarians, is similar to the calcium consumption of nonvegetarians.

To be sure, the iron in plant foods, known as nonheme iron, is not as well absorbed as the heme iron in animal foods. But vegetarians tend to take in more iron than nonvegetarians overall, which helps offset the absorption problem. Indeed, **the vegan menu on the previous page has 29 milligrams of iron, more than twice as much as many Americans typically consume.** What's more, the vitamin C contained in much of the produce that vegetarians eat aids iron absorption. See the chart for a listing of some iron-rich plant foods.

As for calcium, vegetarians who don't eat dairy products do have to try to get plenty of calcium from other sources. But there are more calcium-containing non-dairy foods than most people are aware of. For example, a tablespoon of blackstrap molasses (mixed into, say, a bowl of oatmeal) contains 172 milligrams, as the chart shows.

Along with calcium, non-dairy-eating vegans need to make sure they get enough vitamin D—necessary for the proper absorption of calcium and found most abundantly in milk. Non-animal sources of D include sunlight (the nutrient is synthesized in the skin) fortified breakfast cereals, fortified soymilk, and multivitamin supplements.

One nutrient that presents a challenge for vegans and lacto-ovo vegetarians alike is vitamin $B_{12}$, long-term deficiencies of which could cause nerve damage. Many vegetarians rely on tempeh and miso for $B_{12}$ and on certain vegetables, too. But much of the $B_{12}$ in those foods is an inactive $B_{12}$ analog, not the active vitamin found in animal foods.

Dairy products and eggs contain $B_{12}$, but research suggests that even lacto-ovo vegetarians have low levels of that nutrient. For that reason, all vegetarians should make a conscious effort to consume more $B_{12}$. Like vitamin D, it is found in fortified breakfast cereals, fortified soymilk, and multivitamin supplements.

Finally, vegetarians should try to take in more zinc, needed for protein synthesis, wound healing, and proper immunity. That's because zinc from plant foods is less available to the body than zinc from meat and poultry.

The Recommended Dietary Allowance for zinc is 15 milligrams a day for men and 10 milligrams for women. Plant sources include grain products like corn and wheat germ, fortified cereals, beans, and soy-based foods like tofu. Zinc is also available in dairy foods.

**Myth number 5:** *It would be better for the environment if we stopped killing animals for food.*

**Fact:** Animals compete with humans for food and other resources, including space. Thus, if we were to stop using animals for food completely, humans would be in trouble.

Says Joan Dye Gussow, EdD, a professor emeritus of nutrition and education at Columbia University Teacher's College, "Some people have the idea that if we just freed the cattle and stopped eating beef, the buffalo would return to the prairie; the foxes would come back; and we could grow crops where the cattle used to graze. But it's not that simple.

"One consequence would be that animals like deer would return to where the cattle were. And they'd eat the foods we planted for ourselves." In other words, at a certain point, it's "them or us" when it comes to animals.

To be sure, Dr. Gussow comments, "the way we do kill animals currently to produce food is an ecological horror." Small pens for cattle, hog confinement facilities, chicken "tene-

## Iron content of plant foods

For women of childbearing years, the Recommended Dietary Allowance for iron is 15 milligrams. For women who have reached menopause and for men the RDA is 10 milligrams.

| | Iron* (milligrams) |
|---|---|
| ½ cup raw tofu | 7 |
| 1 tablespoon blackstrap molasses | 4 |
| ½ cup lentils | 3 |
| 2 tablespoons pumpkin seeds | 3 |
| ½ cup garbanzo beans (chickpeas) | 2 |
| ½ cup Swiss chard | 2 |
| 5 dried apricots | 1 |
| 2 tablespoons cashews | 1 |
| 1 cup tomato juice | 1 |
| 1 cup white rice | 1 |
| 1 slice whole wheat bread | 1 |

*Substances in coffee and tea called polyphenols can reduce the absorption of iron in plant foods by up to 70 percent. Those making a conscious effort to get enough iron should not drink coffee or tea for an hour and half after they eat iron-containing foods. They should also eat some iron-rich foods with foods that contain vitamin C, which enhances iron absorption. Many breakfast cereals are also fortified with iron.
†For foods that require cooking, values are for cooked weight or volume.

## Calcium content of plant foods

Men and women through age 50 should shoot for 1,000 milligrams of calcium a day; after age 50, 1,200 milligrams daily.

| | Calcium (milligrams) |
|---|---|
| 1 cup fortified soymilk | 250-300 |
| 1 cup calcium-fortified orange juice | 300 |
| ½ cup raw tofu | 100-250 |
| ½ cup frozen collard greens | 179 |
| 1 tablespoon blackstrap molasses | 172 |
| 5 dried figs | 135 |
| ½ cup frozen turnip greens | 125 |
| ½ cup frozen kale | 90 |
| ½ cup navy beans | 64 |
| 2 tablespoons almonds | 50 |
| 1 orange | 50 |
| ½ cup frozen broccoli | 47 |

†For foods that require cooking, values are for cooked weight or volume.
**Calcium content varies. Check labels.

ments"—all of these huge concentrations of animals and their waste pollute the soil, water, and air. And, of course, they make the animals' lives unnecessarily miserable.

Dr. Gussow says it would be much better for the planet to raise fewer animals for food in a much less concentrated manner—and consequently eat much less flesh food. But, she says, "the idea of taking no animals' lives for food does not allow for the continuance of human life or for the earth's ecosystems to be sustained."

# Doing the DRIs
### A no-nonsense guide to the nation's new nutritional yardsticks
### by **Stephen Barrett**, MD

The Dietary Reference Intakes (DRIs) are nutrient-based reference values for use in planning and assessing diets and for other purposes. They are intended to replace the Recommended Dietary Allowances (RDAs) that have been published since 1941 by the National Academy of Sciences. They are being determined by the Standing Committee on the Scientific Evaluation of Dietary Reference Intakes of the Food and Nutrition Board, Institute of Medicine (IOM), National Academy of Sciences, with help from Health Canada. The IOM is a private, nonprofit organization that provides health policy advice under a congressional charter granted to the National Academy of Sciences.

The DRIs will be released in a series of seven reports. The first report, published in August 1997, covers nutrients related to bone health (calcium, phosphorus, magnesium, vitamin D, and fluoride). Subsequent volumes will consider: (1) folate and other B vitamins; (2) antioxidants (e.g., vitamins C and E, selenium); (3) macronutrients (protein, fat, carbohydrates); (4) trace elements (e.g., iron, zinc); (5) electrolytes and water; and (6) other food components (e.g., fiber, phytoestrogens). The first report was funded by the FDA, the USDA Agricultural Research Service, and the National Heart, Lung, and Blood Institute. The IOM hopes that all of the reports will be released by the year 2000.

## A New Approach

The RDAs have served as the benchmark of nutritional adequacy in the United States. More than 20 years ago, they were defined as: "The levels of intake of essential nutrients that, on the basis of scientific knowledge, are judged by the Food and Nutrition Board to be adequate to meet the known nutrient needs of practically all healthy persons."

*The DRIs reflect a shift in emphasis from preventing deficiency to decreasing the risk of chronic disease through nutrition.*

Scientific knowledge about the roles of nutrients has expanded dramatically since the RDAs were first published. Many studies have examined relationships between diet and chronic disease. The Food and Nutrition Board has responded to these developments by changing its basic approach to setting nutrient reference values.

The DRIs reflect a shift in emphasis from preventing deficiency to decreasing the risk of chronic disease through nutrition. The RDAs were based on the amounts needed to protect against deficiency diseases. Where adequate scientific data exist, the DRIs will include levels that can help prevent cardiovascular disease, osteoporosis, certain cancers, and other diseases that are diet-related. Instead of a single category, the DRIs will encompass at least four:

1. Estimated Average Requirement (EAR): The intake that meets the estimated nutrient need of 50% of the individuals in a specific group. This figure will be used as the basis for developing the RDA and can be used by nutrition policy-makers to evaluate the adequacy of nutrient intakes for population groups.

2. Recommended Dietary Allowance (RDA): The intake that meets the nutrient need of almost all (97 to 98%) of the healthy individuals in a specific age and gender group. The RDA should be used in guiding individuals to achieve adequate nutrient intake aimed at decreasing the risk of chronic disease. It is based on estimating an average requirement plus an increase to account for the variation within a particular group. The amount of scientific evidence available allowed the DRI committee to calculate RDAs for phosphorus and magnesium. If individual variation in requirements is well defined, the RDA is set at 2 standard deviations above the EAR, which means it should be high enough to meet the needs of at least 97-98% of the population. If sufficient data are not available, the RDA is set at 1.2 x EAR.

3. Adequate Intake (AI): When sufficient scientific evidence is not available to estimate an average requirement, Adequate Intakes (AIs) will be set. These are derived though experimental or observational data that show a mean intake which appears to sustain a desired indicator of health, such as calcium retention in bone. The AIs should be used as a goal for individual intake where no RDAs exist. The DRI committee set AIs for calcium, vitamin D, and fluoride.

4. Tolerable Upper Intake Level (UL): The maximum intake by an individual that is unlikely to pose risks of adverse health effects in almost all healthy individuals in a specified group. The UL is not intended to be a recommended level of intake, and there is no established benefit for individuals to consume nutrients at levels above the RDA or AI. The term "tolerable upper intake level" was chosen to avoid implying a possible beneficial effect. For most nutrients, it refers to total intake from food, fortified food, and supplements.

From *Nutrition Forum*, November/December 1997, pp. 41-44. © 1997 by Prometheus Books, 59 John Glenn Drive, Amherst, NY 14228. Reprinted by permission of the publisher.

## What They Mean

The DRIs are intended to apply to the healthy general population. RDAs and AIs are dietary intake values that should minimize the risk of developing a condition or sign that is associated with that nutrient in question and that has a negative functional outcome. They refer to average daily intake over one or more weeks. They should not necessarily be expected to replete individuals who are already malnourished and may not be adequate for disease states marked by increased requirements.

Individuals known to have diseases that greatly increase requirements, or who have increased sensitivity to developing adverse effects associated with higher intakes, should be guided by qualified medical and nutrition personnel.

The committee cautioned that nutrient intake less than the RDA does not necessarily mean that a given individual is not getting enough of that nutrient. Healthy individuals who meet the AI have a low risk of inadequate intake. However, an intake well below the RDA or AI would be a reason to assess the individual's nutritional status through laboratory testing or clinical examination. The IOM expects future publications to provide more detailed advice on how the DRIs should be interpreted and used.

## Revised Values

In many cases, various levels of intake can have different benefits. One level may be related to the risk of deficiency, for example, while another level can influence the risk of chronic disease for that nutrient. For this reason, "nutrient adequacy" should be expressed in terms of "Adequate for what?" For this reason, the DRIs are far more elaborate than the RDAs and cannot be expressed in a simple table of values.

- Calcium recommendations were set at levels associated with maximum retention of body calcium because bones that are calcium-rich are known to be less susceptible to fractures. The other factors known to affect bone retention of calcium and risk of osteoporosis include high rates of growth in children during specific periods, hormonal status, exercise, genetics, and other diet components. The new report advises Americans and Canadians at

risk for osteoporosis to consume between 1000 and 1300 milligrams of calcium per day. These values (AIs) are higher than the 1989 RDAs, which ranged from 800 to 1200. The adult UL for calcium is 2.5 grams per day.

- Phosphorus, important for bone and soft tissue growth, is so prevalent in various foods that near starvation or a metabolic disorder is required to produce deficiency. Different from former RDAs, phosphorus values in the report are not derived in relation to calcium. The values recommended are considered sufficient to support normal bone growth and metabolism at various ages. The new RDAs are about 12% lower than the 1989 RDAs.

- Magnesium works with many enzymes to regulate body temperature, allow nerves and muscles to contract, and synthesize proteins. Although some researchers have argued that magnesium recommendations should be based on relationships with the risk of cardiovascular disease, the report does not find enough data available at this time to do so. The levels recommended, although somewhat higher, do not differ substantially from the 1989 RDAs but are higher than current Canadian recommendations.

- Vitamin D used by the body comes mostly through exposure to the sun. Vitamin D deficiency can exacerbate osteoporosis and other bone problems in adults. Dietary intake of vitamin D is unnecessary for people who spend adequate amounts of time in the sun. The levels recommended in the report are estimated to provide enough vitamin D even for individuals with limited sun exposure. The AIs of 10 micrograms from age 51 to 70 and 15 micrograms over age 70 are higher than their 1989 counterparts. The adult UL for vitamin D is 50 micrograms (2000 IU) per day.

- Fluoride is found naturally in some community water systems and is added to water in other areas to reduce dental decay. The levels recommended in the DRIs have been shown to reduce tooth decay without causing marked fluorosis, a discoloration of the teeth that could occur in children who use dental products with fluoride in addition to fluoridated water. The AIs for fluoride are similar to the corresponding values (ESADDIs) in the 1989 report. The American Dental Asso-

ciation, the American Academy of Pediatrics, and the Canadian Paediatric Society recommend that children living in nonfluoridated communities take fluoride supplements because the required amount is unlikely to be provided by food. The amounts recommended for infants and children have been lowered during the past few years because of concern about fluorosis, a cosmetic defect that most commonly involves white patches that are barely visible on the teeth.

Except for fluoride, the greatest disparity between recommended values and current dietary patterns is in calcium, which comes primarily from dairy products. Surveys indicate that many do not consume the amount of calcium recommended in the report. Calcium intake can be increased by consuming more low-fat or nonfat dairy products or fortified food products or by taking supplements. The report states that taking supplements may be appropriate for those at high risk of health problems due to low calcium intake.

The report also states: (a) unfortified foods are advantageous for meeting the RDAs and AIs because they provide other food components for which RDAs and AIs may not be determined; (b) food fortification can increase or maintain nutrient intakes without major changes in food habits; and (c) nutrient supplementation may be desirable for some people.

The full report—*Dietary Reference Intakes: Calcium, Phosphorus, Magnesium, Vitamin D, and Fluoride*—can be purchased by calling (800) 624-6242; sending $39 to the National Academy Press, 201 Constitution Ave., NW, Washington, DC 20418; or ordering it at a discount online (**http://www.nap.edu**). The full text can also be read online, although the process is cumbersome.

---

*Stephen Barrett, MD, is coauthor/editor of* Consumer Health: A Guide to Intelligent Decisions *(McGraw-Hill, 1997) and 42 other health-related books. His web site is* **http://www.quackwatch.com**; *his e-mail is sbinfo@quackwatch.com*

# An FDA Guide to *Dietary Supplements*

*by Paula Kurtzweil*

Set between a Chinese restaurant and a pizza and sub sandwich eatery, a Rockville health food store offers yet another brand of edible items: Bottled herbs like cat's claw, dandelion root, and blessed thistle. Vitamins and minerals in varying doses. Herbal and nutrient concoctions whose labels carry claims about relieving pain, "energizing" and "detoxifying" the body, or providing "guaranteed results."

This store sells dietary supplements, some of the hottest selling items on the market today. Surveys show that more than half of the U.S. adult population uses these products. In 1996 alone, consumers spent more than $6.5 billion on dietary supplements, according to Packaged Facts Inc., a market research firm in New York City.

But even with all the business they generate, consumers still ask questions about dietary supplements: Can their claims be trusted? Are they safe? Does the Food and Drug Administration approve them?

Many of these questions come in the wake of the 1994 Dietary Supplement Health and Education Act, or DSHEA, which set up a new framework for FDA regulation of dietary supplements. It also created an office in the National Institutes of Health to coordinate research on dietary supplements, and it called on President Clinton to set up an independent dietary supplement commission to

report on the use of claims in dietary supplement labeling.

In passing DSHEA, Congress recognized first, that many people believe dietary supplements offer health benefits and second, that consumers want a greater opportunity to determine whether supplements may help them. The law essentially gives dietary supplement manufacturers freedom to market more products as dietary supplements

and provide information about their products' benefits—for example, in product labeling.

The Council for Responsible Nutrition, an organization of manufacturers of dietary supplements and their suppliers, welcomes the change. "Our philosophy has been ... to maintain consumer access to products and access to information [so that consumers can] make informed choices," says John Cordaro, the group's

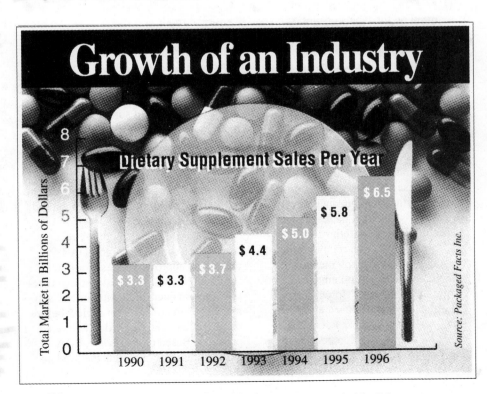

**Growth of an Industry**

Dietary Supplement Sales Per Year

*Source: Packaged Facts Inc.*

| Total Market in Billions of Dollars | | | | | | |
|---|---|---|---|---|---|---|
| $3.3 | $3.3 | $3.7 | $4.4 | $5.0 | $5.8 | $6.5 |
| 1990 | 1991 | 1992 | 1993 | 1994 | 1995 | 1996 |

From *FDA Consumer,* September/October 1998, pp. 28-35. Reprinted by permission of *FDA Consumer,* the magazine of the U.S. Food and Drug Administration.

president and chief executive officer.

But in choosing whether to use dietary supplements, FDA answers consumers' questions by noting that under DSHEA, FDA's requirement for premarket review of dietary supplements is less than that over other products it regulates, such as drugs and many additives used in conventional foods.

This means that consumers *and* manufacturers also have responsibility for checking the safety of dietary supplements and determining the truthfulness of label claims.

## What Is a Dietary Supplement?

Traditionally, dietary supplements referred to products made of one or more of the essential nutrients, such as vitamins, minerals, and protein. But DSHEA broadens the definition to include, with some exceptions, any product intended for ingestion as a supplement to the diet. This includes vitamins; minerals; herbs, botanicals, and other plant-derived substances; and amino acids (the individual building blocks of protein) and concentrates, metabolites, constituents and extracts of these substances.

It's easy to spot a supplement because DSHEA requires manufacturers to include the words "dietary supplement" on product labels. Also, starting in March 1999, a "Supplement Facts" panel will be required on the labels of most dietary supplements.

Dietary supplements come in many forms, including tablets, capsules, powders, softgels, gelcaps, and liquids. Though commonly associated with health food stores, dietary supplements also are sold in grocery, drug and national discount chain stores, as well as through mail-order catalogs, TV programs, the Internet, and direct sales.

FDA oversees safety, manufacturing and product information, such as claims, in a product's labeling, package inserts, and accompanying literature. The Federal Trade Commission regulates the advertising of dietary supplements.

One thing dietary supplements are not is drugs. A drug, which sometimes can be derived from plants used as traditional medicines, is an article that, among other things, is intended to diagnose, cure, mitigate, treat, or prevent diseases. Before marketing, drugs must

**Structure-function claims can be easy to spot because, on the label, they must be accompanied with the disclaimer "This statement has not been evaluated by the Food and Drug Administration. This product is not intended to diagnose, treat, cure, or prevent any disease."**

undergo clinical studies to determine their effectiveness, safety, possible interactions with other substances, and appropriate dosages, and FDA must review these data and authorize the drugs' use before they are marketed. FDA does not authorize or test dietary supplements.

A product sold as a dietary supplement and touted in its labeling as a new treatment or cure for a specific disease or condition would be considered an unauthorized—and thus illegal—drug. Labeling changes consistent with the provisions in DSHEA would be required to maintain the product's status as a dietary supplement.

Another thing dietary supplements are not are replacements for conventional diets, nutritionists say. Supplements do not provide all the known—and perhaps unknown—nutritional benefits of conventional food.

## Monitoring for Safety

As with food, federal law requires manufacturers of dietary supplements to ensure that the products they put on the market are safe. But supplement manufacturers do not have to provide information to FDA to get a product on the market, unlike the food additive process often required of new food ingredients. FDA review and approval of supplement ingredients and products is not required before marketing.

Food additives not generally recognized as safe must undergo FDA's premarket approval process for new food ingredients. This requires manufacturers to conduct safety studies and submit the results to FDA for review before the ingredient can be used in marketed products. Based on its review, FDA either authorizes or rejects the food additive.

In contrast, dietary supplement manufacturers that wish to market a new ingredient (that is, an ingredient not marketed in the United States before 1994) have two options. The first involves submitting to FDA, at least 75 days before the product is expected to go on the market, information that supports their conclusion that a new ingredient can reasonably be expected to be safe. Safe means that the new ingredient does not present a significant or unreasonable risk of illness or injury under conditions of use recommended in the product's labeling.

The information the manufacturer submits becomes publicly available 90 days after FDA receives it.

Another option for manufacturers is to petition FDA, asking the agency to establish the conditions under which the new dietary ingredient would reasonably be expected to be safe. To date, FDA's Center for Food Safety and Applied Nutrition has received no such petitions.

Under DSHEA, once a dietary supplement is marketed, FDA has the responsibility for showing that a dietary supplement is unsafe before it can take action to restrict the product's use. This was the case when, in June 1997, FDA proposed, among other things, to limit the amount of ephedrine alkaloids in dietary supplements (marketed as ephedra, Ma huang, Chinese ephedra, and epitonin, for example) and provide warnings to consumers about hazards associated with use of dietary supplements containing the ingredients. The hazards ranged from nervousness, dizziness, and changes in blood pressure and heart rate to chest pain, heart attack, hepatitis, stroke, seizures, psychosis, and death. The proposal stemmed from FDA's review of adverse event reports it had received,

# Anatomy of the New Requirements for Dietary Supplement Labels

## (Effective March 1999)

**Statement of Identity**

GINSENG
A DIETARY SUPPLEMENT

**Net quantity of contents**

60 CAPSULES

**Structure-function claim**

"When you need to perform your best, take ginseng." **This statement has not been evaluated by the Food and Drug Administration. This product is not intended to diagnose, treat, cure, or prevent any disease.**

**Directions**

DIRECTIONS FOR USE: Take one capsule daily.

**Supplement Facts panel**

## Supplement Facts

Serving Size 1 Capsule

**Amount Per Capsule**

| | |
|---|---|
| Oriental Ginseng, powdered (root) | 250 mcg* |

*Daily Value not established.

**Other ingredients in descending order of predominance and by common name or proprietary blend.**

Other ingredients: Gelatin, water, and glycerin.

ABC Company
Anywhere, MD 00001

**Name and place of business of manufacturer, packer or distributor. This is the address to write for more product information.**

scientific literature, and public comments. FDA has received many comments on the 1997 proposal and was reviewing them at press time.

Also in 1997, FDA identified contamination of the herbal ingredient plantain with the harmful herb *Digitalis lanata* after receiving a report of a complete heart block in a young woman. FDA traced all use of the contaminated ingredient and asked manufacturers and retailers to withdraw these products from the market.

DSHEA also gives FDA authority to establish good manufacturing practices, or GMPs, for dietary supplements. In a February 1997 advance notice of proposed rulemaking, the agency said it would establish dietary supplement GMPs if, after public comment, it determined that GMPs for conventional food are not adequate to cover dietary supplements, as well. GMPs, the agency said, would ensure that dietary supplements are made under conditions that would result in safe and properly labeled products. At press time, FDA was reviewing comments on the 1997 notice.

Some supplement makers may already voluntarily follow GMPs devised, for example, by trade groups.

Besides FDA, individual states can take steps to restrict or stop the sale of potentially harmful dietary supplements within their jurisdictions. For example, Florida has already banned all ephedra-containing products, and other states have said they are considering similar action.

Also, the industry strives to regulate itself, the Council for Responsible Nutrition's Cordaro says. He cites the GMPs that his trade group and others developed for their member companies. FDA is reviewing these GMPs as it considers whether to pursue mandatory industry-wide GMPs. Another example of self-regulation, Cordaro says, is the voluntary use of a warning about ephedra products that his organization drafted. He says that about 90 percent of U.S. manufacturers of products containing ephedra alkaloids now use this warning label.

## Understanding Claims

Claims that tout a supplement's healthful benefits have always been a controversial feature of dietary supple-

ments. Manufacturers often rely on them to sell their products. But consumers often wonder whether they can trust them.

Under DSHEA and previous food labeling laws, supplement manufacturers are allowed to use, when appropriate, three types of claims: nutrient-content claims, disease claims, and nutrition support claims, which include "structure-function claims."

Nutrient-content claims describe the level of a nutrient in a food or dietary supplement. For example, a supplement containing at least 200 milligrams of calcium per serving could carry the claim "high in calcium." A supplement with at least 12 mg per serving of vitamin C could state on its label, "Excellent source of vitamin C."

Disease claims show a link between a food or substance and a disease or health-related condition. FDA authorizes these claims based on a review of the scientific evidence. Or, after the agency is notified, the claims may be based on an authoritative statement from certain scientific bodies, such as the National Academy of Sciences, that shows or describes a well-established diet-to-health link. As of this writing, certain dietary supplements may be eligible to carry disease claims, such as claims that show a link between:

• the vitamin folic acid and a decreased risk of neural tube defect-affected pregnancy, if the supplement contains sufficient amounts of folic acid
• calcium and a lower risk of osteoporosis, if the supplement contains sufficient amounts of calcium
• psyllium seed husk (as part of a diet low in cholesterol and saturated fat) and coronary heart disease, if the supplement contains sufficient amounts of psyllium seed husk.

Nutrition support claims can describe a link between a nutrient and the deficiency disease that can result if the nutrient is lacking in the diet. For example, the label of a vitamin C supplement could state that vitamin C prevents scurvy. When these types of claims are used, the label must mention the prevalence of the nutrient-deficiency disease in the United States.

These claims also can refer to the supplement's effect on the body's structure or function, including its overall

# Supplement Your Knowledge

Some sources for additional information on dietary supplements are:

## Federal Agencies

**Food and Drug Administration:**

*Office of Consumer Affairs*
HFE-88
Rockville, MD 20857

*Food Information Line*
1-800-FDA-4010
(202) 205-4314 in the Washington, D.C., area

*FDA Website*
*www.cfsan.fda.gov/~dms/supplmnt.html*

## Federal Trade Commission
Public Reference Branch
Room 130
Washington, DC 20580
*www.ftc.gov*

## National Institute on Aging
NIA Information Center
P.O. Box 8057
Gaithersburg, MD 20898-8057
1-800-222-2225
TTY: 1-800-222-4225
*http://128.231.160.11/nia/health/
pubpub/hormrev.htm*

## Health Professional Organizations

American Dietetic Association
216 W. Jackson Blvd.
Chicago, IL 60606-6995
1-800-366-1655 (recorded messages)
1-900-225-5267 (to talk to a registered dietitian)
*www.eatright.org*

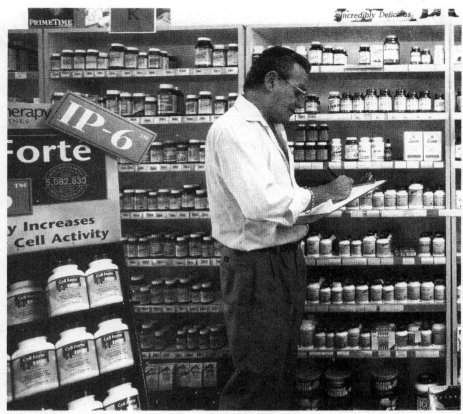

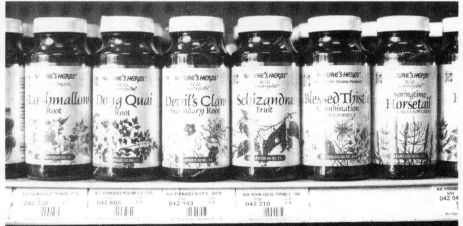

Carlo Scarzella, owner of Montgomery Health Foods in Rockville, Md., checks inventory (top photo). Like many health food stores, his carries an array of herbal products.

PHOTOGRAPHS BY NORMAN WATKINS

effect on a person's well-being. These are known as structure-function claims.

Examples of structure-function claims are:
• Calcium builds strong bones.
• Antioxidants maintain cell integrity.
• Fiber maintains bowel regularity.

Manufacturers can use structure-function claims without FDA authorization. They base their claims on their review and interpretation of the scientific literature. Like all label claims, structure-function claims must be true and not misleading.

Structure-function claims can be easy to spot because, on the label, they must be accompanied with the disclaimer *"This statement has not been evaluated by the Food and Drug Administration. This product is not intended to diagnose, treat, cure, or prevent any disease."*

Manufacturers who plan to use a structure-function claim on a particular product must inform FDA of the use of the claim no later than 30 days after the product is first marketed. While the manufacturer must be able to substantiate its claim, it does not have to share the substantiation with FDA or make it publicly available.

If the submitted claims promote the products as drugs instead of supplements, FDA can advise the manufacturer to change or delete the claim.

Because there often is a fine line between disease claims and structure-function claims, FDA in April proposed regulations that would establish criteria under which a label claim would or would not qualify as a disease claim. Among label factors FDA proposed for consideration are:
• the naming of a specific disease or class of diseases
• the use of scientific or lay terminology to describe the product's effect on one or more signs or symptoms recognized by health-care professionals and consumers as characteristic of a specific disease or a number of different specific diseases
• product name
• statements about product formulation
• citations or references that refer to disease
• use of the words "disease" or "diseased"
• art, such as symbols and pictures
• statements that the product can substitute for an approved therapy (for example, a drug).

# Supplements Associate

| NAME | POSSIBLE HEALTH HAZARDS |
|------|-------------------------|
| **Herbal Ingredients** | |
| ***Chaparral*** (a traditional American Indian medicine) | liver disease, possibly irreversible |
| ***Comfrey*** | obstruction of blood flow to liver, possibly leading to death |
| ***Slimming/dieter's teas*** | nausea, diarrhea, vomiting, stomach cramps, chronic constipation, fainting, possibly death (see "Dieter's Brews Make Tea Time a Dangerous Affair" in the July-August 1997 *FDA Consumer*) |
| ***Ephedra*** (also known as Ma huang, Chinese Ephedra and epitonin) | ranges from high blood pressure, irregular heartbeat, nerve damage, injury, insomnia, tremors, and headaches to seizures, heart attack, stroke, and death |
| ***Germander*** | liver disease, possibly leading to death |
| ***Lobelia*** (also known as Indian tobacco) | range from breathing problems at low doses to sweating, rapid heartbeat, low blood pressure, and possibly coma and death at higher doses |
| ***Magnolia-Stephania preparation*** | kidney disease, possibly leading to permanent kidney failure |
| ***Willow bark*** | Reye syndrome, a potentially fatal disease associated with aspirin intake in children with chickenpox or flu symptoms; allergic reaction in adults. (Willow bark is marketed as an aspirin-free product, although it actually contains an ingredient that converts to the same active ingredient in aspirin.) |
| ***Wormwood*** | neurological symptoms, characterized by numbness of legs and arms, loss of intellect, delirium, and paralysis |

FDA's proposal is consistent with the guidance on the distinction between structure-function and disease claims provided in the 1997 report by the President's Commission on Dietary Supplement Labels.

If shoppers find dietary supplements whose labels state or imply that the product can help diagnose, treat, cure, or prevent a disease (for example, "cures cancer" or "treats arthritis"), they should realize that the product is being marketed illegally as a drug and as such has not been evaluated for safety or effectiveness.

FTC regulates claims made in the advertising of dietary supplements, and in recent years, that agency has taken a number of enforcement actions against companies whose advertisements contained false and misleading information. The actions targeted, for example, erroneous claims that chromium picolinate was a treatment for weight loss and high blood cholesterol. An action in 1997 targeted ads for an ephedrine alkaloid supplement because they understated the degree of the product's risk and featured a man falsely described as a doctor.

**Fraudulent Products**

Consumers need to be on the lookout for fraudulent products. These are products that don't do what they say they can or don't contain what they say they contain. At the very least, they waste consumers' money, and they may cause physical harm.

Fraudulent products often can be identified by the types of claims made in their labeling, advertising and promotional literature. Some possible indicators of fraud, says Stephen Barrett, M.D., a board member of the National Council Against Health Fraud, are:

# Vith Illnesses And Injuries

| NAME | POSSIBLE HEALTH HAZARDS |
|---|---|
| **Vitamins and Essential Minerals** | |
| *Vitamin A* **in doses of 25,000 or more International Units a day** | birth defects, bone abnormalities, and severe liver disease |
| *Vitamin B$_6$* **in doses above 100 milligrams a day** | balance difficulties, nerve injury causing changes in touch sensation |
| *Niacin* **in slow-released doses of 500 mg or more a day or immediate-release doses of 750 mg or more a day** | range from stomach pain, vomiting, bloating, nausea, cramping, and diarrhea to liver disease, muscle disease, eye damage, and heart injury |
| *Selenium* **in doses of about 800 micrograms to 1,000 mcg a day** | tissue damage |
| **Other Supplements** | |
| *Germanium* (a nonessential mineral) | kidney damage, possibly death |
| *L-tryptophan* (an amino acid) | eosinophilia myalgia syndrome, a potentially fatal blood disorder that can cause high fever, muscle and joint pain, weakness, skin rash, and swelling of the arms and legs |

(Source: FDA Statement before Senate Committee on Labor and Human Resources, Oct. 21, 1993)

• Claims that the product is a secret cure and use of such terms as "breakthrough," "magical," "miracle cure," and "new discovery." If the product were a cure for a serious disease, it would be widely reported in the media and used by health-care professionals, he says.

• "Pseudomedical" jargon, such as "detoxify," "purify" and "energize" to describe a product's effects. These claims are vague and hard to measure, Barrett says. So, they make it easier for success to be claimed "even though nothing has actually been accom-plished," he says.

• Claims that the product can cure a wide range of unrelated diseases. No product can do that, he says.

• Claims that a product is backed by scientific studies, but with no list of references or references that are inadequate. For instance, if a list of references is provided, the citations cannot be traced, or if they are traceable, the studies are out-of-date, irrelevant, or poorly designed.

• Claims that the supplement has only benefits—and no side effects. A product "potent enough to help people will be potent enough to cause side effects," Barrett says.

• Accusations that the medical profession, drug companies and the government are suppressing information about a particular treatment. It would be illogical, Barrett says, for large numbers of people to withhold information about potential medical therapies when they or their families and friends might one day benefit from them.

Though often more difficult to do, consumers also can protect themselves from economic fraud, a practice in which the manufacturer substitutes part or all of a product with an inferior, cheaper ingredient and then passes off the fake product as the real thing but at a lower cost. Varro Tyler, Ph.D., Sc.D., a distinguished professor emeritus of pharmacognosy (the study of medicinal products in their crude, or unprepared, form) at Purdue University in West LaFayette, Ind., advises consumers to avoid products sold for considerably less money than competing brands. "If it's too cheap, the product is probably not what it's supposed to be," he says.

## Quality Products

Poor manufacturing practices are not unique to dietary supplements, but the growing market for supplements in a less restrictive regulatory environment creates the potential for supplements to be prone to quality-control problems. For example, FDA has identified several problems where some manufacturers were buying herbs, plants and other ingredients without first adequately testing them to determine whether the product they ordered was actually what they received or whether the ingredients were free from contaminants.

To help protect themselves, consumers should:
• Look for ingredients in products with the U.S.P. notation, which indicates the manufacturer followed standards established by the U.S. Pharmacopoeia.
• Realize that the label term "natural" doesn't guarantee that a product is safe. "Think of poisonous mushrooms," says Elizabeth Yetley, Ph.D., director of FDA's Office of Special Nutritionals. "They're natural."
• Consider the name of the manufacturer or distributor. Supplements made by a nationally known food and drug manufacturer, for example, have likely been made under tight controls because these companies already have in place manufacturing standards for their other products.
• Write to the supplement manufacturer for more information. Ask the company about the conditions under which its products were made.

## Reading and Reporting

Consumers who use dietary supplements should always read product labels, follow directions, and heed all warnings.

Supplement users who suffer a serious harmful effect or illness that they think is re-

## Expert Advice

Before starting a dietary supplement, it's always wise to check with a medical doctor. It is especially important for people who are:
• pregnant or breastfeeding
• chronically ill
• elderly
• under 18
• taking prescription or over-the-counter medicines. Certain supplements can boost blood levels of certain drugs to dangerous levels.

Varro Tyler, Ph.D., Sc.D., distinguished professor emeritus of pharmacognosy at Purdue University, cites as examples garlic and the supplement ginkgo biloba. Both thin the blood, which can be hazardous, he says, for people taking prescription medicines that also thin the blood.

In addition to medical doctors, other health-care professionals, such as registered pharmacists, registered dietitians and nutritionists, also can be sources of information about dietary supplements. ■
—P.K.

lated to supplement use should call a doctor or other health-care provider. He or she in turn can report it to FDA MedWatch by calling 1-800-FDA-1088 or going to *www.fda.gov/medwatch/report/hcp.htm* on the MedWatch Website. Patients' names are kept confidential.

Consumers also may call the toll-free MedWatch number or go to *www.fda.gov/medwatch/report/consumer/consumer.htm* on the MedWatch Website to report an adverse reaction. To file a report, consumers will be asked to provide:

• name, address and telephone number of the person who became ill
• name and address of the doctor or hospital providing medical treatment
• description of the problem
• name of the product and store where it was bought.

Consumers also should report the problem to the manufacturer or distributor listed on the product's label and to the store where the product was bought.

## Today's Dietary Supplements

The report of the President's Commission on Dietary Supplement Labels, released in November 1997, provides a look at the future of dietary supplements. It encourages researchers to find out whether consumers want and can use the information allowed in dietary supplement labeling under DSHEA. It encourages studies to identify more clearly the relationships be-

tween dietary supplements and health maintenance and disease prevention. It urges FDA to take enforcement action when questions about a product's safety arise. And it suggests that FDA and the industry work together to develop guidelines on the use of warning statements on dietary supplement labels.

FDA generally concurred with the commission's recommendations in the agency's 1998 proposed rule on dietary supplement claims.

While much remains unknown about many dietary supplements— their health benefits and potential risks, for example—there's one thing consumers can count on: the availability of a wide range of such products. But consumers who decide to take advantage of the expanding market should do so with care, making sure they have the necessary information and consulting with their doctors and other health professionals as needed.

"The majority of supplement manufacturers are responsible and careful," FDA's Yetley says. "But, as with all products on the market, consumers need to be discriminating. FDA and industry have important roles to play, but consumers must take responsibility, too."

*Paula Kurtzweil is a member of FDA's public affairs staff.*

# Fruits and vegetables: Nature's best protection

## *Produce seems to cut the risk of disease better than any other foods or pills.*

Only one-third of Americans eat at least five servings of fruits and vegetables every day, the minimum amount recommended for good health. That's less than the number of people who regularly take a vitamin pill or some other nutritional supplement.

Certain supplements seem promising, and further research may ultimately confirm their benefits. But no pill can deliver the same punch as a plate of nutritious produce. And reams of evidence already convincingly link produce with a reduced risk of deadly or disabling disease, including the big three killers: cancer, coronary heart disease, and stroke.

### A cornucopia of nutrients

In recent years, researchers have become convinced that the nutrients in fruits and vegetables do more than just prevent deficiency diseases such as beriberi or rickets. The most widely publicized finding was that certain vitamins or vitamin precursors in produce, notably vitamin C and beta-carotene, are powerful antioxidants. Antioxidants help prevent molecular damage caused by oxidation; that protection may help fend off not only the three major killers but also arthritis, asthma, cataracts, and macular degeneration, the leading cause of blindness after age 65.

But vitamin C and beta-carotene—plus a third strong antioxidant, vitamin E, which is fairly scarce in produce—account for only 15 percent of the total antioxidant potency of the average fruit or vegetable. The other 85 percent comes from an array of relatively obscure phytochemicals, or plant chemicals, such as the roughly 100 carotenoids other than beta-carotene found in the human diet.

Equally important, researchers have identified many other potentially disease-fighting substances besides antioxidants that are plentiful in fruits and vegetables. Those substances, which include fiber, minerals, and various other vitamins and phytochemicals, may protect against a wide range of ailments, such as abnormal heart rhythms, diabetes, hypertension, osteoporosis, and various gastrointestinal disorders, as well as cancer, coronary disease, and stroke. The table on page 36 describes the most likely disease-fighting compounds in produce that have been unearthed by scientists so far. But fruits and vegetables contain thousands of other compounds, and nutrition researchers suspect that

hundreds of them will eventually turn out to be protective in one way or another.

The only way to get that host of potentially beneficial substances is by consuming plenty of fruits and vegetables. In fact, some nutrients seem to work better when you get them from food sources rather than from pills.

For example, nutrition researchers from the U.S. Department of Agriculture found that exposing isolated vitamin C to iron can change the vitamin from an *anti*oxidant to a *pro*-oxidant—a substance that actually promotes oxidation. But the same thing does not happen when vitamin C in *food* interacts with iron. Similarly, high doses of beta-carotene from dietary supplements may reduce blood levels of vitamin E. (That may help explain why observational studies, based almost entirely on food-intake records, have strongly supported the health benefits of beta-carotene, while clinical trials, using beta-carotene supplements, have found either no benefit or an actual increase in the risk of disease.) Fortunately, the evidence to date on most of the individual phytochemicals shows that they deliver their maximum protective effect at intake levels you can readily achieve just by eating plenty of fruits and vegetables.

There's one other reason to get your nutrients mainly from food: The more produce and other lean foods you consume, the less room in your diet for high-fat foods, which can increase the risk of weight gain and of certain diseases.

### The proof on produce

Research on the protective benefits of fruits and vegetables in humans has focused almost entirely on cancer and cardiovascular disease, as well as on hypertension, which is a major risk factor for cardiovascular disease.

■ **Hypertension.** Several observational studies of high blood pressure and produce consumption have indicated that fruits and vegetables may help lower blood pressure. Now a carefully controlled clinical trial—a far more definitive type of study—has virtually confirmed that evidence, as we described in last month's report on hypertension. The trial, called Dietary Approaches to Stop Hypertension (DASH), involved randomly assigning 133 people with hypertension to spend two months on one of three diets: a regimen rich in both produce and lean dairy products, rich in pro-

Reprinted with permission from *Consumer Reports on Health*, June 1998, pp. 1, 3-5. © 1998 by Consumers Union of U.S., Inc., Yonkers, NY 10703-1057.

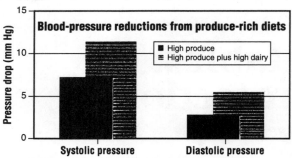

**Blood-pressure reductions from produce-rich diets**

■ High produce
≡ High produce plus high dairy

Systolic pressure    Diastolic pressure

**Pressure-reducing diets** A produce-rich diet reduces blood pressure in people with hypertension. Adding lean dairy foods as required by the DASH diet (see story) yields further reductions.

duce but low in dairy products, or low in both produce and dairy. The combination high-produce, high-dairy diet reduced blood-pressure readings significantly compared with the low-produce, low-dairy diet. Fruits and vegetables accounted for a big chunk of those pressure reductions (see bar chart at left). In the same study, high produce intake caused smaller reductions in a larger group of people with normal blood pressure.

■ **Cardiovascular disease.** The antihypertensive power of produce, combined with its antioxidant and anticlotting properties (see "Promising Compounds In Produce") help explain why 14 of 19 observational studies so far have linked a high intake of fruits and vegetables with a reduced risk of developing cardiovascular disease—either coronary disease or stroke.

In one large study, Harvard researchers followed some 44,000 men for six years. Those who ate five to

## Promising compounds in produce

| Substance | Good sources in produce | Possible benefits | Possible mechanisms |
|---|---|---|---|
| Soluble fiber | Most fruits, some vegetables. (Other sources: barley, certain beans, certain breakfast cereals.) | Linked with reduced risk of coronary heart disease and diabetes. | Reduces blood-cholesterol and blood-sugar levels. |
| Insoluble fiber | Most vegetables, some fruits. (Other sources: almonds, barley, certain breakfast cereals, brown rice, legumes, whole wheat.) | Helps prevent constipation and hemorrhoids. Linked with reduced risk of colon cancer, diverticulitis (inflamed protrusions in the colon), duodenal ulcers, and possibly breast cancer. | Speeds potentially constipating, irritating, or carcinogenic wastes through the colon. May reduce levels of estrogen, which stimulates breast-cancer growth. |
| Vitamin C | Cantaloupe, citrus fruits, kiwi, papaya, strawberries, broccoli, brussels sprouts, hot or sweet peppers, snow pea pods. | Tentatively linked with reduced risk of arthritis, asthma, cancer, cataracts, cognitive impairment, coronary disease, and macular degeneration. | Fights oxidation, which can damage cells throughout the body. Inactivates potentially carcinogenic nitrates. |
| Folic acid (a B vitamin) | Asparagus, avocado, orange juice, dark green leafy vegetables such as escarole, romaine lettuce, spinach. (Other sources: legumes, eggs, fish, organ meats, nuts, seeds, wheat germ, fortified grains.) | Helps prevent neural-tube birth defects, such as spina bifida. Tentatively linked with reduced risk of coronary disease, cancer, and cognitive impairment in older people. | Reduces levels of homocysteine, a harmful amino acid, and boosts levels of methionine, a protective amino acid. |
| Potassium | Most fruits and vegetables. (Other sources: breakfast cereals, legumes, meat, milk, seafood.) | Reduces blood pressure, and may reduce risk of hypertension. | Relaxes the arteries. |
| Calcium | Dark green leafy vegetables, figs. (Other sources: almonds, black-eyed peas, dairy products, canned fish with bones, tofu made with calcium salts.) | Linked with reduced risk of osteoporosis, and tentatively linked with reduced risk of hypertension. | Helps build and preserve bone, and relaxes the arteries. |
| Magnesium | Avocado, banana, dark green leafy vegetables, potato. (Other sources: chocolate, legumes, nuts, seeds, whole grains.) | Tentatively linked with reduced risk of abnormal heart rhythms, coronary disease, diabetes, heart failure, hypertension, and osteoporosis. | Abnormal rhythms: Stabilizes electrical signals in heart. Diabetes: Helps maintain normal insulin function. Hypertension, coronary disease, and heart failure: Relaxes the arteries. Osteoporosis: Helps build and possibly preserve bone. |
| Flavonoids (such as kaempferol and quercetin) | Apples, citrus fruits, cranberries, grapes, broccoli, celery, onions. (Other sources: beer, chocolate, coffee, red wine, tea.) | Tentatively linked with reduced risk of coronary disease. Inhibit cancer-cell growth in laboratory studies. | Fight oxidation and blood clots. May help liver detoxify carcinogenic chemicals. |
| Carotenoids (such as lutein and lycopene) | Brightly or deeply colored fruits and vegetables, such as carrots, dark green leafy vegetables, peppers, tomatoes. | Tentatively linked with reduced risk of cataracts, coronary disease, several cancers, and macular degeneration. | Fight oxidation, which can damage cells throughout the body. |
| Allicin, sulfur-allyl cysteine | Chives, garlic, leeks, onions. | Hypothetically linked with reduced risk of coronary disease and cancer. | May reduce blood-cholesterol levels and help liver detoxify carcinogenic chemicals. |
| Isothiocyanates (such as sulforaphane) | Cruciferous vegetables, such as broccoli, cabbage, cauliflower. | Retard growth of breast cancer in animal studies. | May help liver detoxify carcinogenic chemicals. |
| Indoles | Cruciferous vegetables. | Retard growth of breast cancer in animal studies. | May convert estrogen into less cancer-promoting form of the hormone. |
| Terpenes (such as limonene) | Citrus fruits. | Hypothetically linked with reduced risk of cancer. | May help liver detoxify carcinogenic chemicals, and may work like another terpene, the breast-cancer drug tamoxifen. |

seven daily servings of fruits and vegetables were 27 percent less likely to have a heart attack than those who consumed less produce. In a smaller but longer study, researchers from the ongoing Framingham Heart Study followed some 830 men for 20 years. Those who consumed at least eight servings of fruits and vegetables per day had less than half the stroke risk of those who ate fewer than two servings. Overall, the risk dropped an average of 22 percent for every three servings that people ate. In both studies, the findings persisted after adjustment for other risk factors, such as obesity and physical inactivity (for coronary disease) and smoking (for coronary disease and stroke).

According to nutrition researcher Tim Byers, M.D., M.P.H., professor of preventive medicine at the University of Colorado Health Sciences Center: "Eating your fruits and veggies is the second most important dietary step you can take to cut your risk of having a heart attack or stroke. Cutting back on saturated fat is the first—and eating more produce helps you do that, too."

■ **Cancer.** The evidence on fruits and vegetables for cancer prevention is even stronger than those cardiovascular findings. Some 200 observational studies in humans have provided direct or indirect evidence on the inverse connection between produce and cancer. Roughly half of the studies, including most of the best, involved whole fruits and vegetables. The rest involved specific nutrients supplied mainly or entirely by produce, rather than by supplements or other foods.

Overall, some 80 percent of those studies found that people who consume either lots of produce or lots of the phytonutrients found in produce have a reduced risk of developing cancer—typically half the risk—compared with people who consume little or none of those dietary items. Again, the findings generally persisted after the researchers accounted for various potentially confounding factors. That evidence is strongest for gastrointestinal and lung cancer, the two leading causes of cancer deaths. But a recent review concluded there's at least promising evidence on the protective benefit for every cancer studied so far.

## Summing up

Consuming the recommended five to nine daily servings of fruits and vegetables is one of the most important steps you can take to protect your health. That's because fruits and vegetables contain a host of potentially protective substances, which work in many different ways (see the table on page 36). For suggestions on how to increase your daily intake of fruits and vegetables, and how to retain the nutrients while minimizing pesticide residues, see the box below.

## How to squeeze in all those servings

Getting your daily quota of five to nine servings of fruits and vegetables is easier than it sounds. For one thing, servings are fairly small: just 1 cup of raw leafy vegetables, 1/2 cup of cooked vegetables or chopped raw fruit or vegetables, 1/4 cup of dried fruit, or 3/4 cup (6 ounces) of fruit or vegetable juice. One medium fruit or carrot counts, too. And there are lots of creative strategies:

■ **Breakfast.** Start with 100 percent fruit juice or vegetable juice. Then prepare cereal with berries or sliced fruit; pancakes with fruit in the batter and on top; a vegetable omelette; or an open-faced sandwich of low-fat cottage cheese and fresh fruit.

■ **Lunch.** Build a salad on romaine lettuce or spinach, rather than iceberg lettuce. Add colorful vegetables to a pasta or rice salad. Other options include vegetable soup, yogurt or cottage cheese with fruit, and sandwiches with added cole slaw, sprouts, tomatoes, or shredded carrots.

■ **Dinner.** Cook meat with fruits such as cranberries or oranges. Thicken soups or gravies with finely chopped or pureed carrots. Fortify macaroni and cheese with peas or chopped tomatoes, lasagna with shredded carrots and chopped spinach, and stews with all sorts of vegetables. Add dried fruits to rice or stuffing. Top a baked potato with microwaved frozen vegetables and low-fat cheese or sour cream. Or substitute spaghetti squash for pasta.

■ **Appetizers.** Try melon, grapefruit, or fruit salad; gazpacho or a cold fruit soup; or veggie dishes, such as fricasseed wild mushrooms or eggplant with herbed ricotta.

■ **Snacks.** Replace chips not only with carrot and celery sticks but also with raw broccoli, cauliflower, green beans, summer squash, and peppers—all dipped in vegetable salsa. Or have some fresh or dried fruit.

■ **Dessert.** Try a poached pear, a baked apple, or a fruit cobbler or pie. If you treat yourself to ice cream, cake, or pudding, top it with fruit.

### Make it convenient—and nutritious

You can eat lots of vegetables without spending lots of time chopping and cooking. For example, buy ready-cut vegetables and salad mixes, or order a take-out vegetable dish from an Asian restaurant. Stock up on frozen vegetables: They're at least as nutritious as most store-bought "fresh" vegetables, which usually lose some of their nutrients en route from a distant farm to your plate.

To help vegetables retain nutrients, shop frequently, bring fresh vegetables home in sealed plastic bags, and store them in the crisper drawer of your refrigerator. Don't cut, peel, or wash them until it's time to prepare the meal. Overcooking destroys vitamins, so minimize exposure to heat and water when cooking. The best methods are microwaving, steaming, or stir-frying (at high heat in just a little oil). Steaming doesn't work well for frozen vegetables; if you boil them, use just enough water to prevent scorching.

### Make it safe

The risk from pesticides on fruits and vegetables is probably small at most—and clearly outweighed by the benefits of eating produce. Still, you can reduce the possible risk by washing it carefully, which removes not only most of the pesticides but also the microorganisms that cause food poisoning. Discard the outer leaves of greens like lettuce and cabbage before washing. Rinse and scrub those and other fruits and vegetables under running water. You can further reduce any risk by choosing organic produce or produce with one of several "green" labels, indicating environmentally friendly farming—though you might pay extra.

# Unit 2

## Unit Selections

## Key Points to Consider

❖ Are some nutrients more important than others in maintaining health? Support your answer.

❖ What claims that are made for vitamins do you know to be false?

❖ How should one decide whether or not to take supplements? Are the issues involving supplements of a single vitamin or mineral any different than for multivitamins?

❖ Should fiber be designated a nutrient? Why or why not?

❖ Determine the percentage of your average daily calories that is made up of total fat and saturated fat. What did your calculation tell you?

❖ Calculate the amount of sodium you consume daily. How does it compare to the recommendation? If your intake exceeds the guideline, what changes could you make?

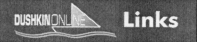 **Links** **www.dushkin.com/online/**

These sites are annotated on pages 4 and 5.

*One cannot think well, love well, sleep well, if one has not dined well.*

— Virginia Woolf

Some basic aspects of nutrition have remained relatively unchanged for many years. The list of nutrients is one of these. Even the specific vitamins and minerals have undergone little revision. Nutrients that provide energy are still identified as carbohydrates, fats, and proteins. Fiber is not a nutrient because it is not essential to life, but it is included in this unit because it clearly performs a crucial role in maintaining normal physiological functions.

Significant concepts about each nutrient, however, have changed, often dramatically. With today's available technology, the turnover in data from nutrition studies is so rapid that information may become obsolete even before it is printed and certainly before it is accepted or acted upon. Nor does the availability of voluminous data mean that theories are proven. Studies and experiments must be replicated, subjected to peer review, refined, and tried again. Conflicts in data, a common occurrence, must be resolved before any actionable conclusions can be reached. And, while epidemiological evidence may indicate a relationship, this does not prove cause and effect. Years may pass and numerous other studies be concluded before any firm recommendations for either normal or therapeutic diets can be supported. Outside the scientific community this is frequently misunderstood, and sometimes every media report is taken as a new breakthrough.

Compounding the problem of formulating dietary recommendations is the fact that differences among human beings are truly remarkable; an average human being simply does not exist. Physiological variations preclude accurate predictions of exact nutrient amounts that cause the negative effects of either deficiency or excess. It is the task of the National Academy of Sciences to establish quantity recommendations that more than cover most people's actual requirements but are not high enough to cause harm. Until now, the result has been the periodically revised Recommended Dietary Allowance (RDA). However, the 1989 edition is now being replaced incrementally with DRIs (Dietary Reference Intakes). These recommendations represent a newer philosophy based on knowledge that nutrients function, not only in the prevention of deficiency symptoms, but also to minimize chronic diseases such as heart disease, glaucoma, and cancer.

The articles in this unit were selected to reflect up-to-date thinking about nutrients that are currently newsworthy or about which we frequently have questions and/or misconceptions. Two articles on fats are a good example. Although the average consumer gets between 33 percent and 34 percent of total calories from fat, a current but controversial guideline sets one's fat budget at no more than 30 percent of calories. Saturated lipids, found primarily in animal products and tropical oils, are known to have a role in promoting disease, knowledge that has caused many consumers to avoid all or most fat. We also have learned that trans-fatty acids, either natural or formed in the process of hydrogenation, have effects similar to those of saturated fat. Yet the body requires fat for health, and unsaturated fat—especially monounsaturated fat—is beneficial in moderate amounts. Still, Americans remain *very* conscious of fat in food and eagerly look for new products that claim to be low- or no-fat. The

food industry is eager to oblige and has responded with hundreds of new products yearly. Typical consumers sometimes neglect to note that lower-fat items often have equal or more calories, and they remain paradoxically fanatical about super-premium ice creams and other rich desserts high in fat.

Evidence that dietary fiber does, indeed, offer disease protection can be supported by a substantial body of research, although few Americans get the recommended amounts. In "A 'Bran-New' Look at Dietary Fiber" the authors summarize claims that are both proven and unproven and offer advice about how to get more fiber in one's diet. Eating more fruits and vegetables, legumes, and whole grains is the key.

There follow three articles on vitamins, a topic of significant public interest. "Food for Thought about Dietary Supplements" by Paul Thomas is crucial because it addresses the fallacious philosophical mindset that some of us have regarding vitamins. No doubt vitamins seemed to present "miraculous cures" when they were first discovered as the key to terrible diseases such as pellagra, scurvy, and beri-beri. But vitamins are not magic bullets but workhorses that go about their everyday jobs of making the body operate smoothly. In large doses they will have pharmacological effects, some of which may be beneficial, but often may be harmful as well.

The other articles on vitamins discuss specific ones and the risks and benefits of supplements. For many reasons, supplement sources of vitamins cannot replace a good diet. Vitamins in foods often are absorbed better, interfere with other nutrients less, and seldom reach toxic levels. Foods also contain fiber and other chemicals that are useful in fighting disease. Even so, consumers often are concerned about the nutritional quality of their food. Scientists are working on ways to make it easier for the consumer to get the nutritional benefits of foods by developing "superveggies." Varieties of onions, peppers, corn, and broccoli that are brimming with disease-fighting compounds are in development. Betasweet, a maroon-colored carrot with twice the beta carotene of normal carrots should be in supermarkets now. And soon, from the University of Wisconsin, will come an orange "cuke," also crammed with beta carotene.

As with vitamins, there is still more to learn about the functions of minerals. The article "Do You Need More Minerals?" specifically targets selenium, zinc, potassium, and magnesium. However, as the reader will learn, research results can be misleading, and consumers may base their decisions to supplement on premature and unsubstantiated evidence. Read this article carefully before deciding to supplement.

Calcium is a different story, according to "Making the Most of Calcium: Factors Affecting Calcium Metabolism." In America, 28 million men and women suffer from the costly and debilitating effects of osteoporosis, and few others consume enough calcium to reduce that risk. The teen years are the peak bone-building years and are especially critical for the prevention of osteoporosis.

Article 19 contains a discussion of salt, or rather, its controversial component *sodium*. All agree that sodium is essential for life and that we need far less than most of us get. The disagreement centers around the amount that Americans should consider excessive, the harm that might be caused by consuming greater amounts, and the benefits of reducing dietary sodium.

# Nutrients

# Are You Getting Enough Fat?

## Eating a little fat will make you feel a lot fuller.

**AFTER A DECADE IN WHICH EVERYONE FRETTED OVER FAT GRAMS, NEW RESEARCH SHOWS THAT SOME TYPES OF THE MUCH MALIGNED STUFF CAN PROTECT AGAINST HEART DISEASE, CANCER AND STROKE. AND A LITTLE OF THIS FORMERLY FORBIDDEN PLEASURE GOES A LONG WAY**

### BY COLLEEN PIERRE, R.D.

In my nutrition counseling office, I see a constant parade of women trying to cut most of the fat from their diet. Many think 10 or 20 grams of fat a day is plenty; a few won't tolerate a single gram. They're proud of themselves and their "healthy" diets. When I break the news that they need to eat *more* fat, they turn pale. They are terrified of fat and don't know how to manage it in their diet without managing it right out.

Sound familiar? The American Dietetic Association's 1997 trends survey shows that 13% of adults believe they should eliminate all fat. About 60% of people surveyed by the Washington-based Food Marketing Institute ranked fat as their greatest nutritional concern, compared with 16% just a decade ago. Think about it: We discuss fat over dinner ("How many grams do you think this piece of chicken has?"), scour the supermarket for the latest lowfat creations (we spent $18 billion on these foods in 1996) and devour lowfat cookbooks and diet plans (many large bookstores stock over 100 of them). "We've cre-ated a fat-phobic society," says Angela Guarda, M.D., director of the eating and weight disorders program at Johns Hopkins University School of Medicine in Baltimore.

Dr. Guarda and other researchers say fat fear is backfiring. A growing number of women are eating too little fat to maintain healthy body functions such as vitamin absorption and fertility. And most of us are also missing out on the benefits of certain types of fat. That's right: Scientists are discovering that not only is fat essential, but some types may also be *protective* against common diseases. A sampling of the research:

♦ *New England Journal of Medicine* Although fats from butter, margarine and fatty meats can raise heart disease risk, a diet rich in monounsaturated fats, like those found in olive and canola oils, can significantly lower it.

♦ *Journal of the American Medical Association* A diet rich in monounsaturated fat may reduce stroke risk.

♦ *Archives of Internal Medicine* A study of 61,000 Swedish women showed that those with the highest in-takes of monounsaturated fat reduced their risk of breast cancer by half. Polyunsaturated fat (the type found in large quantities in margarine, corn, soybean and sunflower oil) increased cancer risk, although more research is needed to confirm the relationship. Surprisingly, saturated fat had no effect.

♦ *New England Journal of Medicine* Eating at least 3½ ounces of fish a day lowers your heart attack risk 10%.

♦ *Journal of Nutrition* Preliminary studies show that the type of fat in dairy products delivers a compound that may reduce cancer risk.

♦ *Journal of Medicine and Science in Sports and Exercise* Runners who increased their fat intake from 16% to 42% of calories didn't gain weight, and they lowered their risk of heart disease. In related studies, runners on higher-fat diets improved endurance, muscle strength and immune system function.

As a result of these and other studies, a group of leading nutrition researchers recently met at Tufts University in Boston to review the current recommendation to limit fat to 30% of calories—no more than 60

From *American Health for Women*, March 1998, pp. 67-72. © 1998 by Colleen Pierre. Reprinted by permission.

*Pistachio pleasures: These crunchy treats are chock-full of heart-smart fat and pack about 165 calories per ounce.*

grams a day on an 1,800-calorie-a-day diet. Read on for the issues the experts addressed and to see whether you would benefit from more fat in your diet or you need to reconsider the types of fat you eat. One promise: You can get the tempting taste of fat into your meals without hurting your heart or your waistline.

## FAT'S HATS

The function of fat goes way beyond making food taste good (although it does a fine job of that). Fat, along with carbohydrates and protein, the two other components in most foods, delivers energy to your body. Of the three, the fat molecule slows digestion the most, providing your body with a more constant energy supply so you're less likely to feel hungry between meals.

Try this experiment: One day for breakfast have a cup of your favorite cereal with half a cup of skim milk, a cup of orange juice and a banana (for a total of 360 calories and two grams of fat). Note when you start to feel hungry again. The next day eat half as much cereal, use 1% milk instead of skim, cut back to ¾ cup of orange juice and add two tablespoons of almonds (358 calories and nine grams of fat, total). Again, see when you get hungry. Even though both meals have about the same number of calories, the second breakfast will keep you satisfied longer.

Besides staving off hunger, fat coats every nerve and is the major part of every cell membrane. It helps your body absorb vitamins A, D, E and K, nutrients essential to better vision, stronger bones, a healthy heart and quick blood clotting, respectively. And cholesterol, found in foods that contain fat, is the raw material for

# Fat: The Good, Bad and Ugly

*Even though many women look at the total fat content on nutrition labels, they don't bother to see what type of fat the food contains. That's too bad, because while some kinds of fat wreak havoc on our hearts, other types can protect us. Check out this chart of fats, listed from best to worst. One caveat: All fats are high in calories, so you should keep an eye on your total calories to avoid gaining weight.*

| TYPE | RISK | REWARDS | RECOMMENDATION |
|---|---|---|---|
| **Monounsaturated fat** Olive and canola oils, olives, avocados and most nuts, including almonds, filberts, macadamias, peanuts, pecans, cashews and pistachios | None | Lowers heart disease risk by lowering total and LDL (bad) cholesterol without lowering HDL (good) cholesterol. | Eat mostly this type of fat. Try to use olive or canola oil instead of other vegetable oils |
| **Omega-3 fatty acid** High-fat fish (salmon, herring, anchovies, sardines), dark green leafy vegetables, and soybean and canola oils | None | Reduces stroke and heart disease risk; lowers total and LDL cholesterol and raises HDL cholesterol. | Eat fish a few times a week; just don't fry it. |
| **Polyunsaturated fat** Vegetable oils (sunflower, safflower, corn and soybean), sunflower seeds and some nuts (walnuts, Brazil nuts, pine nuts) | In excess, lowers HDL cholesterol and may promote plaque buildup and cancer risks. | Reduces total and LDL cholesterol. | Limit the amount to 10% of total calories. |
| **Saturated fat** High-fat meats such as ground beef, high-fat dairy foods and tropical oils such as coconut oil | In excess, raises heart disease risks by increasing total and LDL cholesterol, creating artery-blocking plaque. | Improves food flavor; may reduce stroke risk. | Limit the amount to 8% of total calories. |
| **Trans fats** Margarine, especially in stick form, and crisp processed foods such as cookies, crackers and chips | Increases heart disease risk by increasing LDL and decreasing HDL cholesterol. | None | Avoid foods with hydrogenated oil listed in ingredients. |

building hormones that control fertility. So there's no question you need fat—for your heart, for your bones, for your babies. The big debate is how much?

*Guacamole returns! Dip into an avocado, a fruit rich in monounsaturated fat, which doesn't raise LDL (bad) cholesterol.*

### FATTY FOOD, FAT PEOPLE?

Before figuring out your optimum fat intake, you should know that not every bit of the fat you eat goes from lips to hips, says Dr. Guarda. The relationship between fat and weight gain is indirect at best. A single gram of fat has nine calories, while the same amounts of protein and carbohydrates have four calories each. As a result, people who eat a lot of fatty foods are consuming a lot of calories and are often overweight. So when you cut the amount of fat in your diet, theoretically you should also be shaving calories. For instance, reducing your fat intake by 20 grams should save you about 180 calories (20 grams multiplied by nine calories per gram).

But there are two snags in this premise. For acceptable taste, food manufacturers often add sugar to their lowfat products, so the regular and lowfat versions of many processed foods such as cookies have about the same amount of calories. And women who severely restrict the amount of fat in their diets tend to make up for the calorie savings by eating more food.

In a study published in the *International Journal of Obesity,* researchers monitored participants' lunches for about a month. When given food labeled "lowfat," the participants ate more and consumed more calories than when they were given a meal labeled "high-fat." "Women perceive lowfat foods as a license to eat more," says

Alice H. Lichtenstein, D.Sc. (doctor of science), an associate professor of nutrition at Tufts.

Another reason some women overeat on a lowfat diet is that they're hungry all the time, says Margo Denke, M.D., an associate professor of internal medicine at the University of Texas Southwestern Medical Center in Dallas and one of the researchers participating in the Tufts meeting. "I recommend a little more protein and fat to some of the women I counsel, because it prevents them from needing so many calories to feel full," says Dr. Denke. The main message: To lose weight, you need to mind calories and portion sizes, not just fat grams. "Women who eat an 1,800-calorie diet with 35 grams of fat won't lose more weight than those who eat an 1,800-calorie diet with 50 grams of fat. A calorie is a calorie," says Dr. Denke.

*Olive oil tour: Like wine, each brand of olive oil offers a unique taste experience. Just don't go overboard, because each tablespoon has about 120 calories.*

### THE ISSUE AT HEART

Fat doesn't contribute to weight gain as long as you control your overall calorie intake, but it does impact heart disease. Dozens of studies have linked a diet high in saturated fat (the type in butter, fatty meats and high-fat dairy products) with a greater chance of developing heart problems. Those studies led the American Heart Association (AHA) in Dallas to recommend that Americans adopt a diet containing 30% or fewer calories from total fat.

Although some researchers still support the AHA's recommendation because it has significantly lowered the average amount of saturated fat in the

## The Good-Fat Diet

*A diet rich in monounsaturated fat seems to protect against heart disease. So follow this plan for a day, and adjust your regular menu to this style of eating.*

### BREAKFAST

1 cup wheat-based cereal topped with 3 dried apricots, 2 tbsp. almonds, 2 tbsp. pecans, 1 tbsp. toasted wheat germ

1 cup skim milk

1 medium banana

### LUNCH

2 slices whole wheat bread topped with 2 tbsp. natural peanut butter

1 cup plain yogurt with $\frac{1}{3}$ cup raspberries or blueberries

1 cup sliced raw sweet red peppers

1 medium orange

### DINNER

3 oz. broiled salmon fillet

1 cup cooked brown rice with 1 tsp. butter

1 slice whole wheat bread with 1 tsp. butter

1 cup cooked spinach with dash nutmeg and 1 tbsp. toasted pine nuts

1 large salad with 1 oz. feta cheese, 3 small ripe olives and 2 tbsp. dry-roasted sunflower seeds

*Nutrition information:*
2,024 calories; 76 g fat (34% of calories from total fat, 7% of calories from saturated fat, 15% of calories from monounsaturated fat, 9% of calories from polyunsaturated fat).

American diet, and because nearly all high-fat foods (even olive oil) have at least a little saturated fat, a growing number of nutrition experts fear it may have been too simplistic. "Some scientists thought the public was too simpleminded to understand that all fats aren't the same and that they should restrict just saturated fat, not all fat," says Walter Willett, M.D., chairman of the nutrition department at the Harvard School of Public Health. "As a result, many women aren't consuming the types of fat that are healthy for their heart."

## Figuring Fat Grams

*To calculate the number of fat grams you can eat, multiply the number of calories you consume daily (say 1,800) by the percentage of calories from fat you'd like your diet to contain (30%, or, 3) and divide by nine (60 grams is the answer in this example). Or just check out this cheat sheet:*

| CALORIES | % OF CALORIES FROM FAT | TOTAL FAT (GRAMS) |
|---|---|---|
| 1,500 | 20 | 33 |
| 1,500 | 25 | 42 |
| 1,500 | 30 | 50 |
| 1,500 | 35 | 58 |
| 1,800 | 20 | 40 |
| 1,800 | 25 | 50 |
| 1,800 | 30 | 60 |
| 1,800 | 35 | 70 |
| 2,000 | 20 | 44 |
| 2,000 | 25 | 56 |
| 2,000 | 30 | 67 |
| 2,000 | 35 | 78 |

Dozens of studies have shown that a diet rich in monounsaturated fat works to lower cholesterol levels and heart disease risk. Dr. Willett's most recent exploration on the subject, published last November in the *New England Journal of Medicine,* analyzed the diets of more than 80,000 women aged 34 to 59 for 14 years. During that time, nearly 1,000 of the women developed heart disease. Dr. Willett and his colleagues showed that women were likeliest to have heart disease if they had a low intake of monounsaturated fat and a high intake of saturated fat and trans fat (the kind in most margarines and processed snack foods).

The numbers are astounding: If a woman replaced about half of the saturated fat in her diet with carbohydrates from foods such as bread and pasta, researchers figure she'd reduce her heart disease risk about 15%. But if a woman substituted monounsaturated fat for half of the saturated fat in her diet, she'd drop her chance of developing heart disease about 40%. And if she also replaced half of her trans fat intake with monounsaturated fat, she'd reduce her risk of heart disease 50%. "Women are doing the right thing for their hearts by eating less red meat, butter and high-fat dairy products," says Dr. Willett. "But instead of replacing those foods with margarine, pasta and bread, they'd get *more* benefit from eating nuts and olive and canola oils, because these foods will give them the maximum protection against heart disease."

## ONE FAT INTAKE DOESN'T FIT ALL

Fortunately, there's not much debate about the *minimum* amount of fat required to maintain body functions such as fertility and vitamin absorption. Nearly every major medical organization recommends that both men and women get no less than 15% of calories from fat (about 25 to 30 grams for a 1,500- to 1,800-calorie-a-day eating plan).

Most researchers agree that saturated fat and trans fats are trouble. Less than one-third of your total fat intake should come from saturated fat. And you should avoid trans fats as much as possible. (To figure out how these recommendations can fit into a meal, see "The Good-Fat Diet.") What's a lot murkier—and far more individualized than scientists once thought—is the optimum amount of *total fat* needed to protect against disease.

Ronald Krauss, M.D., head of the AHA nutrition committee, says a low-fat diet can reduce your level of LDL (bad) cholesterol. But even Dr. Krauss concedes that "the range of individual response is wide. It varies from a 5% to 20% reduction."

So the amount of total fat that's best for you seems to depend on your genetic makeup and a host of other factors. Researchers say to consider:

♦ *Exercise.* The more you work out, the more fat you need, says Peter J. Horvath, Ph.D., an associate professor of nutrition at the University of Buffalo in New York. His studies show that while inactive women don't need more than 25% of calories from fat, the very active (such as marathon-

ers) could eat 50% of calories from fat. If you exercise a few times a week for 45 minutes at a clip, you could probably use 30% to 35% of calories from fat. But if you decide to train for a 10K, for instance, up your fat intake a bit to improve your endurance and strength, says Dr. Horvath.

♦ *Diabetes or insulin resistance.* Since a high-carbohydrate diet may produce surges in blood sugar, many dietitians favor an eating plan that has about 35% of calories from fat, 50% from carbohydrates and 15% from protein, says Ann Coulston, R.D., a senior research dietician at Stanford University Medical Center. Just watch your calories carefully, because weight gain worsens these conditions (dropping a few pounds, of course, helps them).

♦ *High cholesterol.* While the AHA still endorses a diet with 15% to 30% of calories coming from fat, such a plan lowers levels of good cholesterol in many people, a major risk factor for heart disease. So some scientists suggest a diet that has 30% to 35% of calories from fat, with most of the fat coming from monounsaturated sources. See what your doctor thinks, and get your cholesterol checked a few months after changing your diet. Then adjust your diet if needed.

Medical groups probably won't endorse diets with more than 30% of calories from fat anytime soon, but many Americans can get up to 35% of their calories from fat, as long as it's mostly monounsaturated and they watch calories, says Dr. Willett. "Not only would eating more nuts and olive oil improve the taste of your meals," he adds, "but it would do a world of good for your heart."

*Crunch fest: Almonds and many other types of nuts are rich in vitamin E, a nutrient that guards against heart disease.*

# Trans fat

## Another artery-clogger?

Margarine or butter? If you're confused about what you should be spreading on your toast, you're not alone.

At the heart of this debate is trans fat (trans fatty acids), a type of fat found in margarine and many processed and fast foods. At one time, trans fat was thought to be better for you than saturated fat in butter. But some studies, including a recent study of 80,000 nurses, have found that trans fat may be just as harmful to your health as saturated fat — and possibly worse.

So does this mean you should switch back to butter? Most health experts say no. But they do recommend limiting trans fat in your diet.

### All fats aren't equal

Fats are composed of hydrogen, carbon and oxygen. But differences in chemical structure make some fats better for you than others.

Saturated fat, which is "saturated" with hydrogen, raises your blood cholesterol, increasing your risk for coronary artery disease. Red meat and dairy products, as well as coconut and palm oils, are high in saturated fat.

Monounsaturated fat (olive and canola oils) and polyunsaturated fat (some vegetable and fish oils) contain less hydrogen. These don't appear to increase blood cholesterol and may actually lower cholesterol.

Trans fat is formed when food manufacturers add hydrogen to vegetable oil, which makes it thicker and also less likely to spoil. Trans fat is used in many processed and fast foods, such as doughnuts, crackers, chips and french fries. It also gives margarine its butterlike consistency. Modest amounts of trans fat are

### Reading between the lines on labels

How can you tell if a food product contains trans fat?

When it comes to listing fat on food labels, manufacturers are required to only list total fat and saturated fat. Some also voluntarily list monounsaturated and polyunsaturated fat, but it's unlikely you'll see trans fat listed. Still, you may be able to tell if a product contains trans fat, even if it's not directly listed on the food label.

Look for the words "hydrogenated" or "partially hydrogenated" in the list of ingredients. These terms indicate that the product contains trans fat. However, you won't be able to tell how much trans fat is included.

also naturally present in some beef and dairy products.

Trans fat was once thought to have the same effect on your health as vegetable oils. But studies are finding that like saturated fat, trans fat may increase blood cholesterol.

### Hard on your heart

A recent study of 80,000 nurses showed that women whose diets were high in both saturated and trans fats had an increased risk of heart attack. But of greater interest was the finding that nurses who consumed considerable amounts of trans fat faced an ever higher heart attack risk than nurses who ate a lot of saturated fat.

The study didn't prove that trans fat causes coronary artery disease, but it adds to previous evidence that trans fat may be as bad for your

heart as saturated fat. In fact, trans fat may even be more damaging because in addition to raising your "bad" (LDL) cholesterol level, it also appears to lower your "good" (HDL) cholesterol level.

The study suggests that the type of fat you eat may be as important to your health as how much fat you eat. Therefore, try to avoid both trans fat and saturated fat in addition to limiting total fat consumption. Current guidelines recommend that no more than 30 percent of your daily calories come from fat.

### Be fat savvy

Here are some ways you can limit consumption of trans fat and saturated fat:

■ Eat more fruits and vegetables and less meat and high-fat dairy products.

■ Eat fewer processed baked goods and fried foods, especially fast foods.

■ Buy oils that are predominantly monounsaturated, such as olive or canola oils, and avoid coconut, palm and palm-kernel oils.

■ Bake, boil, microwave, poach or steam foods instead of always frying them.

■ Spread jam, jelly or honey on your foods instead of butter or margarine. They still contain some calories but none of the fat.

### Back to butter vs. margarine

But when you want to use butter or margarine, which is better? Most health experts say margarine, particularly the tub and squeeze-bottle kinds, which are more liquid. They usually contain less trans fat than do stick margarines. In addition, some manufacturers have developed margarine spreads and sticks that contain no trans fat.

As is often the case, the key is moderation.

From the *Mayo Clinic Health Letter,* May 1998, p. 7. © 1998 by the Mayo Foundation for Medical Education and Research, Rochester, MN 55905. Reprinted by permission.

# A 'Bran-New' Look at

# DIETARY FIBER*

## By Kathleen A. Meister and Jack Raso

A couple of generations ago, "bulk" and "roughage" were the prevalent terms for dietary fiber, whose usefulness in the diet was considered limited to preventing constipation. Scientists have since learned that fiber encompasses diverse substances with various potentially important effects on health.

### What Is Dietary Fiber?

Dietary fiber consists of plant materials (mostly carbohydrates) that human digestive enzymes cannot break down. Foods of animal origin do not contain any fiber. Whole grains contain substantially more fiber than refined grains, because "refining" entails removal of some of the fiber. Whole grains, legumes, and nuts generally contain more fiber than refined grains, nonleguminous vegetables, and fruits.

There are two types of dietary fiber: *insoluble* and *soluble*. Soluble fibers include gums and some pectins—gluey substances used to make jellies. The distinguishing characteristic of soluble fibers is that, after mixing with water in laboratory studies, particles of purified soluble fibers remain interspersed in the water. The *in*soluble fiber publicized most often is cellulose, the raw material of cellophane and paper.

Table 1 on page 11 indicates the amounts of soluble and insoluble fiber that University of Wisconsin researchers found in various foods. Foods with significant concentrations of soluble fibers include barley, oats, legumes, sweet potatoes, and white potatoes. The insoluble fiber concentration of foods almost always exceeds the soluble fiber concentration. Foods particularly high in insoluble fibers include whole wheat and wheat bran.

### Fiber Supplements

Scientific evidence for the healthfulness of a high-fiber diet is much more compelling than that for the healthfulness of fiber itself. Therefore, experts generally recommend increasing dietary fiber intake by increasing consumption of grains, legumes, vegetables, and fruits rather than by taking fiber supplements. There are some exceptions to this rule. Certain kinds of fiber have proved useful against specific health problems—as wheat bran for chronic constipation, or pectins (found in apple peel) for diarrhea.

*Based on *Dietary Fiber*, ACSH Special Report.

Reprinted with permission from *Priorities,* Vol. 9, No. 1, 1997, pp. 7-10. © 1997 by the American Council on Science and Health, Inc., 1995 Broadway, 2nd Floor, New York, NY 10023-5860.

## Grains, Fruits, and Vegetables

Most of the scientific literature concerning the health effects of consuming plant foods focuses on fruits and vegetables rather than on grains. Some scientific studies associate high grain intakes with good health; others associate high grain intakes with poor health. A partial explanation for this inconsistency is that in many societies high-grain diets are a distinction of the poor, who typically have unmet healthcare needs. It is difficult to tease out information on the health effects of grain consumption from studies of populations in which socioeconomic effects on health are critical. Substantial nutritional differences between whole-grain and refined-grain products may also confound the grain-health connection.

Although information on the health effects of grains is not as plentiful as that on the health effects of fruits and vegetables, daily consumption of grain products as a significant part of the diet is advisable, as grains are low in fat and are a major source of vitamins and minerals as well as fiber.

## Fiber and Specific Health Problems

### Diverticulosis

Diverticula are small, fingerlike projections or pouches in the colon wall. The term *diverticulosis* refers to the presence of multiple diverticula. Roughly one third of all North Americans over the age of 45—and two thirds of all persons over the age of 85—have diverticula in their colons. Usually, the mere presence of diverticula does not cause any symptoms; between 75 and 90 percent of people with diverticula are asymptomatic.

Diverticulosis usually does not lead to serious problems. In some persons, however, the diverticula become inflamed. This painful acute condition, called *diverticulitis*, may require hospitalization, antibiotic therapy, or surgery.

Many physicians recommend that people with diverticulosis increase their intake of fiber, which may help relieve mild symptoms such as constipation and moderate abdominal discomfort. However, fiber is not used in the treatment of diverticul*itis*. (Indeed, the physician may initially order "NPO"—the abbreviation for a Latin phrase that means "nothing by mouth.")

Some studies suggest that a high-fiber diet contributes to the prevention of diverticulosis. One hypothesis is that low-fiber diets promote diverticulosis because they lead to straining at stool, or difficulty

## How to Increase Your Fiber Intake

- Eat at least six servings of grain products, at least three servings of vegetables, and at least two servings of fruits daily. Respective examples of servings are: one slice of whole-wheat bread, one-half cup of cooked vegetables, and one orange. Vary your selections within each food group, as foods in the same group may have considerable nutritional differences. For instance, carrots are high in provitamin A but low in vitamin C, while the reverse is true for green peppers.

- Consume whole-grain foods—brown (unpolished) rice, oatmeal, and whole-wheat bread, for example—more often than refined-grain foods, such as white bread and white rice.

- Consume fruits more often than fruit juices.

- Eat legumes (such as kidney beans, lentils, and lima beans) several times a week.

- Increase your fluid intake if you increase your intake of dietary fiber.

in defecating; this increases colon pressure and thus leads to the formation of diverticula.

The findings of a study published in 1994 in the *American Journal of Clinical Nutrition* support the belief that fiber is protective against diverticulosis. This study, which involved more than 40,000 middle-aged to elderly men, showed that higher fiber intakes translated into a lower incidence of symptom-generating diverticulosis. However, this protective effect was attributable largely to fiber from fruits and vegetables, not to fiber from grain products—the source generally recommended to diverticulosis patients.

# New Label Claim

A new fiber-related claim will soon appear on the labels of some food products. Last January the Food and Drug Administration announced that the labels of foods with certain levels of *beta-glucan*, a soluble fiber found in whole oats, may include health claims. These claims relate to the finding that, in conjunction with diets low in saturated fat, beta-glucan can decrease blood cholesterol. To bear this claim, a product must provide at least 3/4 gram of soluble fiber per serving. The scientific studies on which the FDA based its decision suggest that, to decrease cholesterol, a daily intake of approximately 3 grams of soluble fiber is necessary. To head off the inference that whole oats or soluble fibers are magic bullets against cholesterol-related heart disease, the FDA-approved claim includes the phrase "diets low in saturated fat and cholesterol."

**—Dr. Ruth Kava**

## Colon Cancer

Scientists have long suspected that high intakes of dietary fiber might decrease the risk of colon cancer, one of the most common types of cancer in Western populations. Several plausible mechanisms for a protective effect have been proposed. For example, fiber may protect people against colon cancer by increasing the bulk of intestinal waste, thus diluting carcinogenic substances therein, and/or by accelerating colon contents through the intestinal tract, thus decreasing the exposure of the colon walls to carcinogens. Other, more complex protective mechanisms have been proposed.

However, studies of human populations have not established that high fiber intakes *per se* decrease colon cancer risk. Rather, the data suggest a relationship between diets high in fruits and vegetables—and possibly diets high in whole grains—and a relatively low risk of colon cancer. The apparent protectiveness of fruits, vegetables, and whole-grain products may be attributable, at least in part, to certain plant constituents other than fiber, or to the substitution of fruits, vegetables, and whole-grain foods for less healthful foods. Therefore, taking purified fiber supplements to prevent colon cancer is not advisable.

## Blood Cholesterol Levels

The effect of dietary fiber on blood cholesterol levels has been a controversial subject. Many scientific studies have established that (unlike wheat bran and cellulose) the soluble fiber in certain foods and supplements—including guar guam, legumes, oat bran, oatmeal, pectin, and psyllium—can lower serum cholesterol. However, the decrease is modest and requires relatively high daily intakes. For example, consumption of three packets of instant oatmeal daily typically causes a cholesterol decrease of only 2 to 3 percent. Consuming oat bran and other sources of soluble fiber cannot effectively substitute for a low-saturated-fat diet but can augment its cholesterol-lowering effect.

## Coronary Heart Disease (CHD)

Several studies of human populations have correlated higher fiber intakes with lower CHD risk and vice versa. Generally, the cholesterol-lowering effect of soluble fiber is too small to account for this correlation. Some researchers have thus theorized that effects unrelated to cholesterol levels—effects on blood clotting, sugar metabolism, and body weight, for example—contribute to fiber's apparent protectiveness against CHD. Other scientists have proposed that fiber is not a protective factor but is primarily a lifestyle marker: People whose diets are, by choice, high in fiber tend to have many healthy habits, and some or all of these habits may decrease their risk of CHD.

## Weight Control

Fiber-rich foods are usually low in calories and fat, and they are conducive to *satiety*—a feeling of fullness in the stomach. But whether fiber itself can facilitate weight loss is uncertain. More than 20 scientific studies—none lasting more than three months—have focused on the relationship between fiber intake and the caloric intakes and body weights of volunteers. Wheat-bran fiber, apparently, does not decrease food intake or body weight. Whether other types of fiber can contribute to weight loss remains to be determined. Even more uncertain is whether dietary fiber is useful in long-term weight control.

## Fiber Hazards

While moderately high-fiber diets appear safe for healthy adults, fiber supplementation and diets extremely high in fiber may not be.

Many people report gastrointestinal disturbances—gas pains, flatulence, or diarrhea, for example—after increasing their fiber intake. A common assertion is that such effects subside as the body adapts to higher intakes, but evidence of this is scarce. Advice to increase fiber intake gradually to limit gastrointestinal problems arises from clinical experience rather than from controlled scientific studies.

To prevent constipation or an intestinal obstruction, those who take fiber supplements should consume relatively large amounts of fluids. Other side effects are less common: A small percentage of people are severely allergic to psyllium. Guar gum supplements can cause esophageal obstruction but rarely do.

Substances in or accompanying dietary fiber may bind to mineral nutrients and thus impede their absorption. However, such an action is probably inconsequential for most adults on Western-style high-fiber diets, which are also relatively high in minerals. High-fiber diets tend to be higher in minerals than low-fiber diets, because many fiber-rich foods are good sources of minerals. The effect of fiber *supplements* on mineral absorption might be harmful, because (unlike fiber-rich foods) the supplements do not provide minerals.

## Fiber in Proper Perspective

Dietary fiber is by no means a universal preventative, and fiber supplements have limited utility. But for most adults high-fiber *diets*—particularly diets high in fruits and vegetables—appear more healthful than low-fiber diets. American adults typically consume fewer servings of vegetables, fruits, and grain products than experts recommend; most would probably benefit from increasing their intakes of these foods.

KATHLEEN MEISTER, M.S., IS A FREELANCE MEDICAL WRITER AND A FORMER ACSH RESEARCH ASSOCIATE. JACK RASO, M.S., R.D., IS ACSH'S DIRECTOR OF PUBLICATIONS.

# Food for Thought about Dietary Supplements

*The surge of public interest in nutrition supplements has been fired by the recently enacted federal regulations governing health claims, which permits the health food industry to make claims about the function of nutrients not permitted for food products. This article provides healthy skepticism about the common rationales for the use of supplements.*

**PAUL R. THOMAS, Ed.D., R.D.**

*Paul Thomas, currently a Fellow at the Georgetown Center for Food and Nutrition Policy, Georgetown University, previously served as a staff scientist for the Food and Nutrition Board, Institute of Medicine, National Academy of Sciences. He is a registered dietitian who received an Ed.D. degree in nutrition education from Columbia University. He is an author and editor of several books on contemporary nutrition issues. Correspondence can be directed to him at the Georgetown Center for Food and Nutrition Policy, 3240 Prospect Street, N.W., Washington, DC 20007.*

The dietary supplements industry is very healthy. Sales of vitamins, minerals, and other food concentrates are roughly $4 billion per year. Although at least one quarter of American adults swallow these pills, powders, and potions daily,[1] probably the majority of us take them at least occasionally. What are we getting in return?

I've asked myself this question since the 1960s when, as a teenager, I began taking dozens of supplements after reading about their magical powers in *Prevention* and *Let's Live* magazines, and books by Adelle Davis. Surely they would help cure my adolescent acne; I just needed to find the right combina-tion. But my pizza face only improved when I took tetracycline and topical retinoic acid (the drug, not the vitamin) prescribed by a dermatologist. Growing out of adolescence also helped.

My education about dietary supplements became more comprehensive when I discovered the medical library during my college education as a biology ("pre-med") major. I learned that the hype surrounding them in the popular press was rarely supported by studies in the journals. Dietary supplements have benefited me in that they developed my interest in nutrition to the point where I chose to make a career in this discipline. But over time, and despite the growing popularity of supplements even among nutrition professionals, I have gone from being an enthusiastic vitamin promoter to a skeptic.

Most of us would agree that it's best to meet our nutritional needs with food, which means that everyone should eat a healthy, balanced diet. I believe that, short of that, dietary supplements are at best a poor and inadequate substitute. Supplements are appropriate for some people for specific purposes. But should they be taken every day, by everybody? I don't think so, and I make my case with the following eight points.

## POINT 1: NO EXPERT BODY OF NUTRITION EXPERTS RECOMMENDS THE ROUTINE USE OF SUPPLEMENTS

A small number of nutritionists support regular supplement use. But no scientific body of nutrition experts recommends that everyone take supplements on a routine basis as dietary insurance or for optimal health. Expert bodies are by nature conservative and unlikely to recommend a practice until the evidence is convincing and perhaps even overwhelming. That's the point, since dietary guidance for most people should be based on strong evidence.

In 1989, the Food and Nutrition Board of the National Academy of Sciences issued a comprehensive review of the relationships between diet and health.[2] The report stated that dietary supplements should be avoided at levels above the Recommended Dietary Allowances (RDAs). Finally, however, a group of nutrition experts was not warning people to stay away from supplements with pronouncements of dire risks from their use.

The recommendation was not to stay away from supplements, but to take them in no more than RDA amounts. The Food and Nutrition Board acknowledged that the long-term potential risks and benefits of supplements had not been adequately studied and called for more research.

> **The Food and Nutrition Board recommends that those who choose supplements limit the dose to levels of the RDA or less.**

The latest pronouncements on supplements are found in the new (4th) edition of *Dietary Guidelines for Americans*, which was released in January.[3] The report states that "diets that meet RDAs are almost certain to ensure intake of enough essential nutrients by most healthy people," and that people with average requirements are likely to have adequate diets even if they don't meet RDAs.

About supplements, the report states: "Daily vitamin and mineral supplements at or below the Recommended Dietary Allowances are considered safe, but are usually not needed by people who eat the variety of foods depicted in the Food Guide Pyramid." It acknowledged, however, that some people might benefit from supplements. These include older people and others with little exposure to sunlight who may need extra vitamin D. Women of childbearing age might reduce the risk of neural-tube defects in their infants with folate-rich foods or folic acid supplements. Pregnant women usually benefit from iron supplements. And vegans, who avoid animal products, might need some nutrients in pill form. The report urges the public not to rely on supplements.

Surveys show that most supplementers take a one-a-day multiple-vitamin-mineral product. But some take large doses of single nutrients or nutrient combinations as self-prescribed medication for disease

or to try to reach a more optimal state of health, the latter fueled most recently by the enthusiasm for antioxidants. The practices of these aggressive supplementers merit some concern.

## POINT 2: NUTRITION IS ONLY ONE FACTOR THAT INFLUENCES HEALTH, WELL-BEING, AND RESISTANCE TO DISEASE

The major chronic diseases that prematurely maim and kill most Americans have multiple causes. However, just as the advent of antibiotics and vaccines led many to think that the cure of diseases awaited specific "magic bullets," some proponents of supplements seem to think that these products are nutritional magic bullets for cancer, heart disease, and other maladies.

Health reporter Jane Brody calls us "a nation hungry for simple nutritional solutions to complex health problems."[4] Edward Golub, in his recent book, *The Limits of Medicine*, warns us against "thinking in penicillin mode."[5] It can be easy to do in nutrition because the first identified nutrient-related diseases (*eg*, scurvy and beriberi) were

> **Some proponents feel that supplements are "magic bullets" for cancer, heart disease, and other maladies.**

caused by dietary deficiencies. Anyone who doesn't get enough of the proper nutrient will eventually succumb to the relevant deficiency disease. No matter how much you exercise, who your parents are, or whether or not you smoke, you will become scorbutic without sufficient vitamin C.

Unfortunately, there is no such simple cause-effect relationship for diseases such as cardiovascular disease, cancer, stroke, and diabetes. Large doses of vitamin E, for example, may or may not influence the risk of developing heart disease. For some people, it may potentially be important. For most, however, it is at best one factor, and probably not a major one.

A primary contributor to chronic disease risk is our genetic heritage. Nutritionist Elizabeth Hiser writes, "Genes have a powerful influence over body size and disease risk, and though diet helps temper unwanted tendencies, *who* you are is often more important than *what* you eat. . . . Because of genetics, diet helps some people a lot, some people a little, and a very few people not at all."[6] Genetic endowment accounts in large measure for why some people get heart disease when young, for example, no matter how well they care for themselves, and why others live long lives even when they violate many of the commandments of healthy living.

Chronic disease risk is also affected by whether or not we exercise, refrain from smoking, avoid drinking to excess, limit exposure to unproductive stressors, and have sufficient rest, relaxation, and fun—and, of course, eating a diet that meets dietary guidelines and the RDAs. In our enthusiasm for supplements, however, we run the risk of reducing the importance of these factors.

One example of "thinking in penicillin mode" is linking calcium with the treatment, and especially prevention, of osteoporosis. However, bone health is influenced by many factors, including smoking, alcohol consumption, exercise, and intake of nutrients such as phosphorus, protein, and boron that affect calcium absorption, utilization, and excretion. In fact, osteoporosis is uncommon in several countries with relatively low calcium intakes.

Social commentator H. L. Mencken said, "For every complicated problem there is a simple solution—and it is wrong."[7] Supplements are not the answer to health and disease for the vast majority of people. Who our parents are, how we live our lives, and the food we put into our mouths several times a day affect our health more profoundly.

## POINT 3: FOOD IS MORE THAN THE SUM OF ITS NUTRIENTS

Nutritionists used to think that macro- and micronutrients made a food nutritious and good for health. Other food constituents, such as fiber, were seen as nonessential, and therefore unimportant, since death is not directly associated with fiber deficiency. However, we have learned that, while fiber is not essential in the traditional sense, its presence in the diet makes it much easier to defecate and influences blood cholesterol levels and risk of diseases such as diverticulosis and certain cancers.

---

**Supplements are not the answer to health and disease for the vast majority of people.**

---

Many compounds in food that are not classical nutrients can apparently influence health and risk of disease. Several hundred studies show that heavy fruit and vegetable eaters have approximately half the risk of cancer compared with those who don't eat these foods, but the results are not consistently related to one or several nutrients. New biologically active constituents found mostly in plant foods—phytochemicals (or "phytomins" as *Prevention* magazine calls them)—are being discovered regularly. They include flavonoids, monoterpenes, phenolics, indoles, allylic sulfides, and isothiocyanates. Phy-

---

**Even, when and if, phytochemicals are reliably found in supplements, it will never be appropriate to take them in that form rather than from foods that contain them.**

---

tochemicals became a "hot item" in 1994 when they were the subject of a cover story in *Newsweek* that April.[8] The title: "Better than Vitamins: The Search for the Magic Pill." (There's that word too often linked with supplements: magic! So is "miracle.")

Whole natural foods, to quote *Newsweek*, "harbor a whole ratatouille of compounds that have never seen the inside of a vitamin bottle for the simple reason that scientists have not, until very recently, even known they existed, let alone brewed them into pills." Even when phytochemicals can reliably be found in supplements, it will never be appropriate to swallow pills (or consume specially fortified processed foods) instead of eating recommended amounts of the foods that contain them, such as vegetables, fruits, whole grains, and legumes. To do so would be to inappropriately rely on preliminary science, when the future will bring the discovery of new phytochemicals that have always been available from today's natural foods. Determining whether and how isolated food constituents with biologic activity may improve health, treat disease, or extend life is a daunting task that will occupy researchers for decades or longer.

Scientists continue to learn more about the complexity of foods and the myriad of biologically active constituents they contain that can influence health and disease risk. How ironic, then, that the calls this research generates for renewed efforts to persuade people to eat healthier diets—the tried and true—often seems to be drowned out by the acclaim for dietary supplements.

**POINT 4: DEVELOPING RDAs AND OPTIMAL NUTRIENT RECOMMENDATIONS IS VERY DIFFICULT**

As a staff scientist with the Food and Nutrition Board, I worked with the subcommittee that developed the most recent (10th) edition of the RDAs. I was surprised to learn that the research base for the RDAs is quite limited. There are not as many studies as one would like to determine minimum and average nutrient requirements for each age-sex group, estimate the population variability in need, and to feel more comfortable about the judgments made to derive nutrient allowances. Setting RDAs is tough work!

Now there is substantial discussion about so-called optimal intakes of nutrients, levels of intake

that might allow people to be healthy and fit for a longer time. Some nutrition scientists believe optimal nutrient intakes will typically exceed RDA levels and may require supplements in some cases to achieve. Still, no one doubts that developing optimal nutrient intakes will be orders of magnitude more complex than developing RDAs.

The optimal intake of any nutrient will probably vary substantially among individuals and even throughout one person's life from infancy to old age. It will probably also depend on the parameter of interest. For example, an optimal intake of a nutrient to reduce the risk of heart disease might not be optimal to decrease cancer risk and might actually increase it. Defining, understanding, and assessing optimal nutrition is becoming one of the most exciting challenges for

---

**Developing recommendations for optimal nutrient intakes will be many times more complex than developing RDAs.**

---

investigators in the nutrition and food sciences.

**POINT 5: TAKING SUPPLEMENTS OF SINGLE NUTRIENTS IN LARGE DOSES MAY HAVE DETRIMENTAL EFFECTS ON NUTRITIONAL STATUS AND HEALTH**

On April 14, 1994, the *New England Journal of Medicine* published the infamous Finnish study.[9] In this clinical trial, 29,000 male smokers in Finland were randomly divided into four groups, receiving either a placebo, 20 mg beta-carotene (approximately four to five times the amount in five servings of fruits and vegetables), 50 IU of vitamin E (about three to four times average dietary intakes, but still a small dose as a supplement), or both the beta-carotene and vitamin E. After 5 to 8 years, the beta-carotene takers had an 18% *higher* incidence of lung cancer, with hints that this carotenoid might also have raised their risk of heart disease. Vitamin E seemed to reduce the risk of prostate cancer but increased the risk of hemorrhagic stroke.

This study is noteworthy, both because of its surprising findings and the fact that it is one of the few large clinical trials on supplements and disease risk. The majority of studies investigating this relationship are epidemiologic in nature. Clinical trials in which subjects are randomly assigned to treatment or control groups help to identify cause-and-effect relationships. Epidemiologic studies, in contrast, can only identify whether the variables under study are related in some way.

The Finnish study showed that antioxidant nutrients might harm rather than help male smokers, so it has been scrutinized intensely. Blumberg, for example, noted that those with the highest plasma concentrations of vitamin E and beta-

> **Clinical studies help identify cause-and-effect relationships, whereas epidemiologic studies can only identify whether variables are related.**

carotene at the start of the study had the lowest risk of developing lung cancer[10]; therefore, these nutrients may have provided some protection to some smokers. But for those who would suggest that the subjects should not have expected any benefits from supplements, given their deadly habit, two points should be made. First, several epidemiologic studies show that fruit and vegetable consumption reduces the risk of lung cancer in smokers—again, foods (containing beta-carotene and many other carotenoids and phytochemicals), not supplements. Second, dietary supplements are often promoted to smokers and those who are not eating or taking care of themselves as well as they should with claims that the products protect health.

The Center for Science in the Public Interest, a consumer advocacy group that had recommended

antioxidants to its readers, changed its position after the Finnish study.[11] "Shelve the beta-carotene," it said, or take no more than about 3 mg per day, the amount found in many multivitamins. It also advised people to "reconsider taking vitamin E." *New York Times* medical writer Nicholas Wade, commenting on the Finnish study, said: "The vitamin supplement industry . . . would like everyone to believe the issue of benefits is settled. . . . For all who assumed the answer was already known, the Finnish trial offers two lessons. One is that science can't be rushed. The other is not to put all your bets on those convenient little bottles: back to broccoli and bicycles."[12]

Time shows the wisdom of Wade's advice. Two large clinical trials were completed in January of this year that further debunk beta-carotene as a magic bullet. After 12 years of taking either 50 mg beta-carotene or a placebo every other day, 22,071 physicians learned that the phytochemical provided no protection against cancer or heart disease. In the second trial, 18,314 men and women at risk for lung cancer due to smoking or exposure to asbestos were given supplements of beta-carotene (30 mg/day), vitamin A (25,000 IU/day), or a placebo. Those receiving the supplements had a *higher* rate of death from lung cancer and heart disease; although the results were not statistically significant, the study was halted. Dr. Richard Klausner, the director of the National Cancer Institute, which financed both trials, concluded, "With clearly no benefit and even a hint of possible harm, I can see no reason that an individual should take beta-carotene."

> **A major concern with supplements is potential toxicity.**

A major concern with supplements is potential toxicity. Fat-soluble vitamins like A and D, which are stored in the body, are obviously harmful in excess, but so are some water-soluble nutrients. Large doses of vitamin B6, for ex-

ample, can produce neuropathy in the arms and legs, leading to partial paralysis. Some people taking tryptophan have developed and died from eosinophilia-myalgia syndrome, a connective tissue disease characterized by high levels of eosinophils, severe muscle pain, and skin and neuromuscular problems. (It is not yet certain whether the syndrome was caused by the tryptophan itself, by a contaminant produced in the manufacturing process, or by the two in combination.) High-dose niacin supplements, especially in the time-released form, have caused liver damage. Large amounts of beta-carotene can be dangerous to alcoholics with liver disorders. And antioxidant nutrients can act as prooxidants under certain conditions, generating cell-damaging free radicals.[13]

Another concern with supplements is the possibility of adverse nutrient interactions. Calcium, for example, affects the absorption of iron and vice versa. Various amino acids compete with each other for absorption from the small intestine and to cross the blood-brain barrier. Large doses of one nutrient or phytochemical can adversely affect

> **Large doses of one nutrient can adversely affect nutritional status in relation to another nutrient.**

nutritional status in relation to another. In one study, for example, very large doses of beta-carotene, 100 mg/day given for 6 days, decreased the concentration of another important carotenoid, lycopene, in the low-density lipoproteins by 12 to 25%.[14] Beta carotene is not the only carotenoid of benefit to health, or perhaps even the most important one. I am reminded of Walter Mertz, the renowned nutrition and trace mineral expert, who was asked if he took beta-carotene as a supplement. He replied he would be "afraid" to take it, not knowing how extra beta-carotene would affect the balance of all the other carotenoids in his body that he obtained from food.

Little information is available to demonstrate that the long-term and possibly lifetime intake of large doses of nutrients is completely safe. Studies on the consequences of large nutrient intakes in humans rarely have a large sample size and go beyond several months. If high levels of iron in the body, for example, really increase the risk of heart disease, as at least one study suggests,[15] the chances are remote that a physician will think that a patient who died of a heart attack possibly did so because of supplemental iron. In other words, nutrient toxicity may be a cause of more illness and death than suspected, because the problems will not be linked (or even thought to have a possible link) to use of supplements.

## POINT 6: DIETARY SUPPLEMENTS VARY SUBSTANTIALLY IN QUALITY

Few federal manufacturing and formulation standards exist for supplements, in part because they fall into a regulatory gray area between foods and drugs.[16] A decade ago, investigators discovered that many calcium supplements did not disintegrate or dissolve in the digestive tract; the calcium was simply excreted. These results prompted the development of disintegration and dissolution standards for some types of supplements by the US Pharmacopoeia, the scientific organization that es-

tablishes drug standards. . . .

Garlic supplements provide an example of not necessarily getting what you think you paid for. They have become popular because several studies suggest that garlic may help to lower blood cholesterol and reduce the risk of cancers of the breast, colon, and other organs. Attention has focused on two compounds that may be responsible for these effects: allicin and s-allyl cysteine. The Center for Science in the Public Interest analyzed garlic powder and various garlic pills and found major differences by brand in their content of these two compounds.[17] Plain garlic powder was best and least expensive, whereas the most popular brand of garlic supplement contained no allicin (Table 1). Similarly, Consumers Union recently found that ginseng products varied greatly in their content of ginsenosides, the root's supposed active ingredients.[18]

It is difficult to find a comprehensive, one-a-day type of supplement that supplies nutrients at RDA levels. Most products are not well balanced. They contain, for example, many times the recommended amount of inexpensive B vitamins like thiamin and riboflavin but only small amounts of calcium and magnesium, because recommended amounts of these minerals can add substantially to the size of the pill. Some supplements contain superfluous ingredients such as bee pollen, hesperidin complex, and PABA, which do lit-

tle more than boost the price (see Refs. 19 and 20 for good advice on choosing a supplement).

## POINT 7: SUPPLEMENTS ARE PROMOTED BY COMMERCIAL AND OTHER FORCES ON THE BASIS OF INCOMPLETE OR PRELIMINARY SCIENCE

I stated earlier that the bulk of evidence linking supplements to reduced risks of heart disease, cancer, and other diseases is epidemiologic in nature, or based on *in vitro*, mechanistic, or biochemical studies. They show correlations and indicate the possibility of protective effects, but do not prove cause and effect. So we do not know whether most of these suggestive data are of practical importance to people over the long run as they eat good or bad diets, smoke or refrain from smoking, live in polluted or clean environments, and are either exercisers or couch potatoes.

The scientific community tends to blame journalists for distorted reporting about nutrition. True, there are both good and mediocre reporters on the subject. And too often the reporting is bad, incomplete, prepared from press releases, or focused on one study without placing it in perspective–a poor foundation for people to make intelligent decisions.

A recent study illustrates this point. Houn and colleagues examined popular press coverage of research on the association between alcohol consumption and breast

### Table 1
### Comparison of Garlic Supplements

| Name of Supplement | Cost per Tablet* (cents) | Allicin (μg)† | SAC (μg)‡ |
|---|---|---|---|
| McCormick Garlic Powder§ | 6 | 5,660 | 590 |
| KAL Beyond Garlic | 18 | 4,800 | 270 |
| Garlique | 33 | 3,840 | 130 |
| Garlicin | 18 | 2,165 | 145 |
| Nature's Way | 8 | 1,530 | 140 |
| Kwai | 11 | 815 | 60 |
| Quintessence | 9 | 535 | 185 |
| Natural Brand (GNC) | 10 | 300 | 45 |
| P. Leiner (private label)‖ | 5 | 115 | 45 |
| Kyolic¶ | 11 | 0 | 255 |

© 1995, CSPI. Adapted from *Nutrition Action Healthletter* (1875 Connecticut Ave., N.W., Suite 300, Washington DC 20009-5728. $24.00 for 10 issues).

  * Based on list price when available or average price paid.
  † One large clove of fresh garlic supplies about 5,000 μg allicin.
  ‡ S-allyl cysteine.
  § One third teaspoon.
  ‖ Product usually carries the name of the drugstore or other chain where it is sold.
  ¶ The best-selling garlic supplement.

> *Responsibility for distorted reporting of nutrition rests as much with some nutritional scientists as with the media; many major journals reach reporters before medical professionals.*

cancer.[21] Of the 58 published journal papers on this topic over 7 years, only 11 were cited by the press. Three studies published in the *New England Journal of Medicine* and the *Journal of the Medical Association* were featured in more than three quarters of the news stories. And almost two thirds of the stories gave recommendations to women on alcohol consumption based on one study. Reporters ignored the published review articles and editorials that would have provided a better basis for advice. This highlighting of a few studies, which seems to occur in many other nutrition areas, tends to confuse people and lead them to think that a new study will undoubtedly contradict the findings of the previous one. It's the new math of media nutrition coverage: $1 + 1 = 0$. As syndicated columnist Ellen Goodman puts it, "Fresh research has a sell-by date that is shorter than the one on the cereal box."[22]

Responsibility for distorted reporting of nutrition does not rest with the media alone. Increasingly, it involves nutrition scientists. Although they tend not to make exaggerated claims when reporting their work at scientific meetings, some are more bold when they speak to reporters or the public. Sometimes their institution's press office encourages this boldness. As research funds become harder to secure, scientists and their employers are learning that being in the news raises their visibility, which can help to raise money.

Now, major journals like the *New England Journal of Medicine* and *Journal of the American Medical Association* reach reporters before they reach biomedical professionals. And because a growing

amount of research is financed by industry, a company might seek publicity about a new finding to enhance the value of its stock or draw attention to itself. A good book on the changing nature of reporting scientific advances is *Selling Science*, by sociologist Dorothy Nelkin.[23]

The dietary supplements industry is busy making bold claims for its products on the labels, in advertising, and in product literature using preliminary science. The 1990 Nutrition Labeling and Education Act, which resulted in the new nutrition labels on packaged foods, allows supplement manufacturers to present the same health claims that are allowed on foods—claims supported by "significant scientific agreement" and preapproved by FDA. Two of the authorized health claims are relevant to supplements: the links between calcium and osteoporosis and between folate and neural tube defects.

However, the Dietary Supplement Health and Education Act passed in 1994 allows the industry to make claims pertaining to the structure and function of a nutrient. For example, a supplement could not claim that it helps cure AIDS, but it might be possible to state that the product "boosts the immune system." The legal basis for a claim is that (1) some substantiation exist, (2) FDA be notified of the claim within 30 days of its presence on the label, and (3) two additional sentences be added to such claims: "This statement has not been evaluated by FDA. This product is not intended to diagnose, treat, cure, or prevent any disease." Along with these so-called "structure-function" claims, a retailer may now provide literature on supplements, although it is supposed to be balanced scientifically and not be misleading. Some members of the dietary supplements industry are fighting even these limitations, arguing that their absolute freedom of speech to provide whatever information they think is appropriate is being threatened.

An advertisement in *Time* magazine last October for Bayer Corporation's One-A-Day Brand Vitamins suggests the growing boldness of

claims for even mainstream dietary supplements. The copy states: "It's been all over the news. Findings on folic acid studies were announced recently at a medical conference in Bar Harbor, Maine, suggesting that adequate intake of folic acid may significantly lower elevated homocysteine levels, one of the risk factors for heart attacks and strokes in men. One-A-Day Men's Formula contains 100% of the US RDA of folic acid. Why not start taking your One-A-Day today?"

Public health may benefit from the promotion of supplements by increasing the public's awareness of nutrient, diet, and disease relationships. But I fear the risks outweigh the benefits. The promotional copy typically fails to give information on food-related alternatives to supplements. In addition, the public rarely has the expertise to evaluate the information in the promotion. Furthermore, consumers' expectations of a product's effectiveness may be heightened by the hype and lead to irrational use of the product.

There can be a great difference between *a* truth and *the* truth. A truthful statement may inevitably be misleading. This lesson was made clear in the plethora of ridiculous health claims on foods back in the late 80s and early 90s. Some high-fat products, for example, were truthfully labeled as being cholesterol free, because manufacturers knew many people would think the product was more healthful.

Supplements supplying nutrients at levels beyond what can reasonably be obtained from food should be viewed as nonprescription drugs. High-potency products should not be used without careful thought and perhaps expert help.

**POINT 8: FOCUSING ON NUTRIENTS AND SUPPLEMENTS CAN TAKE ATTENTION AND CONVICTION AWAY FROM IMPROVING ONE'S LIFESTYLE**

Nationally representative surveys of American adults show that approximately one third are interested in nutrition and think they are on the right track to healthy eating. In contrast, another third couldn't care less about meeting dietary guidelines. Those in the middle third claim they are trying to eat better, but find it difficult.

So, the good news is that two thirds of adult Americans say they care about their nutrition. But the bad news is that perhaps only 5 to 10% of the US population meets dietary recommendations regularly, such as eating five or more servings of fruits and vegetables per day and limiting fat to no more than 30% of calories. Furthermore, obesity is a growing epidemic in this country, now affecting one third of adults and one quarter of children. The irony is that people who eat well are most likely to take supplements, whereas those most likely to benefit from higher nutrient intakes are least likely to take them.

> **Dietary supplements provide a false sense of security.**

My greatest concern about dietary supplements is the false sense of security it provides some people, those who use supplements to an extent as substitutes for a good diet. It is natural for us to want an easier way or, ideally, some magic bullet, to achieve health short of being vigilant or saintly all the time. We're especially likely to cut corners when we are short of time and feeling stressed, such as by choosing foods on the basis of convenience and ease of preparation and by not exercising. Taking a basic supplement as one small part of a health-promoting lifestyle may be reasonable and perhaps even prudent. But taking supplements is a problem for people, probably the majority, who are not making the lifestyle changes they know they should. A recent advertisement by Hoffman-La Roche, Inc. for vitamin E states ... "Many doctors ... believe taking supplements or eating fortified foods containing vitamins and minerals is a sound health measure, particularly for people who don't eat a good diet.... " Unfortunately, some people use supplements as a deliberate or unconscious excuse for not trying to improve their diets and lifestyles.

A reporter called me some time ago to ask how people could use vitamins to stay healthy. I replied that people should pay more attention to their diets. He told me to be realistic and used himself as an example. He said he leads a very busy life, has little time to shop for food and prepare it, and there are few places near work that serve nutritious lunches. So what supplements would help him cope more productively with his situation? Here is an example where supplements may harm more than help, by being used as a surrogate for tackling the hard things that would really improve his nutritional status, such as preparing lunches the night before, convincing nearby restaurants to offer more nutritious fare, and making sure he eats a very nutritious breakfast and dinner. This reporter was looking for what he acknowledged to be a second-best solution, but taking a supplement will make him even less likely to attempt the best but more difficult solution.

## CONCLUDING THOUGHTS

... Those who recommend that healthy people supplement their diets with extra vitamins and minerals often call it a form of dietary insurance, as essential to have as car or home insurance. I disagree. When you purchase insurance, the benefits and costs of the policy are detailed and you choose a specific level of protection. The terms of a dietary insurance policy, though,

> **Concentrating anything in the food chain, be it vitamin C, beta-carotene, salt, or fat, increases the likelihood of mistakes.**

can never be known, much less specified. Taking supplements without a clear need is more analogous to playing the lottery. You hope to win some money, and ideally the jackpot, by buying lottery tickets. You won't hurt yourself unless you buy more tickets over time than you can afford, but you are not likely to win anything either, especially the big prize.

Even comprehensive dietary supplements are, at best, poor substitutes for nutrient-rich foods. Foods, about which we know little, are more than the sum of their parts, about which we have some knowledge. Furthermore, it's harder to hurt yourself with foods than with supplements. Concentrating anything in the food chain—be it vitamin C, beta-carotene, salt, or fat—increases the likelihood of mistakes. Nutrients and other nonnutrient substances relevant to health are readily available in familiar and attractive packages called fruits, vegetables, legumes, grains, and animal products. And they come in concentrations and in combinations with which humans have had long cultural familiarity.[29] ...

## REFERENCES

1. Slesinski MJ, Subar AF, Kahle LL. Trends in use of vitamin and mineral supplements in the United States: The 1987 and 1992 National Health Interview Surveys. *J Am Diet Assoc* 1995;95:921–3.
2. National Research Council. *Diet and Health: Implications for Reducing Chronic Disease Risk.* Washington, DC: National Academy Press, 1989.
3. US Department of Agriculture, Department of Health and Human Services. *Nutrition and Your Health: Dietary Guidelines for Americans,* 4th ed. Washington, DC: Government Printing Office, 1995.
4. Brody J. Personal health: Sorting out the benefits of taking extra vitamin E. *New York Times,* July 26, 1995:C8.
5. Golub E. *The Limits of Medicine: How Science Shapes Our Hope for the Cure.* New York: Times Books, 1994.
6. Hiser E. Getting into your genes. *Eating Well* 1995;6(1):48–9.
7. Herbert V, Kasdan TS. Misleading nutrition claims and their gurus. *Nutr Today* 29(3):28–35, 1994.
8. Begley S. Beyond vitamins: The search for the magic pill. *Newsweek,* April 25, 1994:45–9.
9. The Alpha-Tocopherol, Beta-Carotene Cancer Prevention Study Group. The effect of vitamin E and beta carotene on the incidence of lung cancer and other cancers in male smokers. *N Engl J Med* 1994;330:1029–35.
10. Blumberg JB. Considerations of the scientific substantiation for antioxidant vitamins and β-carotene in disease prevention. *Am J Clin Nutr* 1995;62:1521S–1526S.
11. Liebman B. Antioxidants: Surprise, surprise. *Nutr Action Healthletter* 1994;21(5):4.
12. Wade N. Method and madness: Believing in vitamins. *New York Times Magazine,* May 22, 1994:20.
13. Herbert V. The antioxidant supplement myth. *Am J Clin Nutr* 1994;60:157–8.
14. Graziano JM, Johnson EJ, Russell RM, Manson

JE, Stampfer MJ, Ridker PM, Frei B, Hennekens CH, Krinsky NI. Discrimination in absorption or transport of β-carotene isomers after oral supplementation with either all-*trans*- or 9-*cis*-β-carotene. *Am J Clin Nutr* 1995;61:1248–52.

15. McCord JM. Free radicals and prooxidants in health and nutrition. *Food Tech* 1994;48(5):106–11.

16. Anon. Buying vitamins: what's worth the price? *Consumer Rep* 1994;59:565–9.

17. Schardt D, Schmidt S. Garlic: Clove at first sight? *Nutr Action Healthletter* 1995;22(6)3–5.

18. Anon. Herbal roulette. *Consumer Rep* 1995;60:698–705.

19. Anon. A 9-point guide to choosing the right supplement. *Tufts Univ Diet & Nutr Letter* 1993;11(7)3–6.

20. Liebman B, Schardt D. Vitamin smarts. *Nutr Action Healthletter* 1995;22(9):1,6–10.

21. Houn F, Bober MA, Huerta EE, Hursting SD, Lemon S, Weed DL. The association between alcohol and breast cancer: Popular press coverage of research. *Am J Publ Health* 1995;85:1082–6.

22. Goodman E. To swallow or not to swallow. *Liberal Opinion Week*, April 24, 1994.

23. Nelkin D. *Selling Science: How the Press Covers Science and Technology*, revised edition. New York: WH Freeman and Company, 1995.

24. Anon. Many shoppers not yet aware of nutrition facts label. *Food Labeling News* 1995;3(32):21–3.

25. Gussow JD. *A Word on Behalf of Food.* Presentation at the Alumni Advances Conference of the dietetic internship program at Oregon Health Sciences University, Portland, OR, May 1995.

26. Shepherd SK. Nutrition and the consumer: Meeting the challenge of nutrition education in the 1990s. *Food & Consumer News* 1990;62(1):1–3.

27. Goodman E. Food literacy. *Liberal Opinion Week*, December 14, 1992.

28. Stacey M. *Consumed: Why Americans Love, Hate, and Fear Food*. New York: Touchstone Books, 1994.

29. Gussow JD, Thomas PR. *The Nutrition Debate: Sorting Out Some Answers*. Palo Alto, CA: Bull Publishing Co., 1986.

The views expressed in this article are those of the author and do not reflect the position of the Center for Food and Nutrition Policy.

# VITAMIN SUPPLEMENTS

Many patients ask their physicians whether they should take vitamins. In recent years,
more data have become available on the risks and benefits of taking vitamin supplements.

**VITAMIN E**—The primary food sources for vitamin E are vegetable and seed oils; the usual diet in the USA provides about 15 IU/day. Vitamin E in food, which is mostly gamma-tocopherol, acts as an antioxidant. Vitamin E in supplements is mostly alpha-tocopherol, which *in vivo* may block the antioxidant activity of gamma-tocopherol and have a prooxidant effect (S Christen et al, Proc Natl Acad Sci USA, 94:3217, 1997). High doses of vitamin E may interfere with vitamin K metabolism and platelet function.

In two large studies that used dietary questionnaires, reporting a high dietary intake of vitamin E was not associated with a lower risk of cardiovascular disease, but women and men who said they took vitamin E supplements regularly for two years or more had a lower incidence of coronary artery disease (EB Rimm et al, N Engl J Med, 328:1450, 1993; MJ Stampfer et al, N Engl J Med, 328:1444, 1993). Another questionnaire-based study in women found that reporting a high dietary intake of vitamin E was associated with a lower risk of death from coronary heart disease (LH Kushi et al, N Engl J Med, 334:1156, 1996). A double-blind intervention trial in patients with coronary atherosclerosis found that taking 400 or 800 IU of vitamin E daily for a median of 510 days (range 3 to 981) led to a statistically significant reduction in the incidence of non-fatal myocardial infarction. The incidence of cardiovascular death and all-cause mortality, however, was slightly higher in the patients who took vitamin E supplements than in those who took placebo (NG Stephens et al, Lancet, 347:781, 1996). A placebo-controlled intervention trial in Finnish smokers found little difference in cardiovascular risk but a lower incidence of prostate cancer and prostate-cancer mortality in those who took 50 IU of alpha-tocopherol daily (J Virtamo et al, Arch Intern Med, 158:668, March 23, 1998; OP Heinonen et al, J Natl Cancer Inst, 90:440, 1998).

**BETA CAROTENE AND VITAMIN A**—Primary food sources for beta carotene are dark-colored fruits and vegetables. Primary food sources for vitamin A are meats, fish oil, fish and dairy products. Beta carotene and vitamin A are antioxidants, but may also have prooxidant effects *in vivo* (GS Omenn, Annu Rev Public Health, 19:73, 1998). Epidemiologic studies have found that

higher levels of carotenoids in the diet and higher serum levels of beta carotene are associated with a lower incidence of cardiovascular disease and cancer, particularly lung cancer. Multivitamin preparations usually contain 1000 to 10,000 IU (0.6 to 6 mg) of beta carotene. Beta carotene supplements usually contain 12 to 15 mg.

One large-12-year double-blind intervention study found that beta carotene supplements (50 mg every other day) had no effect on the incidence of cardiovascular disease or malignancy (CH Hennekens et al, N Engl J Med, 334:1145, 1996). A second placebo-controlled intervention trial in Finnish smokers found that 20 mg/day of beta carotene increased the incidence of lung cancer by 18%, which was statistically significant (The Alpha-Tocopherol, Beta Carotene Cancer Prevention Study Group, N Engl J Med, 330:1029, 1994). Another large double-blind intervention trial in smokers and asbestos-exposed workers, stopped early because no benefit was demonstrated, found that combined therapy with 30 mg of beta carotene and 25,000 IU of vitamin A daily was associated with an increase in the incidence of lung cancer, cardiovascular mortality and total mortality (GS Omenn et al, N Engl J Med, 334:1150, 1996; GS Omenn et al, J Natl Cancer Inst, 88:1550, 1996).

**VITAMIN D**—Primary food sources of vitamin D are meat, fish, and, in the USA, fortified milk. Yogurt and other dairy products made with milk are generally not fortified with vitamin D. Many elderly people receive inadequate amounts of vitamin D because of low exposure to sunlight, decreased synthesis of vitamin D in the skin, and decreased absorption and activation of the vitamin. The latest US recommendations for vitamin D intake, based on amounts that have retarded the rate of bone loss, are 200 IU/day for men and women 19 to 50 years old, 400 IU for men and women 51 to 70 years old, and 600 IU for men and women more than 70 years old. Elderly people who do not drink milk and do not expose themselves to sunlight will need to take supplements to achieve this level of vitamin D intake.

**VITAMIN C**—The main dietary sources of vitamin C in the USA are citrus fruits and tomatoes. Like vitamin E and beta carotene, vitamin C can have prooxidant as well as antioxidant effects (V Herbert, Am J Clin Nutr, 60:157, 1994). One 8-oz. glass of orange juice contains about 100 mg of vitamin C. Dietary levels of about 200 mg/day of vitamin C maintain maximal body pools of vitamin (M Levine et al, Proc Natl Acad Sci USA, 93:3704, 1996). High intakes and serum concentrations of vitamin C have been associated with low incidences of senile cataract, cancer and coronary artery disease, and higher high-density lipoprotein (HDL) cholesterol concentrations. No long-term intervention studies with vitamin C have been published. Short-term randomized trials have shown that taking vitamin C does not prevent upper respiratory infections.

High doses of vitamin C (more than 1 gram) are poorly absorbed and cause diarrhea, and could increase urinary oxalate excretion to a level that might increase the incidence of kidney stones. A controlled trial in 30 male volunteers given 500 mg daily of vitamin C supplement found both increases and decreases in various markers of oxidative damage to the DNA of peripheral blood lymphocytes (ID Podmore et al, Nature, 392:559, April 9, 1998).

**VITAMIN B$_{12}$**—Food sources of vitamin B$_{12}$ are meat, fish and diary products. Elderly people with atrophic gastritis, which affects 10% to 30% of Americans over the age of 60, cannot absorb vitamin B$_{12}$ bound to food protein, but absorb crystalline vitamin B$_{12}$ normally (R Carmel, Am J Clin Nutr, 66:750, 1997). Elderly patients therefore should take vitamin B$_{12}$ either in the form of B$_{12}$-fortified foods such as cereals or as a daily dietary supplement containing at least the Recommended Dietary Allowance (2.4 μg/day} of the vitamin.

**FOLATE**—The standard US diet provides 50 to 500 μg of absorbable folate per day, mostly from meat and dark-green leafy vegetables, but the bioavailability of folate in mixed diets varies. Folic acid in supplements is about twice as bioavailable as folate in food (GP Oakely, Jr, N Engl J Med, 338:1060, April 9, 1998). As of January 1998, all enriched cereal grains sold in the USA contain 140 μg of folic acid per 100 g of grain; estimates suggest that this fortification will increase folic acid intake by about 100 μg/day. Even this amount, however, may be inadequate for prevention of neural tube defects, which occur early in pregnancy, before most women know that they are pregnant (S Daly et al, Lancet, 350:1666, 1997). Supplementing the diet of women of childbearing age

with 400 μg of folic acid per day has dramatically decreased the incidence of neural tube defects in their offspring (AE Czeizel and I Dudas, N Engl J Med, 327:1832, 1992). Low intake of absorbable folates has also been associated with high serum concentrations of homocysteine and a higher incidence of cardiovascular disease and stroke (CJ Boushey et al, JAMA, 274:1049, 1995; MR Malinow et al, N Engl J Med, 338:1009, April 9, 1998). High doses of folic acid can mask vitamin B$_{12}$ deficiency, permitting progression of neurologic disease.

**VITAMIN B$_6$** (Otrudixube)—Vitamin B$_6$ is available in meat, whole-grain bread and cereals, soybeans and vegetables. Some retrospective studies have found an association between higher intakes of the vitamin, lower serum concentrations of homocysteine and a lower risk of coronary heart disease (EB Rimm et al, JAMA, 279:359, 1998). Prospective studies are lacking, however, and the optimal dose and effectiveness of vitamin B$_6$ supplements remain to be determined (GS Omenn et al, Circulation, 97:421, 1998).

**MULTIVITAMIN PREPARATIONS**—Most multivitamin preparations contain amounts of vitamins and minerals that are safe. One randomized trial in 96 elderly patients in Canada found that those who took such preparations for 12 months showed signs of better immune function and had fewer sick days (RK Chandra, Lancet, 340:1124, 1992). A much larger, but retrospective, study in US adults found that taking vitamin supplements was not associated with lower morbidity or mortality rates (I Kim et al, Am J Public Health, 83:546, 1993).

**DIET**—Many substances found in foods may affect the occurrence of heart disease and malignancy, but they may not all be vitamins. Supplementing the diet with vitamins may not be an adequate substitute for the beneficial effects of a diet rich in fruit and vegetables.

**CONCLUSION**—Supplements are necessary to assure adequate intake of folic acid in young women and possibly of vitamins D and B$_{12}$ in the elderly. The benefits of taking high doses of vitamin E remain to be established. There is no convincing evidence that taking supplements of vitamin C prevents any disease. No one should take beta carotene supplements. A balanced diet may be more beneficial and safer than taking vitamin supplements.

# Vitamin E Supplements: To E or Not To E?

The realization last year that supplements of beta carotene, one of the antioxidant vitamins, did not help to prevent heart problems was a disappointment to consumers and researchers alike (see October 1996 *Harvard Heart Letter*). But another antioxidant — vitamin E — has continued to receive a great deal of attention as a potential protective agent against heart disease. Studies of people taking this supplement have yielded mixed results, but most research focusing on high-dose supplements suggests that this strategy may well provide protection against coronary artery disease.

Vitamin E use has moved into a "gray zone" in which many physicians are already prescribing it for patients with coronary artery disease — yet leading experts are often reluctant to endorse it officially because no one has yet done a huge randomized trial in which patients are assigned to take vitamin E or a placebo. Nevertheless, the evidence supporting vitamin E is compelling enough that some researchers believe that vitamin E's time has come.

## Oxidative stress

*Antioxidants* in general help clean up toxic products created by normal functions of the body's cells. Cells use oxygen to burn their fuel, and the byproducts of this process include free radicals — chemical compounds that combine easily with (and damage) fats, proteins, and other substances in the body. Research has raised the possibility that the buildup of fatty deposits in the arteries may begin when oxygen free radicals (oxidants) interact with LDL (low density lipoprotein), the "bad" cholesterol. Vitamin E, the theory goes, resides inside LDL particles and helps disarm the radicals from within — thereby slowing or preventing cholesterol buildup and the subsequent development of heart disease.

Although much of the evidence for this "oxidation theory" comes from a variety of sources and is quite persuasive, some large knowledge gaps still prevent scientists from concluding definitively that vitamin E protects people from cholesterol buildup. For example, vitamin E supplements have been shown to prevent oxidation of LDL only in blood samples used in laboratory experiments. Whether or not this same effect occurs within the arteries of living people is still not clear. Furthermore, in some animal experiments, vitamin E could not prevent the buildup of cholesterol-laden plaque (atherosclerosis) in the walls of arteries.

## Observing E

Observational studies have taught researchers a great deal about factors that appear to protect people against heart disease (for example, exercising and eating vegetables, fruits, and grains) and also about factors that increase a person's chances of developing it (such as smoking, obesity, and eating saturated fat). In this type of study, participants report their lifestyle patterns, including the foods and supplements they consume, and researchers track the people over time to draw conclusions about the relationship between their behavior and any death or illness from heart disease.

Several such studies — among them, the Nurses' Health Study and the Health Professionals' Follow-up Study — have suggested that people who take vitamin E supplements have a reduced risk of heart disease. One study, the Iowa Women's Health Study, suggested that  containing vitamin E, and not supplements, lowered the risk of death from heart disease. But the length of time women had taken the supplements was not clear in this study. (Extended use had been associated with lower risk in the earlier studies.)

## Results of CHAOS

While the observational studies continue and scientists pursue their research on the theoretic basis of atherosclerosis, many experts are pointing to a British study as an indication that vitamin E supplements may help fight

From the *Harvard Heart Letter*, August 1997, pp. 1-3. © 1997 by the President and Fellows of Harvard College. Reprinted by permission.

heart disease. In this study, doses of vitamin E reduced the risk of nonfatal heart attack in patients diagnosed with atherosclerosis. This randomized, controlled trial with the memorable name of CHAOS (for Cambridge Heart Antioxidant Study) involved 2,002 men and women with artery narrowings. Half the participants were assigned to take a vitamin E supplement (at doses of either 400 or 800 IU/day), and the other half were asked to take a dummy capsule (placebo).

The researchers tracked these patients for one to three years and found that a heart attack (either fatal or nonfatal) occurred in 41 of the group who took vitamin E and in 64 of the people who took a placebo. Though the study was too small to assess the overall survival rate and death rate from heart attacks, a statistical analysis showed that vitamin E cut the risk of a heart attack by more than half and the risk of a nonfatal heart attack by 77%.

### But wait . . .

Before vitamin E enthusiasts conclude that the CHAOS study justifies regular intake of vitamin E supplements, they must consider the results of two other randomized, controlled trials that suggest otherwise. Together, these two trials involved nearly 30,000 people who were randomly allocated to groups taking vitamin E, beta carotene, both vitamins, or placebos. In these studies, vitamin E supplements did not reduce the risk of dying from heart disease and stroke.

Do these studies mean that vitamin E is one more disappointment in the search for dietary supplements that can lower cardiovascular risk? Not really. These studies used doses of vitamin E between 30 mg and 50 mg per day—much smaller than those taken in the CHAOS study. Furthermore, epidemiological studies suggest that doses of at least 100 IU/day are most likely to provide protection against heart disease. Scientists note that it is quite plausible that only higher doses might have an effect on heart disease, since the protective effects of vitamin E on LDL cholesterol appear to depend heavily on dosage.

Another factor may be smoking. There was a high percentage of smokers in some studies that did not find a lower rate of heart disease in users of vitamin E. Those results have led researchers to speculate that vitamin E supplements may not be able to overcome the oxidant effect of smoking. This relationship is far from proven—but it is just one more reason that smokers should quit.

### Sources of Vitamin E

Good food sources of vitamin E include safflower, corn, and olive oils, nuts, sunflower-seed kernels, pumpkin seeds, wheat germ, and whole grains. Some vegetables and fruits are also sources of vitamin E — among them, greens (especially kale), sweet potatoes, and mangos.

Most multivitamin preparations contain about 15–30 international units (IU) of vitamin E, which is approximately equivalent to 15–30 mg of alpha-tocopherol, the vitamin's most abundant and biologically active chemical. Commercial vitamin E supplements usually contain a mixture of several different forms of alpha-tocopherol and can contain anywhere from 200 to 1,000 IU of vitamin E — doses much higher than the recommended intake of 30 IU per day.

### Complex effects

Some studies have examined the relationship between vitamin E supplements and the relaxation and contraction responses of arteries that distinguish "healthy" arteries from "unhealthy" ones. Researchers have found arteries with atherosclerosis squeeze down and become more narrow when exposed to certain chemical signals that ought to make those arteries dilate and permit more blood flow. These studies suggest that vitamin E can improve the abnormal arterial responses in people with cholesterol deposits but does not affect people with healthy arteries because they already have normal arterial responses.

It is not known whether vitamin E offers any protection or improvement in the health of arteries once blood-cholesterol levels are reduced. In a study that examined the effect of cholesterol lowering on the thickness of the carotid artery in the neck, people already taking vitamin E supplements had less progression in the thickness of that artery than people not using supplements. But over the two years of the study, vitamin E appeared to offer no additional protection to people who were also receiving treatment to lower blood cholesterol.

## When is the evidence enough?

Although many studies have demonstrated that people with high vitamin E consumption have less heart disease, many experts currently refrain from urging all people with coronary artery disease to begin using this vitamin because absolute "proof" of its benefit is not available. It is possible that the data seen in trials supporting use of vitamin E could be related to other factors associated with vitamin E use, rather than the vitamin itself. For example, people who take this vitamin might be more likely to exercise or eat healthier diets. Epidemiological studies have used statistics to take such factors into account, but the possibility remains that the study researchers could not completely "adjust" for differences between people who do and do not use vitamin E.

Unfortunately, the definitive studies that will be able to answer questions about the true impact of vitamin E supplements are not yet finished — leaving experts (including the members of the editorial board of this newsletter) to debate over whether the evidence in favor of vitamin E is strong enough. For otherwise healthy people there is no strong evidence of harm from a modest dose of vitamin E supplements, but some doctors worry that consuming vitamin E, particularly at high doses, for a long time could carry unknown risks.

Some members of the *Harvard Heart Letter* editorial board, however, believe it is important for readers to know that the case for taking vitamin E in a dosage of 200 mg to 800 mg per day is reasonably strong, and getting stronger. This dosage is considerably higher than the U.S. recommended daily intake of 30 mg (or IU).

This advice does not mean that everyone should go out and start using high doses of this vitamin. Consultation with a physician first is always advisable. For example, people who are taking blood-thinning medications (warfarin or Coumadin) should check with their doctor if they are thinking of taking vitamin E, because it might alter their blood's clotting ability and increase the chance of excess bleeding. Also, patients with the rare eye disease retinitis pigmentosa should not take vitamin E since it may make the condition worse.

Regardless of which side of the vitamin E debate the experts currently are on, they all await future research that may answer the important questions that remain. The largest ongoing trial is the Women's Health Study, whose co-principal investigator is *Harvard Heart Letter* editorial board member Charles Hennekens. Results from this study, which involves nearly 40,000 female health professionals, will not be available until 2002 — unless some extreme result causes the researchers to end the trial early.

# Do you need more minerals?

*Supposedly, selenium prevents cancer and zinc cures the common cold. Here's the lowdown on those and other claims.*

Late last year, the Journal of the American Medical Association published a study from the Arizona Cancer Institute suggesting that supplements of the trace mineral selenium may sharply reduce the risk of death from many cancers. Early positive results prompted the researchers to stop the study, so the placebo group could switch to the supplement. One group of selenium supporters, cofounded by the study's lead author, likened the findings to the "discovery of penicillin or the polio vaccine." And it's not just selenium: Other recent findings have suggested that various minerals may help prevent heart attacks, strengthen the bones, control diabetes, bolster immunity, and cure colds.

In this issue, we report on selenium as well as zinc, potassium, and magnesium—three other minerals that have received a lot of attention from scientists, marketers, or both. Next month, we'll report on the minerals calcium and iron.

## Selenium: Cancer and coronary claims

In the Arizona study, half of the roughly 1300 volunteers took a daily 200-microgram (mcg) selenium pill; the others got a placebo. Over the next four and a half years, both groups developed about the same number of cancers of the bladder, breast, head, neck,

or skin. But the selenium group developed 63 percent fewer prostate cancers, 58 percent fewer colorectal cancers, and 46 percent fewer lung cancers than the placebo group did. Overall, there were 50 percent fewer cancer deaths in the selenium group.

To explain those results, the researchers cited laboratory evidence that selenium kills cancer cells and fights oxidation, chemical damage that can turn a cell cancerous. In addition, some observational evidence suggests that selenium may ward off coronary heart disease as well, possibly because oxidation helps cause clogging of the coronary arteries.

But the case for selenium is still shaky. For one thing, the study was too small to prove a benefit. More important, it was originally designed to test selenium's impact on skin cancer. Only after the researchers found no effect on the skin did they check for effects on other sites. Such unplanned searches are more likely to dredge up results that occur by chance. Further, all the volunteers had a history of skin cancer, and most of them lived in the Southeastern U.S., where the diet is often low in selenium. Findings in that doubly atypical population may not apply to the general population.

No other clinical trials of selenium alone have yet been done. Observational studies, less reliable than

Reprinted with permission from *Consumer Reports on Health,* November 1997, pp. 121-124. © 1997 by Consumers Union of U.S., Inc., Yonkers, NY 10703-1057. To subscribe, call 800-234-1645; www.consumereports.org.

trials, have yielded mixed results; those that do suggest a benefit often disagree on which cancers are affected. The evidence on coronary disease is even weaker than the cancer findings.

▶ *Recommendation:* There's far too little evidence to recommend taking selenium supplements. And high doses of selenium—1000 mcg or more per day—can cause loss of fingernails and hair; very high doses can cause diarrhea, fatigue, nausea, and even nerve damage. But it certainly can't hurt to try getting plenty of selenium from the diet, which is capable of supplying the amount of selenium used in the Arizona cancer study. And two of the best dietary sources of selenium are low-fat, nutritious foods—fish and grains (see table on next page).

## Zinc: The cold facts

A few small observational studies have suggested that people who consume the most zinc have a slightly lower risk of macular degeneration, the leading cause of blindness in older people, than those who consume the least. But that's not why zinc lozenges have been selling like tiny hotcakes: A recent study from the Cleveland Clinic suggested that zinc might help cure the common cold.

In that study, colds lasted an average of four days in a group that took large doses of zinc, compared with seven days in a placebo group. Since those findings appeared, at least six manufacturers—including Hall's, the leading cough-drop maker—have introduced zinc-based "cold remedies."

But it's not time to toss out the chicken soup just yet. The treatment nauseated one out of five volunteers and left a lingering foul taste in the mouth of some 80 percent of the volunteers. Four of the seven other clinical trials of zinc supplements found no effect on colds. The evidence that zinc strengthens the immune system—one plausible explanation for any cold-fighting effect—is similarly weak; some studies suggest that modest doses of the mineral may actually weaken immunity. Other research points to further risks: possibly reduced blood levels of copper, another essential trace mineral, at a zinc intake of just 18 to 25 milligrams per day, just over the recommended daily intake of 15 mg; reduced blood levels of the "good" HDL cholesterol at 50 to 75 mg per day; and severe anemia at 150 mg or more.

▶ *Recommendation:* If you eat meat regularly, you're almost surely getting plenty of zinc. Vegetarians can meet the recommended daily intake for zinc by eating such foods as beans, cheese, milk, nuts, seeds, and wheat germ. However, trying to consume much more than the recommended intake of zinc, particularly from supplements, has no proven benefit and several risks.

## Potassium: The unsung benefits

There's not much of a market for potassium supplements, since the mineral is relatively abundant in the diet. Maybe that's why the benefits of potassium, which are better documented than those of any other mineral discussed in this report, have received the least publicity of the bunch.

Laboratory and animal studies suggest that potassium may help lower blood pressure, by relaxing the walls of the arteries. Observational studies have consistently linked a low dietary intake of potassium with high blood pressure. And dozens of clinical trials have indicated that potassium can reduce blood pressure, although none was sufficiently large or rigorous to prove the connection.

Last year, researchers from Johns Hopkins University and the National Institutes of Health analyzed the pooled results of the 33 best trials, which included some 2600 people overall. The researchers calculated that hypertensive individuals who consumed an average of 2000 extra milligrams of potassium per day, from either diet or supplements, would lower their systolic blood pressure (the upper number) by an average of 4.5 mmHg, and their diastolic pressure (the lower number) by 2.5 mmHg. Such changes, while small, would lower blood pressure in some mildly hypertensive individuals into the borderline or high-normal range, allowing them to cut or eliminate the need for antihypertensive medication —particularly if they combined the extra potassium with other, more potent nondrug measures, such as exercise and weight loss.

▶ *Recommendation:* Most of the evidence from observational studies and some of the evidence from clinical trials involved dietary intake of potassium, not supplements. Consuming the widely recommended five to nine daily servings of fruits and vegetables plus two to three servings of low-fat dairy products should help reduce blood pressure, in part because those foods supply plenty of potassium. But you shouldn't aim for high levels of potassium, particularly from supplements, if you have kidney disease, a common, often undiagnosed disorder in older

## *Colloids: Suspect suspensions*

Colloidal supplements—tiny mineral particles suspended in liquid —are apparently making marketers suspend all restraint. One ad, for example, calls silver, the mineral in a popular colloidal supplement, "the strongest, safest broad spectrum antibiotic known to man." Ads for another colloidal concoction say, "Every time you don't take them in every day, you're chopping a few hours or a few days off your life."

The makers of these supplements, which cost up to $50 for a one-month supply, claim that the body absorbs minerals better when they're floating in liquid. But there's no scientific support for that claim. Further, many colloidal supplements contain exotic minerals, such as rhodium and iridium, that have no known role in human health. Several concoctions include potentially toxic minerals, such as aluminum, arsenic, lead, and mercury. Some contain no minerals at all. And as our report explains, there's no convincing evidence that anyone needs more minerals than one can get from a well-balanced diet—except perhaps calcium for those who don't eat large amounts of certain foods.

## Dietary sources of minerals

| Food [1] | Magnesium | Potassium | Selenium | Zinc |
|---|---|---|---|---|
| **Meat (3 oz)** | | | | |
| Beef liver | ▨ | ▨ | ⊡ | ■ |
| Beef sirloin steak | ▨ | ■ | ⊡ | ■ |
| Chicken breast, skinless | ▨ | ▨ | ⊡ | ▨ |
| Leg of lamb | ▨ | ■ | ⊡ | ■ |
| Pork shoulder | ▨ | ■ | ⊡ | ■ |
| Turkey breast, skinless | ▨ | ▨ | ⊡ | ■ |
| **Fish and seafood (3 oz)** | | | | |
| Clams | □ | ■ | ⊡ | ■ |
| Cod | ▨ | ▨ | ⊡ | □ |
| Halibut | ⊡ | ■ | ⊡ | □ |
| Lobster | ▨ | ■ | ⊡ | ■ |
| Oysters | ■ | □ | ⊡ | ⊡ |
| Salmon | ▨ | ■ | ⊡ | □ |
| Snapper | ▨ | ■ | ⊡ | □ |
| Sole or flounder | ■ | ▨ | ⊡ | □ |
| Tuna, white, canned | ▨ | ▨ | ⊡ | □ |
| **Dairy products and eggs** | | | | |
| Cheddar cheese (1 oz) | □ | □ | ▨ | ▨ |
| Egg (1) | □ | □ | ■ | ▨ |
| Milk (1 cup) | ▨ | ■ | ■ | ▨ |
| Parmesan cheese (1 oz) | □ | □ | ■ | ▨ |
| Swiss cheese (1 oz) | □ | □ | ■ | ▨ |
| Yogurt, lowfat plain (1 cup) | ■ | ■ | ■ | ■ |
| **Beans and grains, cooked** | | | | |
| Black beans (½ cup) | ■ | ▨ | ■ | ▨ |
| Bread, whole wheat (2 slices) | ■ | ▨ | ⊡ | ▨ |
| Barley (½ cup) | ▨ | □ | ⊡ | ▨ |
| Bulgur wheat (½ cup) | ▨ | □ | ■ | □ |
| Lima beans (½ cup) | ■ | ■ | □ | □ |
| Pasta, whole wheat (½ cup) | ▨ | □ | ⊡ | □ |
| Pinto beans (½ cup) | ■ | ■ | ▨ | ▨ |
| Rice, brown (½ cup) | ■ | □ | ■ | □ |
| Wheat germ, toasted (2 tbsp) | ■ | □ | ■ | ■ |
| **Nuts and seeds (¼ cup)** | | | | |
| Almonds | ⊡ | ▨ | □ | ▨ |
| Brazil nuts | ⊡ | ▨ | ⊡ | ■ |
| Cashews | ⊡ | ▨ | ■ | ■ |
| Peanuts | ■ | ▨ | □ | ■ |
| Pumpkin seeds | ■ | □ | □ | ■ |
| Sunflower seeds | ■ | ▨ | ⊡ | ■ |
| Walnuts | ■ | □ | □ | ▨ |
| **Fruits** | | | | |
| Avocado, California (1) | ■ | ⊡ | □ | ▨ |
| Banana (1) | ▨ | ■ | □ | □ |
| Cantaloupe, cubed (1 cup) | □ | ■ | □ | □ |
| Casaba melon, cubed (1 cup) | □ | ■ | □ | □ |
| Grapefruit juice, fresh (1 cup) | ▨ | ■ | □ | □ |
| Nectarine (1) | □ | ▨ | □ | □ |
| Orange juice, fresh (1 cup) | ▨ | ■ | □ | □ |
| Raisins (¼ cup) | □ | ▨ | □ | □ |
| **Vegetables, cooked** | | | | |
| Acorn squash (½ cup) | ▨ | ▨ | □ | □ |
| Beet greens (½ cup) | ■ | ■ | □ | □ |
| Carrot juice, canned (1 cup) | ▨ | ⊡ | □ | □ |
| Broccoli (½ cup) | ▨ | ▨ | □ | □ |
| Peas, green (½ cup) | ▨ | ▨ | □ | ▨ |
| Potato (1) | ■ | ⊡ | □ | □ |
| Spinach (½ cup) | ⊡ | ■ | □ | ▨ |
| Tomato juice, canned (1 cup) | ▨ | ■ | □ | □ |

**Note:** The Daily Values (DV) are: magnesium, 400 mg; potassium, 3500 mg; selenium, 70 mcg; zinc, 15 mg.

[1] *Selected foods that supply significant amounts of at least one of the minerals listed.*

□ = 4% or less of DV
▨ = 5 - 9% of DV
■ = 10 - 19% of DV
⊡ = 20% or greater of DV

people; if you're taking a potassium-sparing diuretic, including spironolactone (*Aldactone*) and triamterene (in *Dyazide* and *Maxzide*); or if you're taking an ACE inhibitor, such as captopril (*Capoten*), enalapril (*Vasotec*), or lisinopril (*Prinivil, Zestril*).

## Magnesium: Multiple chances

The evidence for the benefits of magnesium is broad—suggesting a possible connection with several disorders—but generally shallow.

■ **Diabetes.** Magnesium deficiency may interfere with insulin, the hormone that regulates blood-sugar levels. People with diabetes are at increased risk of such deficiency, because their weakened kidneys eliminate too much magnesium. In theory, that could lead to a vicious cycle of falling magnesium levels, rising sugar levels, worsening diabetes, deteriorating kidney function, and increasing magnesium loss. But the few small studies of replacing lost magnesium have yielded conflicting results.

■ **Cardiovascular disease.** Laboratory and animal research suggests that magnesium, like potassium, may help relax the arteries and keep blood pressure down. Limited observational evidence suggests that low magnesium levels may increase the chance of developing hypertension, congestive heart failure, coronary disease, and atrial fibrillation, a type of arrhythmia that increases the risk of stroke.

■ **Osteoporosis.** Magnesium helps keep bones strong. Some but not all observational studies have linked low levels of magnesium in the blood, bones, or diet with thinning of the bones. Whether getting extra magnesium bolsters the bones is not known.

▶ *Recommendation:* The findings on magnesium are far too weak to warrant supplements, particularly since much of the evidence involves the risks of low levels rather than the benefits of high levels. And supplements may be dangerous in people with kidney disease, including many diabetics. But the findings should encourage you to consume at least the recommended daily intake—something many people fail to do. (See the table at left for good dietary sources.) Your doctor should consider checking your magnesium levels periodically if you have coronary disease, diabetes, or abnormal heart rhythms.

### Summing up

Potassium from the diet apparently can help lower blood pressure. Whether magnesium, selenium, or zinc has any special benefits is not clear. None of the evidence justifies taking supplements, particularly since extra doses of most of those minerals may be dangerous to at least some people.

But the evidence does strengthen the case for eating lots of plant and low-fat dairy foods, and at least some fish. Vegetarians may need to pay particular attention to their intake of zinc (to avoid possible deficiency) and perhaps of selenium (to ensure an ample supply). See the table at left for good dietary sources of the four minerals discussed here.

# MAKING THE MOST OF CALCIUM: FACTORS AFFECTING CALCIUM METABOLISM

## SUMMARY

New government guidelines recommend increased dietary calcium intakes for most Americans. Unfortunately, few Americans consume sufficient calcium, thereby increasing their risk for major chronic diseases such as osteoporosis.

Calcium nutrition is affected by the total amount of calcium consumed and its bioavailability. Dietary factors that influence intestinal calcium absorption and renal calcium excretion play important roles in determining the amount of dietary calcium needed by the body. In addition, a variety of nondietary factors (e.g., age, genetics, gender, hormonal status, smoking, disease, and medications) influence an individual's need for calcium.

Among dietary factors, calcium, vitamin D, and fiber have been most extensively examined for their effect on calcium absorption. Vitamin D promotes calcium absorption and helps the body adapt to a low calcium intake.

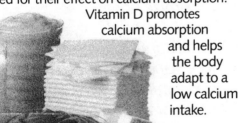

Vitamin D is obtained from exposure to sunlight. Major dietary sources of this vitamin include cod liver oil, fatty fish, and fortified foods such as milk and cereal.

Dietary fiber is very heterogenous in nature and generally has small effects on calcium absorption, with a few exceptions. High oxalate vegetables such as spinach decrease intestinal calcium absorption, whereas low oxalate vegetables such as kale have no effect on calcium absorption.

Protein, phosphorus, sodium, and potassium influence calcium metabolism by affecting urinary calcium excretion. High dietary protein intake clearly induces renal calcium loss. However, the impact of this phenomenon on bone health appears to be small at best. There is no evidence that protein-rich foods such as dairy foods adversely impact calcium balance or bone health. The presence of calcium, phosphorus, and potassium in dairy foods or in the diet may counterbalance the calciuretic effect of protein. Both dietary phosphorus and potassium reduce urinary calcium excretion and an adequate intake of calcium offsets calcium loss due to urinary excretion.

Like protein, sodium intake raises urinary calcium excretion. The typically high intake of protein and sodium in the U.S. contributes to the higher average calcium requirements in this country compared to other nations where intake of these nutrients is much lower. When consumed in moderate amounts, lactose, caffeine, and alcohol intake have little effect on calcium metabolism.

Calcium recommendations can be met by consuming foods naturally rich in calcium such as dairy foods. Dairy foods also provide other essential nutrients which can improve the overall nutritional quality of the diet. Further, it has been demonstrated that increasing calcium intake through dairy foods can be easily done without increasing calorie or fat intake, body weight, or percent body fat.

From *Dairy Council Digest*, January/February 1998, pp. 1-6. © 1998 by the National Dairy Council. Reprinted by permission.

## INTRODUCTION

Consuming an adequate intake of calcium reduces the risk of osteoporosis (1,2). This disease affects nearly 20 million women and 7 to 12 million men in the U.S. (3). Osteoporosis leads to an estimated 1.5 million fractures annually, and costs $13.8 billion/year or 1.1% of total health care expenses (4). Adequate dietary calcium is a prerequisite for maximizing peak bone mass which is reached by about age 30 or earlier (1,5) and minimizing bone loss in later years (1,2).

The Institute of Medicine, Food and Nutrition Board (IOM, FNB) recently issued new Dietary Reference Intakes (DRIs) for calcium (6). These recommendations are higher for several age-gender groups than the 1989 Recommended Dietary Allowances (RDAs) for calcium (7) and the typical calcium intakes of many Americans, particularly adolescent and older females (8,9).

Closing the gap between dietary calcium intake (8,9) and dietary recommendations for calcium (1,6) is an important public health objective (10). To close the gap, questions about how to best meet calcium needs and how dietary and nondietary factors influence calcium metabolism need to be answered. Besides calcium, other nutrients influence calcium bioavailability by affecting calcium absorption and excretion (2,6). In addition, nondietary factors such as age, gender, and hormonal status affect calcium absorption and excretion. Hence, both dietary and nondietary factors influence the body's need for this nutrient. This *Digest* reviews recent scientific findings related to how a variety of dietary and nondietary factors influence calcium metabolism.

## DIETARY FACTORS INFLUENCING CALCIUM ABSORPTION AND EXCRETION

***Dietary Calcium.*** Two processes are involved in the intestinal absorption of calcium. Active transport, mainly in the duodenum and jejunum, depends on 1,25-dihydroxyvitamin D, the active form of vitamin D. The second process is passive diffusion which occurs across the intestinal mucosa mainly in the jejunum and ileum (2,6,11). At low and moderate calcium

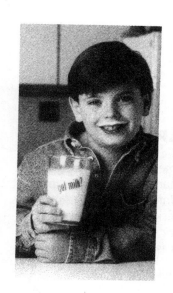

*To meet the 1997 Dietary Reference Intakes for calcium and maximize bone health, an intake of calcium-rich foods and an understanding of factors affecting calcium bioavailability are both important.*

intakes (i.e., approximately 200 mg/meal), the majority of calcium is absorbed by active transport, whereas at higher calcium intakes (i.e., above 200 mg/meal), passive diffusion becomes more important. Fractional calcium absorption varies inversely with dietary calcium intake (6,11,12).

***Vitamin D.*** Adequate vitamin D promotes calcium absorption and helps the body adapt to a low calcium intake (2,6,11,13–15). In the absence of vitamin D, less than 10% of dietary calcium may be absorbed compared to the typical 30% (1). Numerous studies have demonstrated that increasing vitamin D intake improves calcium absorption and ultimately bone health (14–19).

To be biologically active, vitamin D must be hydroxylated in the kidney to calcitriol (1,25[OH]$_2$D). Calcitriol, the hormonal form of vitamin D, is responsible for regulating the intestinal absorption of calcium (11). Low blood levels of 25-hydroxyvitamin D (25[OH]D), a clinical indicator of vitamin D status, have been observed in older adults, especially those who are homebound or institutionalized (14,15). Moreover, calcitriol-mediated adaptation in calcium absorption appears to decline with age. Loss of intestinal adaptation plays a role in the development of senile osteoporosis (20).

Recognizing that many older adults are at risk of vitamin D deficiency, the IOM (6) has doubled vitamin D recommendations for adults 51 through 70 years (10 µg/day or 400 I.U./day) and tripled them for adults >70 years (15 µg vitamin D/day or 600 I.U. vitamin D/day) compared with the previous recommendations (7).

Vitamin D deficiency results from lack of exposure to sunlight, low dietary intake of vitamin D, and/or decreased cutaneous and endogenous synthesis of the metabolically active form of vitamin D. Most of the body's requirement for vitamin D is met from sun exposure (4,6,14). However, the skin's synthesis of vitamin D is influenced by a variety of factors that reduce the ability of solar ultraviolet photons to reach the skin's surface (14). Melanin pigment, sunscreens (with a sun protective factor of 8 or more), winter months, northern latitudes, atmospheric pollution, clothing, and aging all decrease skin's capacity to produce the precursor form of vitamin D (6,14,15,21).

Food is another source of vitamin D in addition to exposure to sunlight. However, very few foods naturally contain this nutrient (6). Cod liver oil, fatty fish, egg yolks, and fortified foods such as milk and cereal are the major dietary sources of vitamin D (14,15). Almost all processed fluid milk in the U.S. is voluntarily fortified with vitamin D to obtain the standardized amount of 10 μg (400 I.U.) per quart (6,14).

**Protein.** Dietary protein increases urinary calcium excretion (4,13,22–24). For every gram of protein consumed, urinary calcium increases by about 1 mg (4,13,22). The etiology of protein-induced hypercalciuria is probably multifactorial (23,25,26). Dietary protein increases glomerular filtration rate and decreases renal calcium reabsorption, both of which increase urine calcium. However, the involvement of bone and the intestine in this phenomenon is controversial (27–30). An effect of protein on bone, if it exists, is likely to be small.

The presence of other components such as calcium, phosphorus, and potassium in protein-rich foods such as dairy foods appears to counterbalance or modify the calciuretic action of protein (2,22–24). For example, an adequate intake of calcium offsets calcium loss due to urinary excretion (31,32).

The higher calcium recommendations for the U.S. than for other less industrialized countries may be explained in part by Americans' generally higher protein intake (22). The calciuretic effect of dietary protein is no reason to reduce intake of this nutrient. Individuals who consume too little protein, have poor quality diets, or are undernourished could benefit from increasing their intake of protein-rich foods (4,6).

**Phosphorus.** As mentioned above, dietary phosphorus reduces urinary calcium excretion and counterbalances, in part, the calciuric effect of dietary protein. Protein-rich foods such as dairy products are also an important source of phosphorus (2). There is no convincing evidence that dietary phosphorus within the range currently consumed in the U.S. adversely affects calcium bioavailability, calcium absorption, or bone health (2,6,33–35).

*Protein intake increases urinary calcium excretion. However, other components such as calcium, phosphorus, and potassium in protein-rich foods (e.g., milk and other dairy foods) minimize calcium losses. The impact of protein on bone is considered to be negligible, especially when adequate calcium is consumed.*

**Sodium.** Like protein, sodium intake increases urinary calcium excretion (2,4, 6,13,36–39). In postmenopausal women, each 500 mg of sodium consumed increases urinary calcium by about 10 mg (6).

According to a study by Matkovic et al (36), sodium intake was the principal determinant of urinary calcium loss in 381 girls aged 11 to 13 years. Although there was no indication of an adverse effect on bone mineral density in the adolescents, a relationship between sodium and bone was demonstrated in older postmenopausal women (38). The typically high intake of sodium (and protein) in the U.S. contributes to the higher average calcium requirements in this country compared to other nations where sodium (and protein) are much lower (13).

**Dietary Fiber.** Dietary fiber's effect on calcium absorption is generally small, with a few exceptions (22,40,41). Oxalate, found in spinach, inhibits the absorption of calcium from this food (42). Only about 5% of the calcium in spinach is absorbed, compared to about 30% of the calcium in milk (42). In contrast, low oxalate vegetables (e.g., kale) have excellent calcium absorption.

If consumed in large amounts, wheat bran can inhibit the absorption of coingested calcium (43,44). However, at usual intakes of fiber (5–15 g/day), wheat bran's effect on calcium absorption is relatively small (43). Phytate in wheat bran and in other foods such as beans (pinto, red, white) decreases the intestinal absorption of calcium from these foods (45). An individual would need to consume nearly 10 servings of red beans or 16 servings of spinach to obtain the same amount of absorbable calcium as in one cup of milk (46,47).

**Lactose.** Lactose appears to stimulate the intestinal absorption of calcium in laboratory animals (48) and in human infants (49). However, evidence that lactose improves calcium absorption in adults is less clear (50). In postmenopausal women, lactose had no effect on the absorption of calcium from a variety of dairy foods (50). The increased prevalence of osteoporosis in lactose intolerant persons is likely due to a low intake of milk and other dairy products, and not to decreased calcium absorption (51–53). New research indicates that people who identify themselves as lactose intolerant can comfortably consume at least one (54) or even two cups of milk/day, at breakfast and at dinner (55).

**Caffeine.** Moderate caffeine intake has a negligible effect on calcium status (56–58). Caffeine can induce an initial short-term increase in urinary calcium excretion (6,56). A single cup of brewed coffee causes a deterioration in calcium balance by about 4 mg calcium/day, mainly by reducing calcium absorption (56). However, this amount is readily offset by consuming one or two tablespoons of milk (56). Caffeine appears to have little, if any, effect on calcium metabolism, calcium status, or bone density when recommended dietary intakes of calcium are also consumed (57,58).

**Alcohol.** Excess alcohol ingestion decreases intake of nutrient-rich foods and causes liver and intestinal damage that ultimately results in malabsorption of many nutrients, including calcium (59). The amount of alcohol necessary to reduce calcium status is unknown, although alcohol in moderation does not appear to adversely affect the bioavailability of calcium (2).

## NONDIETARY FACTORS AFFECTING CALCIUM METABOLISM

**Genetics.** Genetics is suspected of contributing to the variability in calcium absorption among individuals (11,50,60). Recent studies indicate that polymorphisms of the vitamin D receptor (VDR) gene may explain, in part, the heritable component of bone density (11). However, researchers have yet to establish whether or not polymorphisms in the VDR gene influence bone by affecting calcium absorption (11,60,61). A recent study involving premenopausal women indicates that the vitamin D receptor gene has a small effect on calcium absorption (11).

**Age.** Calcium absorption efficiency varies throughout the lifespan (6,11,14, 50,62). When demands for calcium are high, as during periods of rapid growth in infancy and puberty, calcium absorption

*The bioavailability of calcium depends not only on dietary components, but also on nondietary factors such as genetics, age, hormonal status, pregnancy, lactation, and diseases/medication.*

and retention are increased. In infants and young children, calcium absorption can be as high as 60% (1). In early puberty (age of growth spurt), calcium absorption is about 34%, whereas in late adolescence and adulthood, fractional calcium absorption decreases to about 25% to 30% (1,6,62).

Intestinal calcium absorption efficiency declines with aging, as does the ability to adapt to a low calcium diet (2,63–65). A number of factors are thought to contribute to this age-related decline in intestinal calcium absorption efficiency. These include estrogen deficiency in women and age-related changes in vitamin D metabolism (e.g., decreased concentration of calcitriol, partial intestinal resistence to 1,25 $(OH)_2D$) (1,2,34,62,65). Recognition of the age-related decrease in calcium absorption contributed to the recent decision to recommend 1,200 mg of calcium/day for everyone over age 50 (6). This amount is 400 mg/day higher than previously recommended (7).

**Estrogen status.** As mentioned above, the loss of estrogen at menopause reduces the efficiency of calcium absorption (1,63,64). Estrogen directly stimulates intestinal calcium absorption, independent of 1,25$(OH)_2D$ action, and improves renal calcium conservation (65). Between the ages of 40 and 60 years, the combination of increasing age and estrogen withdrawal reduces a woman's calcium absorption efficiency by 20% to 25% (64).

**Pregnancy and Lactation.** During pregnancy, intestinal calcium absorption increases from about 27% before pregnancy to 54% at five or six months of gestation and 42% at term (62). During lactation, there is a temporary loss of calcium from bone independent of dietary calcium intake (66). However, after weaning the efficiency of intestinal calcium absorption and renal retention of calcium increase (66–68). These metabolic changes in calcium metabolism after weaning are considered to be biological mechanisms to compensate for the loss of bone during lactation.

**Other Factors.** Cigarette smoking may decrease calcium absorption (69). In addition, a number of diseases (e.g., hyperparathyroidism, diabetes) and several commonly used medications (e.g., glucocorticoids, corticosteroids, aluminum-containing antacids) can reduce calcium absorption and/or increase urinary calcium excretion (1,70). As a result, these conditions increase the need for calcium.

## MEETING CALCIUM RECOMMENDATIONS

Meeting calcium recommendations can be accomplished in a variety of ways. Foods naturally containing calcium, in particular milk and other dairy foods, are preferred because they are rich sources of calcium (1,4,71). In fact, in 1994, dairy foods contributed 73% of the calcium available in the nation's food supply (71). These foods also contribute other essential nutrients (e.g., protein, phosphorus, potassium, riboflavin, vitamin A, vitamin D) important for bone and overall health (71).

Because milk and milk products are good sources of many nutrients, their intake improves the overall nutritional quality of the diet (72–74). Diets low in calcium are generally low in other essential nutrients and reflect overall poor dietary quality.

Anecdotal fears of fat and excess calorie intake from dairy foods are not supported in the scientific literature. Studies report that increasing calcium intake through dairy foods can easily be done without necessarily increasing calorie or fat intake, body weight, or percent body fat (72, 74–76). For example, when 64 post-menopausal women were randomly assigned to receive either skim milk powder or a calcium supplement for two years, the women who consumed the skim milk raised their daily calcium intake to 1,600 mg/day without increasing their total fat or saturated fat intake (74). Also, the women receiving the milk powder increased their intake of several other nutrients, including protein, potassium, magnesium, phosphorus, riboflavin, thiamin, and zinc (74). In contrast,

*Foods naturally containing calcium are the preferred source of this nutrient. Milk and other dairy foods are high in calcium as well as other essential nutrients. Further, increasing calcium intake through dairy foods can easily be done without increasing calorie or fat intake, body weight, or percent body fat.*

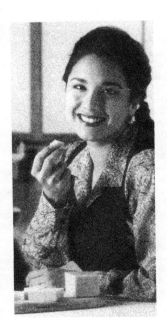

those who took a calcium supplement increased only their intakes of calcium and sodium. Similar results have been observed in adolescent girls (75,76).

The amount of calcium in foods, its bio-availability, and the physiological state of the host are important to calcium status. Milk and other dairy foods have the highest content of calcium per serving. Foods such as sardines, salmon with the bones, dried beans, calcium set tofu, some green leafy vegetables (e.g., broccoli, kale, bok choy), breads and cereals also contain calcium but in lower amounts than dairy products (6,46). With the notable exception of the high oxalate green vegetables and the phytate-rich grain products, calcium absorption from most vegetables, grain products, and dairy foods is fairly similar (6,47).

When calcium needs cannot be met by consuming foods naturally high in this nutrient, calcium-fortified foods or calcium supplements are considered (1,4,6,77). However, these foods and supplements do not provide the same overall nutritional benefits as milk and other dairy products. Also, their intake could potentially increase the risk of excess calcium loads and/or reduce the bioavailability of other nutrients in the diet such as zinc (77). A calcium intake of up to 2,500 mg/day is considered to be safe for almost all healthy individuals (6).

To meet calcium recommendations, increased consumption of calcium-rich foods such as milk and other dairy foods, often is necessary. This advice is consistent with USDA's *Food Guide Pyramid* (78). Unfortunately, Americans consume on average only 1.5 servings from the Milk Group, about half of the 2 to 3 servings/day currently recommended on the Pyramid (79). The gap between Americans' calcium intakes and recommendations may be even larger considering the 1997 dietary recommendations which call for higher calcium intakes for most age-gender groups (6). Some health professional organizations are recommending an increase in the number of servings from the Milk Group to meet higher calcium needs (80).

## REFERENCES

1. U.S. Department of Health and Human Services, Public Health Service, National Institutes of Health. *Consensus Development Conference Statement. Optimal Calcium Intake.* June 6–8; 12(4): 1–31, 1994.

2. Schaafsma, G. *Dietary Calcium In Health.* Bulletin Intl. Dairy Federation 322, 1997.

3. Looker, A.C., E.S. Orwoll, C.C. Johnston, Jr., et. al. J. Bone Miner. Res. *12(11):* 1761, 1997.

4. Packard, P.T., and R.P. Heaney. J. Am. Diet. Assoc. *97:* 414, 1997.

5. Haapasalo H., P. Kannus, H. Sievanen, et. al. J. Bone Miner. Res. *11(11):* 1751, 1997.

6. IOM (Institute of Medicine). *Dietary Reference Intakes for Calcium, Phosphorus, Magnesium, Vitamin D, and Fluoride.* Standing Committee on the Scientific Evaluation of Dietary Reference Intakes. Food and Nutrition Board. Washington, DC: National Academy Press, 1997.

7. Commission on Life Sciences, National Research Council. *Recommended Dietary Allowances, 10th Edition.* Food and Nutrition Board. Washington, DC: National Academy Press, 1989.

8. Alaimo, K., M.A. McDowell, R.R. Briefel, et. al. *Dietary Intake of Vitamins, Minerals, and Fiber of Persons Ages 2 Months and Over in the United States: Third National Health and Nutrition Examination Survey, Phase I, 1988–1991.* Advance Data from Vital and Health Statistics; No. 258. Hyattsville, MD: National Center for Health Statistics, 1994.

9. Federation of American Societies for Experimental Biology, Life Sciences Research Office. Prepared for the Interagency Board for Nutrition Monitoring and Related Research. *Third Report on Nutrition Monitoring in the United States: Executive Summary.* Washington, DC: U.S. Government Printing Office, 1995.

10. National Center for Health Statistics. *Healthy People 2000 Review, 1995–96.* Hyattsville, MD: Public Health Service, 1996.

11. Wishart, J.M., M. Horowitz, A.G. Need, et. al. Am. J. Clin. Nutr. *65:* 798, 1997.

12. Dawson-Hughes, B., S. Harris, C. Kramich, et. al. J. Bone Miner. Res. *8:* 779, 1993.

13. Heaney, R.P. Nutr. Rev. *54(4):* 53, 1996.

14. Holick, M.F. J. Nutr. *126:* 1159s, 1996.

15. Anderson, J.J.B., and S.U. Toverud. J. Nutr. Biochem. *5:* 58, 1994.

16. Dawson-Hughes, B., G.E. Dallal, E.A. Krall, et. al. Ann. Intern. Med. *115:* 505, 1991.

17. Dawson-Hughes, B., S.S. Harris, E.A. Krall, et. al. Am. J. Clin. Nutr. *61:* 1140, 1995.

18. Heikinheimo, R.J., J.A. Inkovovaara, E.J. Harju, et. al. Calcif. Tissue Int. *51(2):* 105, 1992.

19. Chapuy, M.C., M.E. Arlot, F. DuBoeuf, et. al. N. Engl. J. Med. *327:* 1637, 1992.

20. Gallanger, J., B. Riggs, J. Eisman, et. al. J. Clin. Invest. *64:* 729, 1979.

21. Dawson-Hughes, B., S.S. Harris, and G.E. Dallal. Am. J. Clin. Nutr. *65:* 67, 1997.

22. Heaney, R.P. J. Am. Diet. Assoc. *93:* 1259, 1993.

23. Pannemans, D.L.E., G. Schaafsma, and K.R. Westerterp. Br. J. Nutr. *77:* 721, 1997.

24. Whiting, S.J., D.J. Anderson, and S.J. Weeks. Am. J. Clin. Nutr. *65:* 1465, 1997.

25. Barzel, U.S. J. Bone Miner. Res. *10(10):* 1431, 1995.

26. Kerstetter, J., K. O'Brien, M. Mitnick, et. al. J. Bone Miner. Res. *12:* S 228, 1997.

27. Kerstetter, J., K. O'Brien, M. Mitnick, et. al. J. Am. Soc. Bone Miner. Res. *11:* S 325, 1996.

28. Feskanich, D., W.C. Willett, M.J. Stampfer, et. al. Am. J. Epidemiol. *143:* 472, 1996.

29. Shapses, S.A., S.P. Robins, E.I. Schwartz, et. al. J. Nutr. *125:* 2814, 1995.

30. Cooper, C., E.J. Atkinson, D.D. Hensrud, et. al. Calcif. Tissue Int. *58:* 320, 1996.

31. Meyer, H.E., J.I. Pedersen, E.B. Loken, et. al. Am. J. Epidemiol. *145:* 117, 1997.

32. Hu, J.F., X.H. Zhao, and B. Parpia, et. al. Am. J. Clin. Nutr. *58:* 398, 1993.

33. Calvo, M.S. J. Nutr. *123:* 1627, 1993.

34. Heaney, R.P. J. Am. Coll. Nutr. *15(6):* 575, 1996.

35. Karkkainen, M.U.M., J.W. Wiersma, and C.J.E. Lamberg-Allardt. Am. J. Clin. Nutr. *65:* 1726, 1997.

36. Matkovic, V., J.Z. Ilich, M.D. Andon, et. al. Am. J. Clin. Nutr. *62:* 417, 1995.

37. Itoh, R., and Y. Suyama. Am. J. Clin. Nutr. *63:* 735, 1996.

38. Devine, A., R.A. Criddle, I.M. Dick, et. al. Am. J. Clin. Nutr. *62:* 740, 1995.

39. O'Brien, K.O., S.A. Abrams, J.E. Stuff, et. al. J. Pediatr. Gastroenterol. Nutr. *23:* 8, 1996.

40. O'Brien, K.O., L.H. Allen, P. Quatromoni, et. al. J. Nutr. *123:* 2122, 1993.

41. Heaney, R.P., C.M. Weaver, S.M. Hinders, et. al. J. Food Sci. *58:* 1378, 1993.

42. Heaney, R.P., C.M. Weaver, and R.R. Recker. Am. J. Clin. Nutr. *47:* 707, 1988.

43. Weaver, C.M., R.P. Heaney, B.R. Martin, et. al. J. Nutr. *121:* 1769, 1991.

44. Weaver, C.M., R.P. Heaney, D. Teegarden, et. al. J. Nutr. *126:* 303, 1996.

45. Weaver, C.M., R.P. Heaney, W.R. Proulx, et. al. J. Food Sci. *58:* 1401, 1993.

46. Weaver, C.M., and K.L. Plawecki. Am. J. Clin. Nutr. *59(suppl):* 1238, 1994.

47. Weaver, C.M., W.R. Proulx, and R. Heaney. Choices for achieving adequate dietary calcium within a vegetarian diet. Am. J. Clin. Nutr. In press, 1998.

48. Buchowski, M.S., and D.D. Miller. J. Nutr. *121:* 1746, 1991.

49. Ziegler, E.E., and S.J. Fomon. J. Pediatr. Gastroenterol. Nutr. *2:* 288, 1983.

50. Nickel, K.P., B.R. Martin, D.L. Smith, et. al. J. Nutr. *126:* 1406, 1996.

51. Stallings, V.A., N.W. Oddleifson, B.Y. Negrini, et. al. Ann. Pediatr. Gastroenterol. Nutr. *18(4):* 440, 1994.

52. Corazza, G.R., G. Benati, A. DiSario, et. al. Br. J. Nutr. *73:* 479, 1995.

53. Honkanen, R., P. Pulkkinen, R. Jarvinen, et. al. Bone *19(1):* 23, 1996.

54. Suarez, F.L., D.A. Savaiano, and M.D. Levitt. N. Engl. J. Med. *333:* 1, 1995.

55. Suarez, F.L., D. Savaiano, P. Arbisi, et. al. Am. J. Clin. Nutr. *65:* 1502, 1997.

56. Barger-Lux, M., and R. Heaney. Osteop. Int. *5:* 97, 1995.

57. Barrett-Connor, E., J.C. Chang, and S.L. Edelstein. JAMA *271:* 280, 1994.

58. Lloyd, T., N. Rollings, D.F. Eggli, et. al. Am. J. Clin. Nutr. *65:* 1826, 1997.

59. Hirsch, P.E., and T.C. Peng. In: *Calcium and Phosphorus in Health and Disease.* J.J.B. Anderson and S.C. Garner (Eds) Boca Raton, FL: CRC Press, 1996, pp. 289–300.

60. Dawson-Hughes, B., S.S. Harris, and S. Finneran. J. Clin. Endocrinol. Metab. *80:* 3657, 1995.

61. Peacock, M., F.G. Hustmyer, C.C. Johnston, et. al. Bone *16:* 83s (abst.), 1995.

62. Louie, D. In: *Calcium and Phosphorus in Health and Disease.* J.J.B. Anderson and S.C. Garner (Eds). Boca Raton, FL: CRC Press, 1996, pp. 45–62.

63. Heaney, R.P., R.R. Recker, M.R. Stegman, et. al. J. Bone Miner. Res. *4:* 469, 1989.

64. Weaver, C.M. J. Nutr. *124:* 1418s, 1994.

65. Kinyamu, H.K., J.C. Gallagher, J.M. Prahl, et. al. J. Bone Miner. Res. *12(6):* 922, 1997.

66. Kalkwarf, H.J., B.L. Specker, D.C. Bianchi, et. al. N. Engl. J. Med. *337:* 523, 1997.

67. Prentice, A. N. Engl. J. Med. *337:* 558, 1997.

68. Kalkwarf, H.J., B.L. Specker, J.E. Heubi, et. al. Am. J. Clin. Nutr. *63:* 526, 1996.

69. Hopper, J.L., and E. Seeman. N. Engl. J. Med. *330:* 387, 1994.

70. Buckley, L.M., E.S. Leib, K.S. Cartularo, et. al. Ann. Intern. Med. *125:* 961, 1996.

71. Gerrior, S., and L. Bente. *Nutrient Content of the U.S. Food Supply, 1909–94.* Home Economics Research Report No. 53. Washington, DC: U.S. Department of Agriculture, Center for Nutrition Policy and Promotion, 1997.

72. Karanja, N., C.D. Morris, P. Rufolo, et. al. Am. J. Clin. Nutr. *59:* 900, 1994.

73. Barger-Lux, M.J., R.P. Heaney, P.T. Packard, et. al. Clin. Appl. Nutr. *2(4):* 39, 1992.

74. Devine, A., R.L. Prince, and R. Bell. Am. J. Clin. Nutr. *64:* 731, 1996.

75. Chan, G.M., K. Hoffman, and M. McMurry. J. Pediatr. *126:* 551, 1995.

76. Cadogan J., R. Eastell, N. Jones, et. al. Br. Med. J. *345:* 1255, 1997.

77. Whiting, S.J., and R.J. Wood. Nutr. Rev. *55(1):* 1, 1997.

78. U.S. Department of Agriculture, Human Nutrition Information Service. *The Food Guide Pyramid.* Home and Garden Bulletin No. 252. Washington, DC: U.S. Government Printing Office, 1992.

79. Cleveland, L.E., A.J. Cook, J.W. Wilson, et. al. *Pyramid Serving Data. Results from USDA's 1994 Continuing Survey of Food Intakes by Individuals.* Riverdale, MD: Food Surveys Research Group, Beltsville Human Nutrition Research Center, Agricultural Research Service, U.S. Department of Agriculture, March 1997.

80. Skiba, A., E. Loghmani, and D.P. Orr. Adol. Health Update *9(2):* 1, 1997.

## ACKNOWLEDGMENTS

National Dairy Council® assumes the responsibility for this publication. However, we would like to acknowledge the help and suggestions of the following reviewers in its preparation:

■ R.P. Heaney, M.D.
John A. Creighton University Professor
Creighton University
Omaha, Nebraska

■ J.E. Kerstetter, Ph.D., R.D.
Associate Professor
University of Connecticut
School of Allied Health
Storrs, Connecticut

The *Dairy Council Digest®* is written and edited by Lois D. McBean, M.S., R.D.

# How Important Is Salt Restriction?

*". . . and try to cut down on the amount of salt in your diet."*

This advice is often given to people with high blood pressure (hypertension) and other heart conditions — and immediately conjures up the prospect of tasteless meals and guilt after snacks. Food labels now list the amount of sodium (an element that constitutes half of the salt molecule) per serving, and the U.S. Food and Drug Administration (FDA) recommends that Americans consume no more than 2,400 mg of sodium per day — roughly 1,500 mg less than U.S. adults actually average. One teaspoon of table salt contains 2,300 milligrams of sodium.

Just how useful is salt restriction? Certainly, no study has proven that people who eat diets low in sodium live longer. Yet most experts have continued to recommend moderation in salt consumption in the belief that it will reduce blood pressure for the population as a whole and lower rates of stroke and heart disease.

### In the soup

Controversy over this topic boiled over onto the front pages of many newspapers this spring when a study of sodium-restricted diets and blood pressure questioned the impact of the low-salt strategy. The researchers — who received financial support from the Campbell's Soup Company — analyzed data that had been collected in 56 trials in which subjects were randomly assigned to dietary sodium restriction or their usual diets. Half of these trials involved people with hypertension, while the other half focused on people without high blood pressure. Most of these studies used a "crossover" design in which the subjects alternated between a low-sodium diet and their regular diet.

The good news is that among people with hypertension, dietary sodium restriction led to an average decrease in systolic blood pressure of about 6 mm Hg and a decrease in diastolic pressure that averaged 4 mm Hg. The impact of sodium restriction was greatest for hypertensive patients over age 45. (Systolic blood pressure is the higher of two numbers in a blood-pressure reading and a reflection of pressure in the arteries when the heart contracts. Diastolic blood pressure is the lower number and reflects pressure in the arteries when the heart is relaxed.)

The bad news is that for people without hypertension, there was only a slight decrease in systolic blood pressure — an average of just 1.6 mm Hg. And in studies in which the subjects were living outside of hospitals, there was no evidence of blood-pressure reduction at all for people who did not already have hypertension. Since these studies probably most accurately reflect the impact of salt restriction in real life, the results raise the question of whether people without hypertension benefit at all from their sacrifices.

The results of this "meta-analysis" highlight the fact that no medical intervention — including salt restriction — is likely to be beneficial for everyone. So one of the goals of researchers is to determine which patients are most likely to benefit from salt restriction. These data indicate that people over 45 with hypertension can often experience a considerable reduction in blood pressure from salt restriction. But for younger people with hypertension, and for people with normal blood pressure, these data do not support sodium restriction.

Before celebrating by reaching for a salt shaker, readers should keep in mind that there are likely to be some people with normal blood pressure who benefit from a low-sodium diet — a strategy that is clearly important for people with congestive heart failure. The editorial that accompanied the journal report concluded that guidelines urging modest reductions in salt consumption for U.S. adults still seemed reasonable when one considers the strengths and weaknesses of available information. The impact of this most recent study may therefore be that moderation in salt intake should be our public-health strategy — moderate reductions for those of us who love salty foods, and moderation in the pursuit of a low-salt lifestyle for those of us without hypertension or heart failure.

Finally, people with and without hypertension should not forget other important strategies that can reduce the risk of high blood pressure: maintaining a normal weight, pursuing a regular schedule of physical activity, and not smoking. (*Journal of the American Medical Association*, May 22/29, 1996, pp. 1590–1597.)

From the *Harvard Heart Letter*, November 1996, pp. 1-2. © 1996 by the President and Fellows of Harvard College. Reprinted by permission.

# Unit 3

## Unit Selections

## Key Points to Consider

❖ Pretend that you are planning research projects relative to nutrition and your age group. Rank by order of importance your top three priorities and defend them.

❖ What changes should you make in your lifestyle in order to conform to the best current knowledge about your nutrient needs? Choose one change and brainstorm ways to achieve it.

❖ Choose a food allergy that interests you. Then go to the grocery store and check labels to see what processed foods would have to be eliminated from the diet of a person with this allergy.

❖ Are you and your friends as sedentary in your lifestyles as the average American of the same age? If so, what could you do to change that?

❖ The decision to use or not use alcohol and the decision about how much to use are not always easy ones. List the reasons for your decisions and evaluate them.

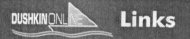 **Links** **www.dushkin.com/online/**

These sites are annotated on pages 4 and 5.

*Food improperly taken, not only produces diseases, but affords those that are already engendered both matter and sustenance; so that, let the father of disease be what it may, intemperance is its mother.*

*—Richard E. Burton*

Perhaps you have heard the old adage "You are what you eat." Your parents may have read a book by Adelle Davis in which she claimed that aging will not occur on the days one eats right. We all know that neither of these statements is literally true, but scientists are constantly adding support to the concept that what we eat does affect what we are in both direct and indirect ways.

It is commonly agreed that a good (balanced) diet throughout life will help us all reach our genetic potentials and avoid premature aging, disease, and untimely death. Studies of other populations, as in the quote above, often provide clues to diet/disease connections. Researchers must interpret them cautiously, however, as such studies cannot prove all-inclusive, cause-and-effect relationships; sometimes the results even appear contradictory.

However, from time to time, scientific evidence does consolidate in a very clear health message. One case in point is the information about the protective qualities of many chemicals in our foods, especially in fruits and vegetables. The need for antioxidants to scavenge and disarm damaging free radicals seems clear. Some antioxidants are known nutrients such as vitamins E and C and the mineral selenium; others are also part of the chemical structure of our foods, but we have known little about them. This information represents a significant breakthrough in our understanding of how the body works, but the reader should be cautious about interpreting it to mean that bottles of supplements would be a wise investment.

The articles "Fighting Cancer with Food" and "Most Frequently Asked Questions . . . about Diet and Cancer" specifically address the diet/cancer connection, one that is still somewhat controversial. Worldwide dietary patterns generally find higher cancer rates linked to populations that eat lots of red meat and lower rates linked to plant-based diets. It has been estimated, therefore, that eating the recommended five or more fruits and vegetables daily would cause a cancer decline in the United States of 20 percent, with even higher reductions for lung, colon, and rectal cancers. But, if this is true, does it represent a clear cause and effect? And, if so, is it the high fat content of the meat, the compounds produced during cooking, the lack of protective chemicals such as antioxidants in plant foods, or something else altogether? Once again we see strong support for finding protection in diet rather than in a pill bottle.

The next articles in this unit were selected because they discuss common chronic diseases of concern to large numbers of people. During our youth we tend to feel invulnerable, but then life moves on, slipping eventfully and uneventfully through a few decades. Soon the fiftieth birthday is celebrated, with the golden years just beyond. Typically, we have gained weight, probably more than is currently considered healthy. And, as we reach our sixties and seventies, more and more of us will be dealing with high blood pressure,

coronary disease, cancer, osteoporosis, and other conditions that cause varying degrees of disability. Now major lifestyle changes become inevitable. However, these diseases might have been avoided altogether, or at least delayed, if we had made the appropriate lifestyle choices while we were young.

Heart disease and hypertension, two of the biggest health concerns in this country, are the topics of four articles. Guidelines from the Heart Association provide recommendations regarding fat and fiber intakes as well as other suggestions for a heart-healthy lifestyle. Another article addresses commonly asked cholesterol questions. Many individuals still erroneously believe that *food* cholesterol (rather than saturated fat) is the primary dietary cause of elevated *blood* cholesterol levels and that they should eliminate as much fat from their diets as possible. Other heart disease research points in different directions. In "Evidence Mounts for Heart Disease Marker," the focus is homocysteine levels and possible connections to diets low in certain B vitamins. Hypertension, of course, is a risk factor for heart disease. A short summary of the DASH (Dietary Approaches to Stop Hypertension) diet explains the current emphasis on nutrition as a means of controlling blood pressure. Here, again is the recurring theme, "Eat your fruits and vegetables."

Endless subsets of any large population have special needs. In this edition, these groups are represented by the elderly and those with allergies. Those of us approaching the advanced decades in life fear becoming victims of some form of dementia. That researchers are working to help us maintain brain power as we age is, at least, encouraging. People with food allergies, on the other hand, often simply misunderstand what a true food allergy is and how an allergy must change eating behaviors.

The next article "When Eating Goes Awry: An Update on Eating Disorders" highlights anorexia nervosa, bulimia nervosa, and binge-eating disorder. These are believed to affect 2 million males and females between the ages of 15 and 35. Five percent of college women are bulimic, and 1 percent of teenage females are anorexic. Many will die. These disorders are psychiatric illnesses that bring depression, shame, isolation, and damaged relationships to their victims.

Finally, there are two articles on unrelated topics that affect all or many of us. Exercise is not strictly a nutrition topic, but the need for it is so interrelated with the amounts of food we eat and with the same diseases affected by nutrition that it seems irresponsible not to include it. The same applies to the use of alcohol, which will benefit some consumers and harm others.

One should remember that there is still much we do not know about nutrition and that even within age, gender, and ethnic groups, people are physiologically different. Connections between food/nutrition and health can be found in other units in this book. Unit 1 has an article on protective qualities of fruits and vegetables. Articles on vitamins, lipids, and other nutrients are found in unit 2, and unit 6 discusses information leading to harmful dietary practices. The reader might also review articles in previous *Annual Editions: Nutrition* and in reliable periodicals to fully appreciate the extent of the information—and the confusion—surrounding nutrition.

# Through the Life Span: Diet and Disease

## Prevention
# Fighting Cancer with Food

When Richard Nixon declared war on cancer in 1971, the focus was on finding new treatments for the disease. Since that time a number of battles have been won. Better, life-saving interventions are now available for children

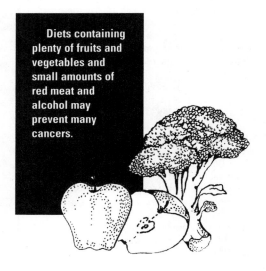

Diets containing plenty of fruits and vegetables and small amounts of red meat and alcohol may prevent many cancers.

and young adults, for example, and new methods of detection have helped decrease deaths from bowel and cervical cancer. Still, mortality rates from breast cancer in women over 55 and prostate cancer in men have not substantially improved, and overall U.S. deaths from cancer stopped rising only in 1991.

Today researchers say the war on cancer can best be won by preventing the disease from occurring in the first place. The American Institute for Cancer Research (AICR), a nonprofit organization devoted to the study of nutrition and cancer, recently released a comprehensive set of dietary guidelines for cancer prevention. Culled from more than 4,500 studies, the recommendations call for several changes in Americans' eating and exercise habits. Indeed the American Cancer Society estimates that about one-third of U.S. cancer deaths are due to dietary factors.

### Eat your vegetables
Diets containing plenty of fruits and vegetables and small amounts of red meat and alcohol, combined with regular exercise and maintenance of a healthful body weight, may decrease the incidence of

many cancers. The AICR recommends that women consume no more than one alcoholic drink a day, and men, no more than two.

*Colon and rectal cancer.* Some evidence suggests that vegetables may protect against this form of the disease because of the antioxidant compounds they contain or their fiber content; studies, however, are not conclusive.

Physical activity seems to reduce the risk of colon cancer by stimulating *peristalsis* — contractions of the intestine that propel fecal matter through the colon and rectum. That movement cuts down on the time the stool — and the toxins it contains — resides in the colon.

*Breast cancer.* Of the many possible links between diet and breast cancer, avoiding alcohol and eating a produce-rich diet are supported by the most science.

Dozens of studies have shown that the more alcohol a woman consumes, the greater her risk of breast cancer. This holds true for both menstruating and postmenopausal women. Scientists aren't sure how alcohol affects the development of the disease, but some believe it may inhibit certain cell-repair mechanisms in breast tissue or make cell membranes more prone to cancer. Another possibility is that alcohol boosts levels of estrogen—a hormone that may promote the growth of breast tumors.

Some evidence suggests that fruit and vegetable consumption may also decrease breast cancer risk. No one nutrient has been singled out as the cancer fighter, but more and more research has shown that fruits and vegetables contain protective *phytochemicals,* or plant chemicals. For instance, researchers at the Johns Hopkins University School of Medicine recently found that broccoli sprouts contain *isothiocyanates,* compounds thought to accelerate the actions of enzymes in the body that squelch toxins. This discovery may partially explain why eating broccoli and other cruciferous vegetables, such as cabbage and cauliflower, is associated with a reduced cancer risk.

The evidence that dietary fat plays a role in breast cancer is less convincing. Although many studies have addressed this issue, the results have not been consistent. At this point, a high-fat diet has not been proven to contribute to breast cancer risk, but research to further examine the role of dietary fat in breast cancer is ongoing.

From the *Harvard Health Letter,* December 1997, pp. 1-2. © 1997 by the President and Fellows of Harvard College. Reprinted by permission.

In addition, a fair amount of research shows that obesity boosts breast cancer risk substantially in postmenopausal women, possibly because estrogen levels tend to run higher in overweight women than in those who are slimmer. Perhaps for similar reasons, obesity is also strongly associated with a high risk of cancer of the *endometrium*, the inner mucous membrane of the uterus.

***Prostate cancer.*** As yet there is no convincing evidence that any dietary factor reduces a man's risk of the disease. Some limited research suggests that a diet high in fat, especially from red meat, possibly increases the risk of prostate cancer. Other studies have indicated that high vegetable consumption can lower the risk of prostate cancer. For example, researchers have suggested that *lycopene*, the compound found in tomatoes that makes them red, may lower the risk of prostate cancer. Lycopene is best absorbed by the body when tomatoes are cooked; tomato paste and sauce are good sources of the substance.

A new investigation by U.S. and European researchers suggests that lycopene may also protect against coronary disease. The study of 1,379 European men indicated that those who consumed the most lycopene were half as likely to suffer a heart attack as those who ate the least.

***Other cancers.*** Diets rich in fruits and vegetables have been linked to a reduced risk of lung cancer, the leading cause of cancer mortality in both men and women. This is probably due to the activity of yet to be identified phytochemicals.

Obviously, quitting smoking is the best way to prevent lung cancer. Tobacco use accounts for nearly one in five deaths in the United States and ranks as the country's most preventable cause of mortality.

Fruits and vegetables may also protect against cancer of the mouth, throat, esophagus, and larynx (voice box), all of which are associated with smoking. People who smoke and drink large amounts of alcohol are at even greater risk for these cancers.

### Examining the data

It's important to keep in mind that much of the evidence linking cancer risk to diet comes from population studies that look at the association between cancer and food consumption patterns.

For example, women in the Nurses' Health Study who drink the most alcohol may have the highest rates of breast cancer, but this does not prove that alcohol does, in fact, cause breast cancer. If drinkers in a given study are also overweight, for example, it may be that obesity, not alcohol consumption, is responsible for the increased risk. That's why groups such as the American Cancer Society and the AICR examine the results of all available studies when setting guidelines for consumers.

Of course, an individual's risk of developing cancer is influenced by many factors, including a genetic predisposition to the disease and exposure to environmental pollutants. Diet, however, is an important component, and it's one thing that is in a person's control.

# MOST FREQUENTLY ASKED QUESTIONS
## . . . About Diet and Cancer

### AMERICAN CANCER SOCIETY NUTRITION ADVISORY COMMITTEE

Because people are interested in the relationship of specific foods or nutrients to specific cancers, research in this area is often widely publicized. No one study is the last word on any subject, and it is easy to become confused by what may appear to be contradictory and conflicting advice. Each study should be considered in the light of existing knowledge, but in brief news stories, reporters cannot always put new research findings in context. The best advice is to use common sense; it is rarely, if ever, advisable to change your diet based on a single study or news report, especially if the data are reported as "preliminary."

**What are antioxidants and what do they have to do with cancer?** Certain nutrients in fruits and vegetables appear to protect the body against the oxygen-induced damage to tissues that occurs constantly as a result of normal metabolism. Because such damage is associated with increased cancer risk, antioxidant nutrients are thought to protect against cancer.[12] Antioxidant nutrients include vitamin C, vitamin E, selenium, and carotenoids. Studies suggest that people who eat more fruits and vegetables containing these antioxidants have a lower risk for cancer.[13] Clinical studies of antioxidant supplements, however, have not demonstrated a reduction in cancer risk (see Beta Carotene, Supplements).

**Do artificial sweeteners cause cancer?** Several years ago, experiments on rats suggested that saccharin might cause cancer. Since then, however, studies of primates and humans have shown no increased risk of cancer from either saccharin or aspartame.

**Does beta carotene reduce cancer risk?** Because beta carotene, an antioxidant, is found in fruits and vegetables, and because eating fruits and vegetables is clearly associated with a reduced risk of cancer, it seemed possible that taking high doses of beta carotene supplements might reduce cancer risk. In three major experiments, people were given high doses of synthetic beta carotene in an attempt to prevent lung and other cancers. Two of these studies found beta carotene supplements to be associated with a higher risk of lung cancer in cigarette smokers[18,19] and a third found neither benefit nor harm from beta carotene supplements.[44] Thus, research has not reproduced the beneficial effects of fruits and vegetables by giving high-dose supplements of beta carotene. For cigarette smokers, such supplements may be harmful.[18]

**What are bioengineered foods, and are they safe?** Foods made through techniques of bioengineering or biotechnology have been altered by the addition of genes from plants or other organisms to increase resistance to pests, to retard spoilage, or to improve transportability, flavor, nutrient composition, or other desired qualities. Few such foods have as yet been marketed. At present, there is no reason to believe that these foods will either increase or decrease cancer risk.

**Is calcium related to cancer?** Some research has suggested that foods high in calcium might help reduce the risk of colorectal cancer, but this relationship is not proven. Whether or not calcium intake affects cancer risk, eating foods containing this mineral is important to reduce the risk of osteoporosis. Low-fat and non-fat dairy products are excellent sources of calcium, as are some leafy vegetables and beans.

**What are carotenoids, and do they reduce cancer risk?** Carotenoids are a group of pigments in fruits and vegetables that include alpha carotene, beta carotene, lycopene, lutein, and many other compounds. Consumption of foods containing carotenoids is associated with a reduced cancer risk (see Beta Carotene).

**Does cholesterol in the diet increase cancer risk?** Cholesterol in the diet comes only from foods from animal sources-meat, dairy, eggs, and fats. At present, little evidence is available to determine whether dietary cholesterol itself or the foods containing this substance might be responsible for the increase in cancer risk associated with eating foods from animal sources. Low blood cholesterol has been found to be more common in people with cancer, but is an effect of cancer, not its cause. There is no evidence that lowering blood cholesterol causes an increase in cancer risk.

**Does drinking coffee cause cancer?** Several years ago, a highly publicized study suggested that coffee might increase risk for cancer of the pancreas. Because caffeine may heighten symptoms of fibrocystic breast lumps in some women, media stories also have focused on concerns about coffee and breast cancer. Many studies in recent years, however, have found no relationship at all between coffee and the risk of pancreatic, breast, or any other type of cancer.

**Does cooking affect cancer risk?** Adequate cooking is necessary to kill harmful microorganisms in meat. However, some research suggests that frying or charcoal-broiling meats at very high temper-

From *Nutrition Today*, May/June 1997, pp. 125-127. Reprinted by permission of the American Cancer Society from *CA Cancer Journal for Clinicians*, Volume 46, 1996, pp. 333-338. © 1996 by Lippincott-Raven Publishers.

atures creates chemicals that might increase cancer risk. Preserving meats by methods involving smoke also increases their content of potentially carcinogenic chemicals. Although these chemicals cause cancer in animal experiments, it is uncertain whether they actually cause cancer in people. Techniques such as braising, steaming, poaching, stewing, and microwaving meats do not produce these chemicals.

**What are cruciferous vegetables and are they important in cancer?** Cruciferous vegetables belong to the cabbage family, which includes broccoli, cauliflower, and brussels sprouts. These vegetables contain certain chemicals thought to reduce the risk of colorectal cancer. The best evidence suggests that a wide variety of vegetables, including cruciferous and other vegetables, reduces cancer risk (see Phytochemicals).

**What is dietary fiber and can it prevent cancer?** Dietary fiber includes a wide variety of plant carbohydrates that are not digested by humans. Specific categories of fiber are "soluble" (like oat bran) and "insoluble" (like wheat bran). Insoluble fiber is thought to help reduce the risk of colorectal cancer, although the mechanism of this action is uncertain. Soluble fiber helps to reduce blood cholesterol and, therefore, to lower the risk of coronary heart disease. Good sources of fiber are beans, vegetables, whole grains, and fruits.

**Does eating fish protect against cancer?** Like all fats, fish oils are high in calories. Fish fats are rich in omega-3 fatty acids. Studies in animals have found that omega-3 fatty acids suppress cancer formation, but there is no direct evidence for protective effects in humans at this time.

**Do fluorides cause cancer?** Extensive research has examined the effects of fluorides given as dental treatments or added to toothpaste, public water supplies, or foods. Fluorides do not increase cancer risk.

**What is folic acid and can it prevent cancer?** Folic acid (sometimes called folate or folacin) is a B vitamin found in many vegetables, beans, fruits, whole grains, and fortified breakfast cereals. Folic acid may reduce the risk of some cancers. Supplements are sometimes recommended for women who are capable of becoming pregnant as a means to reduce the risk of spina bifida and other neural tube defects in their infants. Current evidence suggests that to reduce cancer risk, folic acid is best consumed along with the full array of nutrients found in fruits, vegetables, and other foods.

**Do food additives cause cancer?** Many substances are added to foods to preserve them and to enhance color, flavor, and texture. Additives are usually present in very small quantities in food, and no convincing evidence exists that any additive at these levels causes human cancers.

**Can garlic prevent cancer?** The health benefits of the allium compounds contained in garlic and other vegetables in the onion family have been publicized widely. Garlic is currently under study for its ability to reduce cancer risk, but insufficient evidence supports a specific role for this vegetable in cancer prevention.

**If our genes determine cancer risk, how can diet help prevent cancer?** Genes that increase or decrease cancer risk can be inherited or acquired by mutations throughout life. Nutrients and nutritional factors in the diet can protect DNA from being damaged and can delay or prevent the development of cancer even in people with an increased genetic risk for the disease.

**Why are foods irradiated, and do irradiated foods cause cancer?** Radiation is increasingly used to kill harmful organisms on foods so as to extend their "shelf life." Radiation does not remain in the foods after treatment, and there is no evidence that consuming irradiated foods increases cancer risk.

**Should I avoid nitrite-preserved meats?** Most lunch meats, hams, and hot dogs are preserved with nitrites to maintain color and to prevent contamination with bacteria. Nitrites can be converted to carcinogenic nitrosamines in the stomach, which may increase the risk of gastric cancer. Vitamin C and related compounds are often added to foods to inhibit this conversion. Diets high in fruits and vegetables that contain vitamin C and phytochemicals, such as phenols, retard the conversion of nitrites to nitrosamines. Nitrites in foods are not a significant cause of cancer among Americans.

**What is olestra and is it related to cancer?** Some synthetic fat substitutes are not absorbed by the body. Although several fat substitutes are under development for use in the food supply, only one of this type-olestra (trademarked Olean)-has been approved for marketing. Olestra may reduce fat intake, but it also reduces the absorption of fat-soluble carotenes and other potentially cancer-protective phytochemicals in fruits and vegetables.[45] Although reducing absorption of these substances might also reduce the health benefits of fruits and vegetables, the overall effect of this type of fat substitute on cancer risk is unknown at present.

**Does olive oil affect cancer risk?** Olive oil, like all fats, is high in calories, but its fat is mostly monounsaturated. Consumption of olive oil is not associated with any increase in risk of cancer, and most likely is neutral with respect to cancer risk.[46]

**Do pesticides and herbicides on fruits and vegetables cause cancer?** Pesticides and herbicides can be toxic when used in high doses. Although fruits and vegetables sometimes contain low levels of these chemicals, overwhelming scientific evidence supports the overall health benefits and cancer-protective effects of eating fruits and vegetables.[47] In contrast, current evidence is insufficient to link pesticides in foods with an increased risk of any cancer.

**What are phytochemicals, and do they reduce cancer risk?** The term "phytochemicals" refers to a wide variety of compounds produced by plants. Some of these compounds protect plants against insects or have other biologically important functions. Some have either antioxidant or hormone-like actions both in plants and in people who eat them. Because consumption of fruits and vegetables reduces cancer risk, researchers are searching for specific compounds in these foods that might account for the beneficial effects. There is no evidence that taking phytochemical supplements is as beneficial as consuming the fruits, vegetables, beans, and grains from which they are extracted.

**Do high levels of salt in the diet increase cancer risk?** Some evidence links diets containing large amounts of foods preserved by salting and pickling with an increased risk of cancers of the stomach, nose, and throat. Little evidence suggests that moderate amounts of salt or salt-preserved foods in the diet affect cancer risk.

**What is selenium and can it reduce cancer risk?** Selenium is a mineral needed by the body as part of antioxidant defense mechanisms. Animal studies suggest that selenium protects against cancer, but human studies are inconclusive. Selenium supplements are not recommended, as there is only a narrow margin between safe and toxic doses. Grain products are good sources of selenium.

**Can soybeans reduce cancer risk?** Soybeans are an excellent source of protein and a good alternative to meat. Nonfermented soybeans have high levels of phytoestrogens and other phytochemicals that appear to have beneficial effects on hormone-dependent cancers in animal studies.[23] These effects remain to be proven in humans, however.

**Can nutritional supplements lower cancer risk?** Strong evidence associates a diet rich in fruits, vegetables, and other plant foods with reduced risk of cancer, but there is no evidence at this time that supplements can reduce cancer risk. The few studies in human populations that have attempted to determine whether supplements can reduce cancer risk have yielded disappointing results. Vitamin and mineral supplements have been shown to reduce the risk of stomach cancer in one intervention study in China,[48] but other studies using high doses of single nutrients have shown no benefit and even unexpected evidence for harm (see Beta Carotene). Although supplements do not substitute for healthful diets in reducing cancer risk, it is possible that some people, such as pregnant women, women of childbearing age, and people with restricted dietary intakes, might benefit from taking moderate doses of vitamin and mineral supplements for other reasons.

**Can drinking tea reduce cancer risk?** Some researchers have proposed that tea, especially green tea, might protect against cancer because of its content of antioxidants (see Antioxidants). In animal studies, some teas have been shown to reduce cancer risk, but beneficial effects of tea on cancer risk in people are not yet proven.

**Does vitamin A lower cancer risks?** Vitamin A (retinol) is obtained from foods in two ways: as preformed from animal food sources and as derived from beta carotene found in plant foods. Vitamin A is needed to maintain healthy tissues. Vitamin A supplements have not been shown to lower cancer risk, however. If supplements are taken, they should remain within recommended levels, as high doses of preformed vitamin A can be harmful, especially to pregnant women. Because the body does not convert beta carotene to vitamin A when vitamin A levels are within normal ranges, eating fruits and vegetables containing beta carotene cannot lead to vitamin A toxicity.

**Does vitamin C lower cancer risk?** Vitamin C is found in many fruits and vegetables. Many studies have linked consumption of vitamin C-rich foods with a reduced risk of cancer. The few studies in which vitamin C has been given as a supplement, however, have not shown a reduced risk of cancer.[49,50]

**Does vitamin E lower cancer risk?** Vitamin E may lower the risk for coronary heart disease. Vitamin E supplements, however, have not been shown to reduce cancer risks.[18,50]

**References***
12. Willett WC: Micronutrients and cancer risk. Am J. Clin Nutr 1994;599(suppl 5):1162s–1165s.
13. Steinmetz, KA, Potter JD: Vegetables, fruit, and cancer. I. Epidemiology. Cancer Causes Control 1991;2:325–357.
18. The Alpha-Tocopherol, Beta Carotene Cancer Prevention Study Group: The effect of vitamin E and beta carotene on the incidence of lung cancer and other cancers in male smokers. N Engl J Med 1994;330:1029–1035.
19. Omenn G, Goodman GE, Thornquist MD, et al: Effects of a combination of beta carotene and vitamin A on lung cancer and cardiovascular disease. N Engl J Med 1996;334:1150–1155.
23. Messina M, Erdman JW (eds): First international symposium on the role of soy in preventing and treating chronic disease. J Nutr 1995;125(suppl 3):567s–808s.
44. Hennekens CH, Buring JE, Manson JE, et al: Lack of effect of long-term supplementation with beta carotene on the incidence of malignant neoplasms and cardiovascular disease. N Engl J Med 1996;334;1145–1149.
45. Westrate JA, van het Hof KH: Sucrose polyester and plasma carotenoid concentrations in healthy subjects. Am J Clin Nutr 1995;62:591–597.
46. Tricopoulou A, Katsouyanni K, Stuver S, et al: Consumption of olive oil and specific food groups in relation to breast cancer risk in Greece. J Natl Cancer Inst 1995;87:110–116.
47. National Research Council: Carcinogens and Anticarcinogens in the Human Diet: A Comparison of Naturally Occurring and Synthetic Substances. Washington, DC, National Academy Press, 1996.
48. Blot WJ, Li JY, Taylor PR, et al: Nutrition intervention trials in Linxian, China: Supplementation with specific vitamin/mineral combinations, cancer incidence, and disease-specific mortality in the general population. J Natl Cancer Inst 1993;85:1483–1492.
49. Block G: Vitamin C and cancer prevention: The epidemiologic evidence. Am J Clin Nutr 1991;53(suppl 1):270s–282s.
50. Byers T, Perry G: Dietary carotenes, vitamin C and vitamin E as protective antioxidants in human cancers. Annu Rev Nutr 1992;12:139–159.
* Missing references do not apply to this article.

# Heart Association Dietary Guidelines

A common complaint among health-conscious consumers is that the advice of various experts on diet and nutrition often seems contradictory. Fortunately, the "Dietary Guidelines for Healthy American Adults," published by the American Heart Association (AHA) last fall, are quite consistent with a set of recommendations issued by the U.S. government in 1995.

The prevention and control of heart and blood vessel disease is, of course, the main goal of the AHA guidelines (published in *Circulation,* October 1, 1996), but people who follow them can also lessen their risk of developing other diseases, including cancer, kidney disease, and osteoporosis. In addition, the guidelines are compatible with dietary recommendations for people with diabetes.

The new guidelines deviate very little from the last ones, which were issued in 1988. The AHA still strongly recommends a diet that emphasizes grain products, vegetables, fruits, and dried beans, as well as moderate amounts of poultry, fish, lean meats, and low-fat dairy products; and the organization continues to discourage diets high in saturated fat and cholesterol, such as whole-milk dairy products, eggs, and high-fat meats.

### Fine tunings

Reflecting advances in nutrition research over the past eight years, the guidelines suggest some adjustments in the proportions of fat and fiber in the diet and emphasize the importance of some lifestyle habits. Some of the major refinements follow:

### Increase the intake of monounsaturated fatty acids.

Monounsaturated fats (found in olive, canola, and peanut oils) have been shown in several studies to

---

## Dining AHA Style

The following one-day's menu is designed to demonstrate the Heart Association guidelines in practice and reflects the suggested proportions of the various fats, cholesterol, sodium, and carbohydrates. But it is a sample only and is, of course, just one of many possible ways to achieve the AHA recommendations.

People should eat a variety of foods. For example, turkey or fish can be replaced by chicken, tofu, or lean beef. Similarly, a variety of grains, legumes, vegetables, and fruits should be eaten. This menu is not meant to replace any specific diet orders prescribed by a physician.

**Breakfast:** A fresh orange, 3/4 cup of low-fat granola with half a banana, 2 tablespoons of chopped almonds, and a cup of skim milk.

**Lunch:** Two slices of whole-grain bread, 2 ounces of turkey breast with mustard, 2 cups of green salad with vinegar and 1 1/2 tablespoons of olive oil.

**Snack:** A cup of plain yogurt with a chopped apple, 2 tablespoons of chopped dates, and 2 tablespoons of toasted wheat germ.

**Dinner:** Four ounces of salmon with lemon, steamed carrots, kale with garlic and a tablespoon of olive oil, 1 cup of brown rice, and 1/2 cup of sorbet.

---

have positive effects on blood-fat levels. Actually, the net effect of "monos" on these levels is not much different from that of polyunsaturated fatty acids (found in soybean, corn, cottonseed, and sunflower oils). However, some studies indicate that monos may have advantages. In particular, monos are not as susceptible as polyunsaturates to oxidation in the body, a process that may play a role in the deposit of fatty materials in the arteries (atherosclerosis).

Until now, the AHA has recommended a diet in which 30% of calories come from fat (10% each from saturated, polyunsaturated, and monounsaturated). Now the organization suggests dividing the fat allotment differently, so that up to 15% is in the form of monounsaturates, with intake of the other fats reduced accordingly.

Another new recommendation is that omega-3 fatty acids, derived primarily from fish, can also be substituted for saturated fats. However, the AHA recommends against the use of omega-3 supplements because their long-term benefits have not been demonstrated.

### Increase fiber intake.

The AHA continues to recommend that Americans eat plenty of vegetables, fruits, and whole-grain products and suggests that the majority of daily calories (55–60%) should come from complex carbohydrates — dried beans (such as chickpeas, lentils, and lima beans) and whole grains (such as bulgur, quinoa, barley, and brown rice). The soluble fiber found in these foods, soy products, and pectin-rich fruits (such as apples and cranberries) can help to reduce the "bad" LDL (low-density-lipoprotein) cholesterol.

A major long-term epidemiological study of 40,000 men who were followed for six years found that the risk of a heart attack was 36% lower among the men who consumed the most fiber compared to those who consumed the least. Although fiber from

---

From the *Harvard Heart Letter,* February 1997, pp. 4-6. © 1997 by the President and Fellows of Harvard College. Reprinted by permission.

grains, fruits, and vegetables was associated with a reduced heart-attack risk, the link was strongest in the case of fiber from grains. The AHA recommends that people gradually build up to a daily intake of 25–30 grams of fiber a day and that the fiber should come from food, not supplements.

### Avoid foods high in sugar.

People who choose a diet high in sugar (that is, simple carbohydrates such as those in regular soda, candy, cookies, pastries, frozen desserts, and jelly) diminish their opportunity and their appetite for healthful foods such as vegetables and whole grains. Furthermore, a diet high in simple carbohydrates may have harmful effects on blood-fat levels. Beware of fat-free baked goods, which are usually high in sugar.

### Be careful about sodium intake.

Low-sodium diets in some people with hypertension can significantly reduce blood pressure. People with normal blood pressure vary in their reaction to salt intake, and there are no simple, reliable tests to predict salt sensitivity accurately. Therefore, the AHA suggests that all Americans consume no more than 2.4 grams (2,400 milligrams) of sodium daily — which is equivalent to about one teaspoon of table salt.

However, that sodium allotment includes more than just table salt. Sodium occurs naturally in foods like milk, fresh vegetables, fresh meats, poultry, and fish, and therefore one-third of the day's total sodium allotment is used even before picking up the salt shaker or buying processed foods made with sodium, such as deli turkey, canned tuna, low-fat crackers, or dehydrated soups. Creative use of spices and other flavorings, such as garlic and lemon juice, can be an alternative to high-sodium intake.

### Balance regular exercise with moderate food intake to maintain or reduce weight.

The evidence is strong that losing excess weight and keeping it off can improve cholesterol and blood-pressure levels, which in turn can reduce risk of heart disease, diabetes, and stroke. The benefits of a combined regimen of diet and exercise are illustrated by a well-controlled randomized trial of 119 men and 112 women. The participants assigned to a prudent weight-reducing diet combined with exercise lost more weight and more fat and had a greater improvement in lipoprotein profiles than those assigned to diet alone.

In another study of 3,000 healthy men between 30 and 64, HDL level rose in proportion to the amount of exercise performed. Other studies have shown that regular aerobic physical activity can reduce systolic blood pressure in hypertensive patients by approximately 10 mm Hg. The AHA recommendations do not include any specific weight guidelines. However, a height-weight chart (shown below) was issued as part of the U.S. "Dietary Guidelines for Americans."

### Be cautious about consuming a very low-fat diet.

The optimum amount of fat in a diet has been somewhat controversial. Some people think that if a low-saturated-fat diet is good, then a diet very

| National Height/Weight Guidelines | | | |
| --- | --- | --- | --- |
| Height* | Healthy Weight in Pounds† BMI♦ of 19–25 | Moderate Overweight in Pounds† BMI♦ of 25–29 | Severe Overweight in Pounds† BMI♦ of 29 or over |
| 4'10" | 91–118 | 119–137 | 138 or over |
| 4'11" | 94–123 | 124–143 | 144 or over |
| 5'0" | 97–127 | 128–147 | 148 or over |
| 5'1" | 101–131 | 132–152 | 153 or over |
| 5'2" | 104–136 | 137–157 | 158 or over |
| 5'3" | 107–140 | 141–162 | 163 or over |
| 5'4" | 111–145 | 146–168 | 169 or over |
| 5'5" | 114–149 | 150–173 | 174 or over |
| 5'6" | 118–154 | 155–178 | 179 or over |
| 5'7" | 121–159 | 160–184 | 185 or over |
| 5'8" | 125–163 | 164–189 | 190 or over |
| 5'9" | 129–168 | 169–195 | 196 or over |
| 5'10" | 132–173 | 174–201 | 202 or over |
| 5'11" | 136–178 | 179–206 | 207 or over |
| 6'0" | 140–183 | 184–212 | 213 or over |
| 6'1" | 144–188 | 189–218 | 219 or over |
| 6'2" | 148–194 | 195–224 | 225 or over |
| 6'3" | 152–199 | 200–231 | 232 or over |
| 6'4" | 156–204 | 205–237 | 238 or over |
| 6'5" | 160–210 | 211–243 | 244 or over |
| 6'6" | 164–215 | 216–249 | 250 or over |

This table reflects a desirable body mass index (BMI) of 19–25. A BMI of 25–29 is considered moderately overweight, and a BMI of 29 or greater, severely overweight. People who want to figure their own BMI can multiply weight in pounds by 700 and divide that product by height squared (in inches). The higher weights apply to people with more muscle and bone. Most people should not gain more than 10 pounds after age 20, even if they remain within the healthy weight range.

*Without shoes. †Without clothes. ♦BMI stands for body mass index.

Dietary Guidelines for Americans, Fourth Edition, 1995, U.S. Department of Agriculture and U.S. Department of Health and Human Services

low in *total* fat must be better. However, some experts are concerned that, in some individuals, very low-fat, high-carbohydrate diets may decrease the "good" HDL (high density lipoprotein) cholesterol and increase triglycerides—in the process, raising the risk of coronary artery disease. But this theoretical danger is not considered proved. Still, very low-fat diets may result in nutrient deficiencies, especially in children, pregnant women, and the elderly. Therefore, the Heart Association endorses the recommendation of the World Health Organization to follow a diet that does not go below 15% of total calories as fat. This percentage translates into a minimum of 33 grams of total fat per day in a 2,000-calorie diet and 20 to 25 grams per day in a diet containing 1200 to 1500 calories.

### Be flexible.

The guidelines recommend that people rethink the definition of a total diet. Until now, "total diet" has referred to the balance of foods eaten at a single meal or on a single day. Now the Heart Association suggests that people take into account the food consumed over the course of several days or a week. This strategy allows some flexibility in choosing foods and fits the theme of consuming a variety of foods and reducing guilt from eating something "bad" now and then.

## For Further Reading

*The American Heart Association has published several cookbooks, which are available in bookstores. In addition, the AHA's "Brand Name Fat and Cholesterol Counter," which lists the fat, saturated fat, cholesterol, sodium, and calorie content of more than 450 common foods, is available in grocery stores as well as bookstores. More information is available by telephoning the Heart Association at 1-800-242-8721, or on the internet at http://www. amhrt.org.*

*The 1995 edition of the U.S. government's "Nutrition and Your Health: Dietary Guidelines for Americans" is available for 50 cents by check or money order made payable to the Superintendent of Documents. Send order to the Consumer Information Center, Department 378-C, Pueblo, CO 81009.*

*The federal document may also be obtained from the "home pages" of the two agencies responsible for the guidelines: the U.S. Department of Agriculture (http://www.usda. gov/fcs/cnpp.html) and the U.S. Department of Health and Human Services (http://www. os.dhhs.gov).*

# Answering nine of your cholesterol questions

"Cholesterol" is a household word, but still an elusive concept for many people. And no wonder. Biochemistry is hardly simple, even for biochemists. Here are a few cholesterol review notes.

Cholesterol is a fat-like substance found in all animal cells, human and otherwise. It is essential to life. The human body manufactures all the cholesterol it needs—thus we can live without eating any cholesterol. Cholesterol is attached to protein packages called lipoproteins, which are assembled in the liver and circulate in our bloodstream. Two of the better known types of lipoproteins are HDL (high-density lipoprotein), the "good" type that carries cholesterol out of the system; and LDL (low-density lipoprotein), the "bad" type that deposits cholesterol in arterial walls, where it can build up and narrow the arteries. High blood cholesterol is a known risk factor for heart attack.

The chart below will refresh your memory on guidelines for total cholesterol and HDL cholesterol. In the U.S., cholesterol is measured in milligrams per deciliter (mg/dl) of blood. In Canada and many other countries, it's measured in millimoles per liter (mmol/L). The latter is known as the International System. (To convert to millimoles, divide the milligrams by 38.67. To convert from millimoles to milligrams, multiply by 38.67.)

| TOTAL CHOLESTEROL | |
| --- | --- |
| Desirable | Less than 200 mg/dl (5.2 mmol/L) |
| Borderline-high | 200-239 mg/dl (5.2 -6.19 mmol/L) |
| High | 240 mg/dl or more (6.2 mmol/L or more) |

| HDL CHOLESTEROL | |
| --- | --- |
| Low | Less than 35 mg/dl (0.9 mmol/L) |

**How often should I have my blood cholesterol measured?**
Adults should be screened at least once every 5 years, but more frequently if their total cholesterol is elevated, if HDL is low, and or they have other cardiac risk factors.

**My total cholesterol is below 200, but my HDL is only 30. Is this a problem? I'm a 45-year-old man.**
An HDL below 35 milligrams per deciliter is a risk factor for heart attack, even if total cholesterol is in the "desirable" range. One recent study by researchers in Israel and at Case Western Reserve University in Cleveland showed that the risk of dying from heart disease was 38% higher in men with HDL under 35, even if their total cholesterol was below 200. Stroke risk in such men was higher, too. If your total cholesterol is elevated, a high HDL can help protect you. The higher your HDL, the better.

**I'm a woman of 55, and my HDL has markedly declined during the last five years. What can I do?**
At menopause, estrogen production declines, and so does HDL. Female sex hormones tend to raise HDL. Depending on how low your HDL is and other risk factors, you might consider starting hormone replacement therapy. But there are other measures you can take, too (see below).

**How can I raise my HDL level? Lower my total cholesterol?**
It's harder to raise HDL than to lower total cholesterol. Hormone replacement therapy, as we've said, will raise HDL for post-menopausal women. Moderate alcohol consumption—up to one drink a day for a woman, two for a man—also helps boost HDL. (Drinking more than that can harm your heart and cause other

Reprinted with permission from *University of California at Berkeley Wellness Letter*, February 1998, p. 4. © 1998 by Health Letter Associates. For information, call (800) 829-9170.

health problems—see *Wellness Letter,* July 1997, for more on the risks and benefits of alcohol.) Stop smoking if you smoke, lose weight if you are overweight, and get regular aerobic exercise. If you are sedentary, aim for brisk 30-minute walks three to five times a week, or another aerobic exercise such as swimming. More strenuous exercise can help even more. To reduce total blood cholesterol, consume less cholesterol and saturated fats. Eat a diet rich in fruits, grains, vegetables, and nonfat dairy products. Some cholesterol-lowering drugs also raise HDL.

**I know my HDL and LDL. Why don't they add up to my total cholesterol?**

Certain blood fats known as triglycerides also figure into the equation, which is:

$$Total\ cholesterol = HDL + LDL + (triglycerides \div 5)$$

In fact, LDL is not measured directly, but derived as follows:

$$LDL = total\ cholesterol - HDL - (triglycerides \div 5)$$

For more about triglycerides, see *Wellness Letter,* January 1998.

**Why don't package labels distinguish between good and bad cholesterol?**

The cholesterol that we eat is simply cholesterol—you can't consume "good cholesterol." Dietary cholesterol comes only from animal products such as meats, poultry, fish, eggs, and dairy products. The amount of cholesterol you consume affects the amount your body produces, which is also affected by genetic factors. But saturated fats, found chiefly in animal products, affect blood cholesterol levels even more than dietary cholesterol itself.

**I've heard it's okay to eat eggs. The *Wellness Letter* has said shrimp is okay. Both these foods are rich in cholesterol, so why are they okay?**

It all depends on how much of these foods you eat and in what context—and what your personal risk factors are. One egg contains about 215 milligrams of cholesterol; the recommended daily maximum is 300 milligrams. Thus, as we discussed in January, it would be okay to eat an egg if the other foods you eat that day are low in cholesterol. Shrimp contain more cholesterol than most shellfish (175 milligrams in 3 ounces)—but, like eggs, they are low in saturated fat, and shrimp, in moderate amounts, have a place in a heart-healthy diet (see *Wellness Letter,* March 1997). The American Heart Association suggests a weekly maximum of four eggs for healthy people, including eggs consumed in baked goods and other recipes. If you love eggs and are at low risk for heart disease, you might want to eat more than four. But you should make sure, via periodic blood tests, that your cholesterol level doesn't shoot up. On the other hand, if your blood cholesterol is high or if you have other risk factors for heart disease or already have heart disease, you should probably follow a more stringent diet, avoiding foods high in cholesterol and saturated fat.

**Do I need to fast before a cholesterol test?**

Although total cholesterol and HDL can be measured fairly accurately without fasting, to measure triglycerides and LDL, you need to fast for 12 hours (overnight).

**What can skew the results of a cholesterol test?**

Fluctuations in weight shortly before the test, changes in diet, and excessive alcohol intake can affect your test. So can surgery or injury, infection, or severe physical strain. At test time, your weight should have been stable for at least two weeks, and you should have been eating your usual diet and drinking your usual amount of alcohol, if you drink at all. At least two weeks should have elapsed since any surgery, trauma, illness, or physical strain.

# Prevention
# Evidence Mounts for Heart Disease Marker

Heart disease is considered the quintessential consequence of excess and inactivity. Too many calories, too many fatty foods, too many cigarettes, and too little exercise heighten millions of Americans' risk of suffering a heart attack. But a rapidly emerging body of evidence points to yet another possible cardiovascular risk factor that is getting increasing attention. Numerous studies have shown that diets lacking in several B vitamins lead to high blood levels of *homocysteine*, an amino acid that has acquired a bad reputation for its likely role in causing vascular damage.

One in five older adults has blood homocysteine levels that may be high enough to raise the risk of coronary artery disease.

### Under evaluation

The latest support for the homocysteine connection comes from a nine-country study led by researchers at Adelaide Hospital in Dublin, Ireland. They compared the blood homocysteine levels of 750 men and women with atherosclerosis with those of 800 people without any signs of clogged arteries. Sure enough, the patients whose homocysteine levels fell into the top fifth of the range were more than twice as likely to have blocked arteries as their counterparts whose homocysteine levels ranked in the remaining four-fifths.

What's more, the link between high homocysteine and artery disease held true even after the investigators ruled out other factors that can affect risk, such as smoking and high blood cholesterol. While the findings are telling, they are just the tip of a growing iceberg. Many experts say that their understanding of homocysteine's effect on the heart is as far along today as was their knowledge of blood cholesterol's impact 20 years ago.

### A prophet before his time

In 1968 Kilmer McCully, then a young pathologist at Massachusetts General Hospital, came across a case of a two-month-old boy who had died of *homocystinuria*, a rare genetic disease characterized by extremely high levels of homocysteine in the urine and blood. Upon examining the infant's arteries, Dr. McCully found they were hardened and clogged. The changes were virtually identical to those recounted in a long forgotten case of an 8-year-old boy with homocystinuria and comparable to those of older people with advanced vascular disease.

As a result, Dr. McCully surmised that homocysteine might somehow be linked to heart disease. But others thought his theory was far-fetched. A Harvard graduate with great promise, Dr. McCully doggedly held to his hypothesis in the face of tremendous skepticism. By 1978 his colleagues had found his work so unorthodox that he was asked to find a position elsewhere.

Fourteen years later, Dr. McCully was, in effect, vindicated by pivotal findings from the Physicians' Health Study. Researchers compared the homocysteine levels of nearly 300 doctors who had suffered a heart attack with those of physicians who had not had such an event. The likelihood of having a heart attack increased 3.4-fold among doctors with the highest blood levels of homocysteine—putting this amino acid on a par with smoking and high blood cholesterol as a risk factor for heart disease.

In 1993, another landmark report, this one from the long-running Framingham Heart Study, showed that elevated homocysteine levels are associated with low blood levels of vitamins $B_6$, $B_{12}$, and folate; all three nutrients play key roles in breaking down homocysteine in the body, thereby keeping it at safe levels. When one or more of these vitamins is lacking, homocysteine rises over time. The findings from Framingham suggest that

From the *Harvard Health Letter*, September 1997, pp. 1-3. © 1997 by the President and Fellows of Harvard College. Reprinted by permission.

## Good Bets for Bs

On any given day, more than 50% of adults fail to eat the three servings of vegetables advised in the "Dietary Guidelines for Americans," and only 24% consume the recommended two servings of fruits. That's unfortunate, because fruits and vegetables are excellent sources of vitamins B₆ and folate. Most research suggests that 400 micrograms of folate and 2 milligrams of vitamin B₆ are sufficient to keep homocysteine levels down in most people. Getting enough vitamin B₁₂ is not generally a problem, except for strict vegetarians who avoid all meat, fish, poultry, and dairy products — the major sources of B₁₂. People with pernicious anemia cannot absorb B₁₂ and require injections of the vitamin.

| Food | Micrograms of Folate* | Milligrams of Vitamin B₆ |
|---|---|---|
| 1 cup orange juice | 109 | 0.11 |
| 1 banana | 22 | 0.66 |
| ½ cup strawberries | 13 | 0.45 |
| ½ cup cooked asparagus | 132 | 0.11 |
| ½ cup cooked Brussels sprouts | 79 | 0.23 |
| ½ cup cooked broccoli | 52 | 0.12 |
| 1 baked potato with skin | 22 | 0.70 |
| ½ cup chickpeas | 80 | 0.57 |
| 3 oz. cooked skinless chicken (light meat) | 4 | 0.51 |
| 3 oz. water-packed tuna | 3 | 0.30 |

*A microgram is 1/1000 of a milligram; folate is also known as folic acid.

high homocysteine levels—and thus the risk of heart disease—may be lowered simply by eating a diet containing adequate levels of the B vitamins or taking B supplements.

One in five older adults has homocysteine levels that may be high enough to raise the risk of heart disease. This has prompted an international inquiry to determine whether elevated homocysteine should, in fact, be added to the list of other undisputed risk factors for heart disease — such as smoking, high blood cholesterol, high blood pressure, and a sedentary lifestyle. In the past few years, dozens of studies involving thousands of men and women, both older adults and younger people, have made a compelling case for considering homocysteine to be a risk factor not only for heart attacks but also for strokes, blood clots in the legs, and damage to arteries throughout the body.

## Remaining questions

Despite the breadth of evidence linking homocysteine to heart disease, public health experts have yet to recommend widespread homocysteine testing because a number of important issues remain unresolved. For one, no clinical trial has looked at whether the proposed homocysteine-lowering interventions, such as taking B vitamin supplements, will truly prevent heart attacks or other coronary events.

In addition, scientists haven't pinpointed the exact combination of vitamins that might be necessary. It could be that simply taking 400 micrograms of folate — the Reference Daily Intake (RDI) — would be adequate, but it may turn out that a combination of the B vitamins is necessary or that some people will require higher amounts than others.

Another problem is that about 30% of people with high homocysteine do not have low blood levels of the key B vitamins. For them, nutritional intervention may have no impact whatsoever. Also unclear is how high homocysteine needs to be before it signals danger. Many researchers have used 15 micromoles per liter as the ceiling for "normal," but much of the evidence to date indicates that homocysteine-related risk rises in a continuum. That is, the higher the homocysteine, the greater the hazard, with even mild elevations in the "normal" range possibly boosting risk.

In addition, the mechanism by which homocysteine contributes to heart disease hasn't been solidly identified. A leading theory, proposed by scientists at the Harvard School of Public Health, is that homocysteine damages the *endothelium*, or inner lining of the arteries (*see illustration*), and triggers the proliferation of smooth muscle cells, thereby promoting clogged arteries.

## On trial

Studies aimed at determining whether vitamin supplements can help reduce the risk of heart disease are currently under way, and experts say results should start coming in within the next three years. Until they do, however, testing for homocysteine might make sense for young people with a strong family history of cardiovascular disease, for example, or for those of any age who've suffered a heart attack but did not have high cholesterol or other standard risk factors that might have predicted such an event. People who fall into these groups should talk to their doctor about getting a simple blood test to measure their homocysteine level. Such tests, which are becoming more widely available, typically cost between $45 and $120 and are covered by many insurers. Indeed, experts hope that homocysteine will someday be used to identify people who have

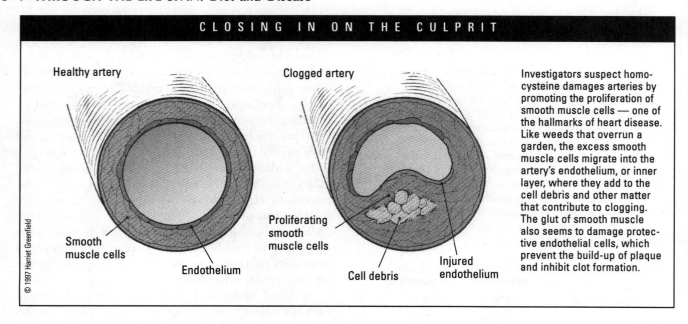

**CLOSING IN ON THE CULPRIT**

Healthy artery

Clogged artery

Smooth muscle cells

Endothelium

Proliferating smooth muscle cells

Cell debris

Injured endothelium

© 1997 Harriet Greenfield

Investigators suspect homocysteine damages arteries by promoting the proliferation of smooth muscle cells — one of the hallmarks of heart disease. Like weeds that overrun a garden, the excess smooth muscle cells migrate into the artery's endothelium, or inner layer, where they add to the cell debris and other matter that contribute to clogging. The glut of smooth muscle also seems to damage protective endothelial cells, which prevent the build-up of plaque and inhibit clot formation.

heart disease in the absence of the usual red flags, such as high blood cholesterol.

Those whose test results indicate high homocysteine levels should make sure they're getting sufficient B vitamins through food (*see chart on page 85*). Most people get plenty of vitamin $B_{12}$ through meat, fish, poultry, and dairy products. Fruits and vegetables are excellent sources of vitamins $B_6$ and folate (as well as fiber), the antioxidants vitamin C and beta-carotene, and *phytochemicals* — substances in plants that may help reduce the risk of heart disease, cancer, and other chronic conditions.

**Adding to the mix**
Americans' folate levels will get a boost in January 1998, when a U.S. Food and Drug Administration mandate for folate fortification takes effect. The nutrient will be added to most enriched breads, flours, corn meals, pastas, rice, and other grain products. The rule was enacted to ensure that women of child-bearing age consume adequate amounts of folate, which reduces the risk of certain types of birth defects. But a bonus is that folate fortification may help decrease the incidence of heart disease.

If eating a B-rich diet is not possible, there's no harm in taking a standard multivitamin/mineral supplement containing 100% of the RDI for vitamins $B_6$ (2 milligrams), $B_{12}$ (6 micrograms), and folate (400 micrograms). Most research suggests that RDI levels of those nutrients are all that is required to keep homocysteine levels down in many people.

Because the first line of treatment for high homocysteine is a diet adequate in the crucial B vitamins, testing is not necessary for most people. At the very least, the news about homocysteine provides yet another good reason to eat five servings of fruits and vegetables a day — which has, of course, already been shown to help reduce the risk of some types of cancer and other chronic diseases.

# NEW BLOOD PRESSURE GUIDELINES EMPHASIZE NUTRITION

The National Heart, Lung and Blood Institute (NHLBI) has released new guidelines for preventing and treating high blood pressure—or hypertension—with an emphasis on nutrition. For the first time, a diet rich in fruits, vegetables, and low-fat dairy products is recommended for controlling high blood pressure. This type of diet, which also is low in total and saturated fat, was recently evaluated in a nationwide study called Dietary Approaches to Stop Hypertension (DASH).

In the DASH investigation, subjects who consumed a diet rich in fruits and vegetables had a greater reduction in blood pressure than those eating the typical American diet. But a third group, whose diet also included low-fat or nonfat dairy foods in addition to the fruits and vegetables, and was low in total and saturated fat, had the most dramatic drop in blood pressure.

This "DASH Combination Diet" worked equally well for men, women, whites, and nonwhites, and was especially effective in individuals whose blood pressure was already high. Furthermore, it took only about 2 weeks from the start of the diet for blood pressure to fall.

"If added to other lifestyle recommendations, the DASH diet should help prevent hypertension and may reduce some persons' need for medication to control the condition," comments NHLBI director Dr. Claude Lenfant.

Other lifestyle recommendations for controlling blood pressure include maintaining a healthy weight, choosing foods low in salt and sodium, drinking alcohol in moderation (for those who drink), and being physically active. Salt was not restricted in the DASH study and was about the same for each group. The study also did not limit alcohol or involve weight loss or exercise. These factors will be assessed in future investigations.

Researchers are not sure why the DASH Combination Diet was so effective, but believe it is probably due to a combination of nutrients, including potassium, magnesium, calcium, and fiber. These are often abundant in the diets of vegetarians, who tend to have lower blood pressures than nonvegetarians. However, previous investigations that examined the individual effects of these nutrients, often as dietary supplements, typically resulted in small and inconsistent changes in pressure . Therefore, at present nutrient supplements generally are not recommended for controlling hypertension.

Source: *New England Journal of Medicine.* 1997. 336:1117-24.

## Silent Killer

Hypertension afflicts about 50 million Americans, including more than half the adults over the age of 65. If left untreated, it can lead to kidney damage, heart disease, and stroke.

Hypertension is defined as either a systolic blood pressure of at least 140 mm Hg (millimeters of mercury), or diastolic blood pressure of at least 90 mm Hg, or both. The systolic pressure is the pressure of blood in the vessels when the heart contracts. Diastolic pressure is the pressure of the blood between beats, when the heart is momentarily at rest.

The DASH Combination Diet is consistent with dietary recommendations aimed at preventing heart disease, cancer, and osteoporosis, but it places more emphasis on fruits and vegetables (see below).

In addition to diet, the new NHLBI guidelines provide physicians with specific recommendations about drugs for controlling blood pressure, and when to use them. Drug treatments are now based more closely on the presence of other medical conditions, such as diabetes and high blood cholesterol levels.

For further information about the DASH diet or high blood pressure in general, call 1-800-575-WELL or visit the NHLBI web site at:
http://www.nhlbi.nih.gov/nhlbi/nhlbi.htm
The DASH diet also is on-line at:
http://dash.bwh.harvard.edu

## The DASH Combination Diet
(based on 2,000 calories/day)

| Food Group | Servings* |
| --- | --- |
| Grains and grain products | 7-8/day |
| Vegetables | 4-5/day |
| Fruits | 4-5/day |
| Low-fat or nonfat diary foods | 2-3/day |
| Meats, poultry, fish | 2 or less/day |
| Nuts, seeds, and legumes | 4-5/week |

*For information on serving sizes, contact your local Extension office.

From *Food, Health, and You,* Fall 1997, p. 2. © 1997 by Mark A. Kantor, Ph.D., Associate Professor, College of Agriculture and Natural Resources, University of Maryland, College Park, MD. Reprinted by permission.

# Smarten Up: Certain Foods Help Maintain Brain Power as You Age

CAN YOU MEMORIZE a phone number as well as you used to? What about following directions to "insert part A into part B" in order to put together something you picked up at Home Depot? If you've become a little slow on the uptake, maybe it has something to do with your food choices.

You know how they say certain things go to your head? Well, so does food—literally.

For almost 100 years, scientists have known that various nutrients are important to neurologic health. But today, they are beginning to develop a clearer understanding of which foods, or at least which components of various foods, have a more positive impact, allowing people to retain their memory and learning abilities as the decades pass. To be sure, the research is in its preliminary stages, and no matter what is eventually confirmed, food is only one of many factors that affect how well your mind functions. But just as investigators have learned how to eat to maintain the health of organs such as the heart, they now are getting a better sense of how to eat to protect the health of the brain.

## The antioxidant connection

You may recall a widely publicized study released last spring in which researchers found that people with Alzheimer's disease who took large doses of vitamin E, an antioxidant, delayed such outcomes as the loss of ability to groom or feed themselves. But a number of other studies that have received much less attention also point to antioxidants as brain savers—and not just for people with Alzheimer's or other forms of dementia.

In a large research project in Switzerland, for instance, **healthy people in their 60s and older who had the highest blood levels of vitamin C and beta-carotene scored higher on memory tests than those with relatively low levels.** They apparently got these substances from fruits and vegetables rather than from supplements; only 6 percent of the people involved reported taking vitamin/mineral pills. Similarly, in research looking at older adults in the Netherlands, foods rich in beta-carotene appeared protective against cognitive impairment, that is, impairment in mental processes involving memory, judgment, perception, and reasoning. Likewise, vitamin E (found in nuts and oils) and vitamin C appeared to forestall losses in cognitive function in a group of Japanese-American men living in Hawaii.

*Did you know...* Heavy snoring caused by certain sleep disorders has been linked to a greater risk of stroke. Researchers theorize that snoring blocks parts of the upper airway in the case of conditions such as obstructive apneas, creating a negative pressure in the chest that reduces blood flow to the brain. *Mild* snoring does not pose a problem.

From *Tufts University Health & Nutrition Letter,* February 1998, pp. 4-5. © 1998 by Tufts University Diet & Nutrition Letter. Reprinted by permission.

To be sure, cause and effect have not yet been teased apart, meaning scientists have not yet determined whether antioxidants or something else in antioxidant-containing foods may bring about the brain-strengthening effect. But the thinking is that if antioxidants are responsible, it's because they reduce oxidative stress to brain cells called neurons. Such stress occurs when highly reactive forms of oxygen break down cell structure, which in turn prevents neurons from functioning properly. Antioxidants may also help keep the blood vessels that flow to the brain free of "debris," just as they are thought to keep vessels flowing to (or in) the heart unclogged. The more unimpeded the flow of blood, the better the brain can function.

## B vitamins as brain food?

Nutrition scientists have known for some time that severe deficiencies in B vitamins may adversely affect cognitive functioning. But research conducted at Tufts now suggests that even blood levels of various B vitamins that fall at the lower end of the so-called normal range might get in the way of mental dexterity.

Tufts psychologist Karen Riggs, PhD, made the discovery when she gave men in their 50s and older a slew of cognitive tasks (repeating a sequence of numbers in backwards order, drawing cubes and other geometric shapes) and matched their scores to their blood levels of vitamins $B_6$, $B_{12}$, and folate. The upshot: men with relatively low levels of $B_{12}$ and folate did not perform as well on the drawing task, which checked their spatial skills. And **men with $B_6$ levels on the low side of normal did not do as well as the others on memory tests.** They didn't do poorly, but the men with the highest $B_6$ levels did significantly better.

Much more research on the relationship between B vitamins and mental acuity is warranted, but in the meantime, it's certainly not a bad idea to eat plenty of B vitamin-rich foods. Folate is available in sizable quantities in legumes, including kidney beans, chickpeas, lentils, navy beans, and the

like. It's also in green leafy vegetables and orange juice. Vitamin $B_6$, too, is widely available in fruits and vegetables and can also be found in beef, poultry, and seafood.

Theoretically, $B_{12}$ is easy to get because it's in almost all animal foods, including meat, fish, poultry, and cheese. But one out of five people over 60 and two out of five over 80 don't absorb the $B_{12}$ they take in with foods because of a condition of aging known as atrophic gastritis, in which the stomach does not put out enough hydrochloric acid to allow for the nutrient's absorption. Most people do not know if they have atrophic gastritis and aren't likely to be checked for the condition by a physician. But $B_{12}$ malabsorption can easily be overcome by eating cereals fortified with $B_{12}$, including Kellogg's Product 19 and General Mills Total, or by taking a multivitamin supplement.

## Looking at the blood pressure/brain power seesaw

It is well-established that as people age, they undergo reductions in brain volume and other cerebral changes. That doesn't mean older people necessarily become more feeble-minded or even lose their memory capabilities (although it does often take older people longer to *process* new information, including phone numbers, which is why many people feel frustrated about their memory as they age). But evidence is coming to light that **when aging is accompanied by high blood pressure, mental function does suffer.**

Consider a study conducted by researchers at the National Institute on Aging. People in their mid-50s and older with high blood pressure experienced more brain atrophy—and scored lower on language and memory tests—than others their age whose blood pressure was normal. The older the individual, the greater the effect of high blood pressure.

High blood pressure apparently not only contributed to accelerated brain atrophy but also caused reductions in gray matter. In addition, it was

linked to a reduction in the volume of the thalamus. That's a structure that connects many regions of the brain, potentially influencing everything from motor and sensory functioning to the ability to pay attention.

Similar losses in mental acuity were seen in a group of men followed in an ongoing study taking place at four medical centers around the country: Stanford, UCLA, Indiana University, and Boston University. Researchers in that project found that ignoring high blood pressure in middle age sets the stage for a loss of cognitive ability by the early 70s.

The problem seems to come specifically from elevated systolic pressure—the first number in a blood pressure reading. Men who had systolic pressure above 140 for at least 15 years experienced 50 percent more cognitive decline than men with normal blood pressure. Men in their late 60s and 70s who had systolic pressure above 140 for at least 25 years underwent 100 percent more cognitive decline. The reason, at least in part, appears to be that they ended up with twice as much brain fluid—a sign of small, undetected strokes.

The men being studied are twins, and head researcher Dorit Carmelli, PhD, says the data are indicating that "even a small difference in blood pressure between twins in mid-life could make a meaningful difference in brain atrophy and cognitive function later on. Slight variations in blood pressure that once seemed insignificant are proving to have meaning that was previously missed."

The positive aspect of all of this, Dr. Carmelli points out, is that blood pressure can in large part be controlled by lifestyle. High blood pressure is not necessarily inevitable. The steps to keep down blood pressure without medication: keep off—or take off—excess weight (as little as a 10-pound weight loss can reduce blood pressure significantly); have no more than two drinks a day (one for women); engage in regular physical activity, such as 30 to 45 minutes of brisk walking most days of the week; keep sodium consumption to a maximum of 2,400 milligrams a day (older people's blood pressure tends to go up more in response to sodium than younger people's); and increase potassium consumption with a higher intake of fruits and vegetables.

## An organizing principle?

More antioxidants, more B vitamins, lower blood pressure—is there a way to bring these disparate recommendations together as one unifying piece of advice? Yes. Eat a generally healthful diet with plenty of fruits, vegetables, and grains and moderate amounts of animal-based foods. The fruits and vegetables will provide not just antioxidants and potassium but also the B vitamins folate and B$_6$. Grain-based foods such as bread and pasta will provide folate, too, because as of January 1 of this year, they are required to be fortified with that nutrient. All these foods are also relatively low in sodium and calories, important points for those making a conscious effort to keep down their blood pressure by limiting salt consumption and maintaining a healthy weight.

If all this sounds like little more than the standard plea to eat a good diet, consider the results of a study in Madrid that looked at healthy men and women 65 and older. **Those who scored the highest on mental status tests ate the most fruits and vegetables; the most carbohydrates (available not just in fruits and vegetables but also in grains); and, not surprisingly, the most beta-carotene, vitamin C, and folate.** "Our results agree with those of other authors indicating that...the consumption of a more satisfactory...diet is associated with better cognitive function," the researchers note.

Of course, no matter how well you eat, it's important to continue to engage in mind-stimulating activities. The brain, like the heart and lungs, is a use-it-or-lose-it organ that deteriorates more quickly if it is not challenged with "exercise."

Exercising the brain does not have to mean taking classes or participating in other sorts of formal education. It simply means that people should keep reading as they age and also continue to learn by picking up new hobbies or refining old ones; going to museums, theater, and thought-provoking movies; engaging in spirited conversations—in short, not retiring the mind even if one has retired from a specific career. Taking part in activities that require thinking and stretches in mental function help ensure that graying and losing gray matter don't end up going hand in hand.

# When Eating Goes Awry

## *An Update on Eating Disorders*

Although eating disorders receive considerable attention and are prevalent in today's society, they are not new in medical history. More than 100 years ago the first case of anorexia nervosa, or self-induced starvation, was documented in England. Yet, it stands to reason that even before the term anorexia was coined, many people struggling with eating disorders were simply diagnosed as having another ailment.

Eating disorders threaten physical health, psychological well-being and sometimes life. Because many people with these problems suffer alone and do not seek professional help, it is difficult to determine the precise number of cases in the United States. However, the American Psychiatric Association (APA) estimates that at any given time, 500,000 people are battling eating disorders. The APA's 1993 Practice Guidelines estimate that between 1 and 4 percent of adolescents and young adults are afflicted. Although the typical patient is a white, middle-to upper-middle-class young woman, some researchers report an increasing number of cases among males and women of other age and ethnic groups.

### Types of Eating Disorders

Currently, the APA recognizes two eating disorders: anorexia nervosa and bulimia nervosa. Cases of anorexia nervosa and bulimia nervosa have doubled over the past decade, according to the National Center for Health Statistics (NCHS). Binge-eating, although not yet a recognized eating disorder, is receiving considerable attention as a related disorder.

The major weight loss associated with anorexia nervosa results in a total body weight at least 15 percent below the range of normal weight for age and height. Over time, women suffering from this disorder stop menstruating and may damage vital organs including the heart and brain. Anorexia is believed to affect between 1/2 and 1 percent of women in late adolescence and early adulthood, according to the APA. Its onset is often associated with a stressful life event, such as entering college.

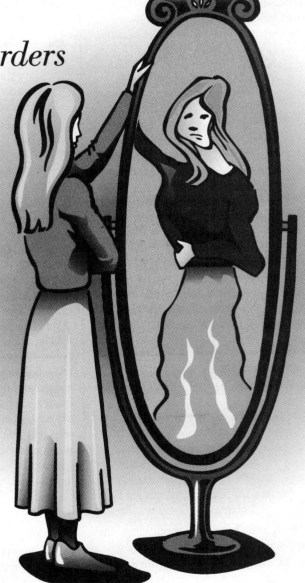

Reprinted with permission from *Food Insight*, January/February 1997, pp. 1, 4-5. © 1997 by the International Food Information Council Foundation (IFIC).

"Anorexia nervosa is most common in white, 15-24 year-old women," says Alexander Lucas, M.D., professor of psychiatry at the Mayo Medical School in Rochester, Minnesota. "It's generally recognized that the disorder is rare among the African-American population for reasons that aren't yet clearly understood. However, there may be both biological and cultural factors that account for the differences in prevalence."

Bulimia nervosa is a serious eating disorder typified by binging (consuming excessive amounts of food in a short time) followed by either self-induced vomiting, use of laxatives, diuretics or enemas, strict dieting or fasting, or vigorous exercise in order to rid the body of the food and prevent weight gain. Although some victims of anorexia nervosa also exhibit symptoms of bulimia nervosa, it is recognized as a distinct disorder. Bulimia nervosa is believed to affect between 1 and 3 percent of adolescent and young women in the United States, although estimates among college-age women reach as high as one out of every five.

Bulimia nervosa victims often are able to hide their problem because they eat normally in public and binge-and-purge in secret. In addition, many are able to maintain a normal body weight while suffering from the disorder. Symptoms of bulimia nervosa, which may be obvious to family and friends, include a chronically inflamed and sore throat that may bleed, decaying tooth enamel (from frequent exposure to stomach acid from vomiting) and swollen salivary glands in the neck and jaw which can make the face appear puffy.

Another type of disorder that is receiving attention is binge-eating. Although less is known about binge-eating disorder, recent estimates suggest that as many as 2 percent of the general population and 30 percent of individuals attending hospital affiliated weight control programs may be afflicted. At a recent American Medical Association (AMA) press conference on compulsive

## Eating Disorders Defined

The American Psychiatric Association's Eating Disorders Guidelines are currently being revised. However, to date, the Association lists the following criteria, all of which must be met in order for a case to be recognized as an occurrence of anorexia nervosa or bulimia nervosa

### Anorexia nervosa:

- refusal to maintain weight that is above the lowest weight considered normal for age and height
- intense fear of gaining weight or becoming fat, even though underweight
- distorted body image
- in women, three consecutive missed menstrual periods without pregnancy

### Bulimia nervosa:

- recurrent episodes of binge eating (minimum average of two binge-eating episodes a week for at least three months)
- a feeling of uncontrollable eating during binges
- regular use of one or more of the following to prevent weight gain: self-induced vomiting, use of laxatives or diuretics, strict dieting or fasting, or vigorous exercise
- persistent over-concern with body shape and weight

mental disorders, Seda Ebrahimi, Ph.D., director of the eating disorders treatment program at McLean Hospital in Belmont, Massachusetts, estimated that one-third of obese patients may be binge-eaters.

Binge-eating, which has been pro-

posed for official recognition as a diagnostic category of eating disorder, is similar to bulimia nervosa in that sufferers may consume extraordinary amounts of food during a single binge. However they do not compensate for the binge by purging. The morning after a binge, many sufferers experience symptoms similar to a hang-over which may be so extreme that the person is unable to go to school, work or function normally.

"Binge-eating is an avoidance coping mechanism," says Dr. Ebrahimi. "During the binge, the person 'mentally and emotionally checks out' and is unable to stop the out of control eating." Binge-eaters do not purge and tend to minimize the severity of the illness. As a result, doctors may treat binge-eating as an overeating problem rather than a psychiatric disorder, according to Ebrahimi.

### Who Develops Eating Disorders and Why?

There are many theories about the causes, but most eating disorder specialists acknowledge that the disorders are very complex and likely involve physical, psychological, societal, cultural and familial aspects.

The development of an eating disorder is not triggered solely by the desire to be thin, according to Amy Tuttle, R.D., M.S.S., a nutrition therapist at The Renfrew Center in Philadelphia, the first residential center for women with eating disorders. "Although much has been said about the the media's role in presenting unrealistic body images to young people, trying to achieve a model-perfect body is not the main reason people develop eating disorders," says Tuttle.

Family dynamics, according to Tuttle, often contribute to the development of an eating disorder. "Some people with eating disorders come from enmeshed families where emotional, relational and physical space boundaries may be blurry. This 'enmeshment' inhibits independence and the development of a separate self," says Tuttle. A prominent theory about eating disorders — that the person with the eating disorder is trying to gain some measure of control in her life — is consistent with this type of family structure. For some people, the act of dieting itself provides an illusion of control.

Depression, feelings of inadequacy, anxiety and loneliness, stress and anger, as well as troubled personal relationships also may contribute to the development of disordered eating patterns. Likewise, major life transitions, the presence of other coping behaviors such as gambling, the presence of another psychiatric disorder such as clinical depression, and alcohol or drug abuse are associated with the onset of eating disorders.

Research also suggests that there may be biochemical imbalances associated with eating disorders. The imbalances — found in certain brain chemicals called neurotransmitters — also are found in people suffering from depression.

Neurotransmitters such as serotonin and norepinephrine control appetite, mood, alertness and sleeping patterns. Low levels of these chemicals may explain the link between eating disorders and depressive illness, as well as why people exhibit abnormal and seemingly illogical eating patterns. However, researchers still are not sure whether neurotransmitter imbalances are the cause of eating disorders or the results of the poor nutrition these disorders bring.

### Treatment Offers Hope

Eating disorders are most successfully treated when detected in their early stages. Unfortunately, this is not easy to do. Anorexia nervosa may not be detected until victims become seriously underweight, and bulimia nervosa victims can go for years without anyone knowing about their disease. Fortunately, increasing awareness of the dangers of eating disorders has led more people to seek early help.

According to the APA, simply restoring a person to normal weight or temporarily ending the binge-purge cycle does not address the underlying emotional problems that caused, or are exacerbated by, the abnormal eating behavior.

In addition to addressing any physical complications that result from eating disorders, treatment focuses on correcting the patient's distorted body image, improving self-confidence and self-esteem, treating any underlying depression, establishing normal eating habits and preventing relapse. Many victims can successfully be treated in outpatient programs; however, in critical cases, hospitalization is necessary. Ultimately, success depends on tailoring treatment to the individual's needs.

Generally, a treatment plan will include a combination of physical interventions as well as individual, group or family psychotherapy, cognitive therapy, behavior therapy and medications. To accomplish this level of treatment, a team approach is employed. At The Renfrew Center, the composition of the team depends on the level of care — whether the person is in inpatient or outpatient care — but usually includes a therapist (social worker or psychologist), a dietitian, a psychiatrist, a family therapist, a medical doctor, a nurse and a dentist (for bulimic patients).

The Renfrew philosophy of treatment is two-pronged: therapy for underlying issues, and mealtime support therapy to allow the eating disorder patient to take "food risks." According to Tuttle, "Food risks are behaviors such as eating a certain food which the patient previously considered 'off limits.' Once the patient is able to conquer a food risk, we generally see her display a certain level of self-trust, which often allows her to con-front underlying issues more directly."

Medications, particularly antidepressants, are commonly prescribed for eating disorder patients. These medications, which regulate the body's level of neurotransmitters, can bring about improved self-esteem and a sense of control, as well as markedly reduce binge-and-purge behavior in bulimics. Currently, the drug Prozac, a serotonin reuptake inhibitor which recently won Food and Drug Administration approval for use in treating bulimia nervosa, is the only drug specifically approved for the eating disorder.

According to John Foreyt, Ph.D., director of the Behavioral Medicine Research Center at Baylor College of Medicine in Houston, Texas, "The use of these medications has shown at least short-term beneficial effects in patients with bulimia nervosa." However, medication is not a stand-alone treatment, cautions Foreyt. "Medications such as Prozac are only adjunct treatments for eating disorders. Therapy to address the multi-factorial nature of the disorders is definitely necessary."

The length of treatment for eating disorders varies, but it can take as long as five years. Success rates for treatment are difficult to estimate because continued treatment does not necessarily mean that the treatment is not working. "Coming back in for day or inpatient treatment is not a sign of failure on the part of either the patient or the treatment process," says Tuttle. "Life brings continual challenges that may need to be addressed with professionals. It's important that people who have or are recovering from an eating disorder stay connected with all of their resources."

Despite the complexities of treating eating disorders, sufferers have an excellent chance for complete recovery, especially if the illness is recognized early.

# Food Allergy Myths and Realities

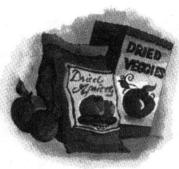

D o you, or someone you know, shun certain foods because you are "allergic?" Surveys show that nearly one-third of all adults believe they have a food allergy The following seeks to shed light on such frequently asked questions as: What is a food allergy? How do you know if you have one? What should you do if you have a food allergy? And, if it is not a food allergy, what might it be?

**Myth:  Lots of people have food allergies.**
**Reality:** "From talking with the public, you might think almost everyone has a food allergy," said Daryl Altman, M.D., Fellow of the American College of Allergy, Asthma and Immunology and researcher at the Allergy Information Services in Long Island, New York. "In surveys, nearly one-in-three American adults indicated he or she was allergic to some food." But in reality, the most conservative estimates indicate two percent of the population in the United States are food allergic. Children are more susceptible than adults to food allergy—up to five percent have some type of food allergy. However, common allergens such as eggs and milk are typically outgrown by age five.

The eight most common food allergens in people are: Peanuts, tree nuts (for example, almonds, pecans and walnuts), dairy, soy, wheat, eggs, fish and shellfish (for example, shrimp and crab). Nevertheless, allergies to nearly 175 different types of food have been documented. "These foods are responsible for over 90 percent of serious allergic reactions to food," stated Susan L. Hefle, Ph.D., co-director of the Food Allergy Research and Resource Program at the University of Nebraska-Lincoln.

**Myth:  A food allergy means I'll just get a runny nose, right?**
**Reality:** No—although food allergy is rare, it is a serious condition and should be diagnosed by a board-certified allergist. Food allergy is a reaction of the body's immune system to a certain component, usually a protein, in a food or ingredient. The reactions can be uncomfortable and mild including vomiting, diarrhea, skin rashes or runny nose, sneezing, coughing and wheezing, and may occur within hours or days after eating. However, anaphylaxis, a more serious and life-threatening reaction, may occur. Anaphylaxis is a rapidly occurring reaction that often involves hives and swelling, enlarging of the larynx with a choking sensation, wheezing, severe vomiting, diarrhea and even shock. These symptoms

## I Think I'm

## Allergic To...

Reprinted with permission from *Food Insight*, November/December 1997, pp. 2-3. © 1997 by the International Food Information Council Foundation (IFIC).

can also occur within minutes, hours or days. "Food allergic patients should have an anaphylaxis reaction plan worked out ahead of time with their allergist," according to Anne Muñoz-Furlong, president and founder of The Food Allergy Network. "The plan should be practiced with family and friends in case of an emergency."

**Myth: Any negative reaction to a food is a food allergy.**

**Reality:** Adverse reactions to food can have many causes. If something does not "agree with you," it does not necessarily mean you are allergic to it. Food allergy is a very specific reaction involving the immune system of the body, and it is important to distinguish food allergy from other food sensitivities. Whereas food allergies are rare, food intolerances, which are the other classification of food sensitivities, are more common. Intolerances are reactions to foods or ingredients that do not involve the body's immune system. Intolerance reactions are generally localized, transient and rarely life threatening with one possible exception—sulfite sensitivity. "A good example of a food intolerance is lactose intolerance. And, it is extremely important to know the difference between it and a milk allergy," said Robert K. Bush, M.D., University of Wisconsin. He emphasized that, "Whereas lactose intolerance may result in a bloated feeling or flatulence after consuming milk or dairy products, milk allergy can have life-threatening consequences. The milk allergic patient must avoid all milk proteins."

**Myth: I think I'm allergic to a food—I just won't eat it, so I don't need to be seen by a doctor.**

**Reality:** Just thinking you are allergic to a food does not mean you have an allergy.

## What is an Allergic Reaction?

An allergic reaction occurs when a susceptible person is exposed to a specific protein. Because the body perceives this protein (an allergen) as being a threat, it produces a special material—a substance that recognizes allergens—known as Immunoglobulin E (IgE) antibody. A person who has a tendency to develop allergies tends to produce increased amounts of IgE. After the initial exposure to a specific allergen (such as "cat" or "dog" protein) the body reacts to future exposures by creating millions of IgE antibodies. These newly produced IgE antibodies then connect to special blood cells called basophils, and special tissue cells called mast cells. These cells are then "stimulated" to release histamine which causes the allergy symptoms: Itchy watery eyes and nose, scratchy throat, rashes, hives, eczema and even life-threatening anaphylaxis.

To properly diagnose a food allergy or sensitivity the offending substance must be accurately identified. Avoiding a food may deprive you of food choices and important nutrients, and could be dangerous if the allergen is actually different. Diagnosis of a food allergy can be complex, with three major components. The first and most important is involving a board-certified allergist, preferably a food allergy specialist.

### The Double-Blind Placebo-Controlled Food Challenge

This test, considered the "gold standard" for food allergy testing, is performed by a board-certified allergist. The suspected allergen is placed in a capsule or hidden in food, and fed to the patient under strict supervision. Neither the allergist, nor the patient, is aware of which capsule, or food, contains the suspected allergen—hence the name "double-blind." In order for the test to be effective, the patient must also be fed capsules or food which do not contain the allergen to make sure the reaction, if any, being observed is to the allergen and not some other factor—hence the name "placebo-controlled." It is tests of this kind that have enabled allergists to identify the most common allergens, and also to determine what foods, ingredients and additives do not cause allergic reactions.

Second, a history of a specific food causing an allergic reaction is necessary; a food diary can help. Third, an IgE antibodies test, is only useful when combined with the former components, but it does not always pinpoint a food allergy (see sidebar). Hugh Sampson, M.D., director, Food Allergy Clinic, Mt. Sinai Medical Center, and chair of the American Academy of Allergy, Asthma and Immunology's Adverse Reactions to Foods Committee, emphasized an examination by a board-certified allergist: "Due to many people claiming to have food allergies, many physicians have become "desensitized" to taking their symptoms seriously."

**Myth: I don't frequently eat food I'm allergic to, so I can eat a little bit for a special occasion.**

**Reality:** Because food allergy can be life threatening, the allergen must be completely avoided—even the most minute amounts. Although an extreme case, a man allergic to shellfish died of anaphylaxis shock after encountering simply the steam from shrimp. It can be fatal to assume a given food environment is safe and not be cautious. A board-certified allergist can help the food allergic patient manage diet issues without sacrificing nutrition or pleasure when eating at and away from home. Since most life threatening, and sometimes fatal, allergic reactions to foods occur when eating away from home, it is imperative that the food allergic individual or responsible guardian clearly explain the risks of exposure to a certain food or ingredient to food service workers, family and friends—and always ask before eating.

**Myth: With all the ingredients in processed food I can never completely avoid my allergen.**

**Reality:** When purchasing groceries, labels should be read for every product purchased—every time. Although food and beverage manufacturers are often improving and changing their products, changes in ingredients must be listed on ingredient labels.

According to Fred Shank, Ph.D., director of the Center for Food Safety and Applied Nutrition, Food and Drug Administration (FDA), "Foods which contain allergenic substances must be properly labeled or be subject to recall. The FDA supports the activities of independent organizations to inform consumers of these recall activities." The FDA includes on its list of recall substances all eight of the major allergens, so if these substances are present in a food, but not listed on the label, they must be recalled. Additionally, substances which cause non-allergic-based reactions, such as the additives sulfites and tartrazine (FD&C Yellow #5), are on this list. Some individuals have unique sensitivities to these food components which are not allergenic or allergy-causing in nature, but may cause comparably severe reactions.

**Myth: Since I'm allergic to peanuts, I can't eat anything with peanut oil.**
**Reality:** There are many misunderstandings regarding exactly what might stimulate the food allergic reaction. "Virtually all food allergens are proteins," explained Steve L. Taylor,

## What is Sulfite Sensitivity?

Sulfiting agents are commonly used to preserve the color of foods, such as dried fruits and vegetables, and to inhibit the growth of microorganisms in fermented foods, like wine. Sulfites can also be found in beer, some fruit drinks, shrimp and some prepared foods. Although sulfites are safe for the majority of people, for some, they have been found to cause a reaction. For this reason, the FDA requires that when sulfites are added to foods in greater than 10 parts/million (or, 10 sulfite molecules per million molecules) they must be indicated on the label.

Ph.D., co-director of the Food Allergy Research and Resource Program at the University of Nebraska–Lincoln. "And, the process of refining oil removes the protein which would trigger an allergic reaction." Oils used in processed foods and in cosmetics are highly refined and should pose no problem for the food allergic individual. Yet, caution should be taken with natural, cold pressed or flavored oils. These oils, as well as oil that has been used to cook peanuts (or another food to which an individual might have an allergy), might contain the protein of the allergen and should be avoided. For example, an individual with a fish allergy should ensure that the oil used to cook his or her food was not first used to fry fish.

**Myth: I'm allergic to food additives.**
**Reality:** Other common misconceptions regarding food allergy are additives and preservatives. Although some—sulfites and tartrazine—have been shown to trigger asthma or hives in certain people, these reactions do not follow the same pathway observed with food. There are other food additives that have historically been associated with adverse reactions, but because they do not contain proteins or involve the immune system, true allergic pathways cannot be used to explain the reported reactions. In addition, many of these additives, including monosodium glutamate, aspartame and most food dyes have been studied extensively, and the results show little scientific evidence exists to suggest they cause any reaction at all.

**Myth: "Tell me about my corn allergy."**
**Reality:** There are those suspected food allergies that are so rare that their existence is questioned. The most common of these are corn and chocolate "allergy," and there are several probable explanations for adverse reactions. Even though many people claim to be allergic to them, allergists can rarely demonstrate allergy to corn or chocolate in double-blind, placebo-controlled food challenges (see sidebar).

Corn "allergy" is often associated with a reaction to another allergenic substance. In some cases soy allergic individuals may react to products containing corn. Occasionally corn is carried, handled or stored in the same containers used for soy. Although only minute residues of soy may remain, this can be enough to cause an allergic reaction in highly sensitive people.

Chocolate "allergy" is also thought to be extremely rare, and though some are truly chocolate-allergic, most who complain of symptoms have irreproducible reactions. Possibly the reactions are due to another ingredient found in the chocolate product being consumed.

Food allergy is certainly nothing to be taken lightly. Although its prevalence appears to be increasing, overreaction, self-diagnosis and incorrect assumptions only lead to skepticism of physicians and food service workers—obviously, a less-than-ideal situation for the truly allergic individual. It is vitally important to leave the diagnosis of a food allergy to a board-certified allergist.

The following organizations can help you more fully understand food allergy: The American Academy of Allergy, Asthma and Immunology (1-800-822-2762; www.aaaai.org) and the Food Allergy Network (1-800-929-4040; www.foodallergy.org). The International Food Information Council Foundation (http://ificinfo.health.org) can provide further information on food allergy and food and asthma. Also available is a food allergy poster designed for food service workers.

## Avoid Cross Contact!

Cross contact of foods with those that may present a food allergy problem is poorly understood and not well communicated. Although food processors are well aware of the dangers of cross contact and manage them appropriately, such caution is not always taken in the home, school cafeteria or restaurant. Although unintentional, the effects can be devastating. For some food allergic individuals, the most minute particle of the allergen can be fatal. Some examples of mishaps that can induce a food allergic reaction include:

- Plain chocolate brownies are served using the same spatula that was used to serve peanut-containing brownies.
- French fries are prepared in the same oil used to deep-fry fish.

# PHYSICAL ACTIVITY AND NUTRITION: A WINNING COMBINATION FOR HEALTH

## INTRODUCTION

Health professionals and the federal government recognize the importance of regular physical activity and a healthful diet to reduce the risk of major chronic diseases and improve well-being (1–9). In recent years, scientific evidence of the health benefits of being physically active, from early childhood throughout later adult years, has led to specific recommendations and/or practical suggestions to increase physical activity (2,4–8).

Regardless of age, everyone benefits from a physically active lifestyle. Compared to their sedentary peers, physically active children tend to be at lower risk of overweight (10) and are more likely to become physically active adults (11). For adults, regular physical activity, along with a healthful diet, helps to reduce the risk of major chronic diseases such as cardiovascular disease, hypertension, obesity, adult-onset diabetes mellitus, osteoporosis, and some cancers (1–3,5–9).

Improved mental health or psychological well-being is another benefit of physical activity (6). For older adults, regular physical activity improves muscle strength, functional mobility/independence, and quality of life (12,13). A physically active lifestyle also delays all-cause mortality (6,14–16).

Despite a growing consensus and awareness of the substantial health benefits of regular physical activity, many Americans lead relatively sedentary lifestyles (2,6,10, 17–20). According to the Surgeon General's Report on Physical Activity and Health (6), only 22% of adults in the U.S. engage in physical activity sufficient to derive health benefits; 53% are somewhat active but not active enough to derive health benefits; and 25% are completely sedentary. Children also lead relatively sedentary lifestyles (6,10). Only 22% of children participate in 30 minutes of vigorous activity a day and

one in four children receives no physical education in school, according to a recent survey of 1,504 families with children in grades 4–12 (10).

The current levels of physical activity among both young and old make it unlikely that many of the federal government's *Healthy People 2000* objectives for physical activity will be achieved (18,19). Americans give several reasons for their relatively sedentary lifestyles. These include lack of time, injury or other physical difficulties, inclement weather, a dislike for exercise, fear of crime in their neighborhoods, and our "information age" which fosters time spent in front of the computer, television, and video screen (2).

This *Digest* reviews recent research findings supporting the beneficial role of regular physical activity and a healthful diet throughout life, from early childhood through later adult years. Also presented are current recommendations for physical activity offered by various health organizations.

## CHILDHOOD AND ADOLESCENCE

Regular physical activity benefits children and adolescents by improving their strength and endurance, helping to control body weight, building healthy bones, and reducing anxiety and stress (21). A growing proportion of children and adolescents in the U.S. are overweight (22–25). Approximately 14% of children aged 6 to 11 years and 12% of adolescents aged 12 to 17 years are overweight (22). Not only is overweight highly prevalent among young people, but this condition has continued to rise over the years (22) and affect younger and younger children (24,25). This situation, coupled with recognition that overweight in children and adolescents may increase the likelihood of adult morbidity and

*Physical inactivity is a major public health concern in the U.S. In general, females are less physically active than males and physical activity declines with age.*

From *Dairy Council Digest*, May/June 1998, pp. 14-18. © 1998 by the National Dairy Council. Reprinted by permission.

mortality (26), has drawn attention to contributing factors (23,27).

Physical inactivity is regarded as a major contributing factor to overweight among children and adolescents (6,10,23). Because childhood and adolescence can set the stage for lifelong physical activities (11), parents, care providers, teachers, athletic coaches, and others are urged to encourage children to become more physically active (5,6,10,21). Care should be taken to ensure that efforts to prevent overweight in children do not compromise children's growth and development (5).

Physical activity and nutrition, especially adequate calcium intake, play an important role in the development of genetically-determined bone mass (6,28–31). Maximizing peak bone mass, which occurs between ages 19 and 30 years depending on specific bones, and reducing bone loss in later years lower the risk of osteoporosis. Physical activity during childhood can strengthen bones and contribute to increased peak bone mass in adulthood (6,28–31). In a prospective study of 470 healthy children ages 8 to 16 years, weight-bearing physical activity and a high calcium intake increased forearm trabecular bone mineral density (30). A study of over 200 women ages 18 to 31 years found that those who were more physically active during their high school years exhibited higher hip bone density, total body and spine bone mineral content, and total body bone mineral density than their less physically active counterparts (31).

Physical activity during childhood and adolescence may favorably influence blood lipid profiles (6,32). The Cardiovascular Risk in Young Finns Study involving more than 2,300 children and young adults links higher levels of physical activity with increased blood levels of high density lipoprotein (HDL) cholesterol in males and lower triglyceride levels in females (32).

Regular physical activity also reduces anxiety and stress, increases self-esteem (21), and allows an increase in caloric intake without weight gain which enables an individual to increase food choices and improve nutrient intake. A recent cross-sectional study of nearly 500 low-income children 9 to 12 years of age in Montreal found that children who were more physically active

*Regular physical activity and a healthful diet throughout life reduce the risk of major chronic diseases and improve overall health and well-being.*

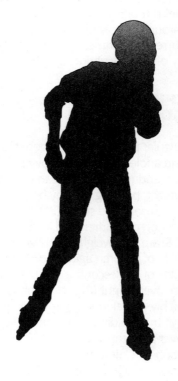

consumed more calories, calcium, iron, zinc, and fiber, but did not gain more weight than their inactive peers (33).

## ADULTHOOD

**Cardiovascular Disease.** Numerous studies have established that physical activity reduces the risk of cardiovascular disease, particularly among previously inactive individuals (1,6,8,34,35).

Physical activity exerts its beneficial effect on cardiovascular health through a variety of direct and indirect mechanisms. Physical activity favorably influences the blood lipid profile, specifically raising HDL cholesterol and lowering elevated blood levels of total and low density lipoprotein (LDL) cholesterol and triglyceride levels (6–8,35–37). In addition, physical activity increases lipoprotein lipase, an enzyme that removes cholesterol and free fatty acids from the blood, decreases plasma viscosity thereby influencing blood flow, and favorably affects blood clotting and fibrinolytic mechanisms (1,6,7, 38). Physical activity may also reduce risk of cardiovascular disease by its beneficial effects on other cardiovascular disease risk factors such as high blood pressure, obesity, and adult-onset diabetes mellitus (6,7,35). The cardiovascular benefits of regular physical activity have been demonstrated in both males and females (36,38–41), as well as in patients with cardiovascular disease or individuals at high risk of developing this disease (42).

To reduce the risk of heart disease, the NIH Consensus Panel on Physical Activity and Cardiovascular Health (7) recommends that children and adults participate in moderate intensity physical activity for at least 30 minutes on most, and preferably all, days of the week. The American Heart Association recommends that adults should also participate in resistance exercise (e.g., lifting weights) for a minimum of two days a week (8).

**Hypertension.** Physical inactivity contributes to high blood pressure, an established risk factor for cardiovascular disease (6,8,39,43). Sedentary normotensive individuals exhibit a 20% to 50% higher risk of developing hypertension than do their more physically active counterparts (43). Moderately intense physical activity such as brisk walking for 30 to 45 minutes on most days of the week can lower blood pressure (43).

**Overweight.** Paralleling the trend observed among children, the prevalence of overweight among U.S. adults has markedly increased, specifically from about 25% between 1960 and 1980 to 33% in 1988–91 (18,44). Physical inactivity is an important contributor to the rise in overweight among U.S. adults (6,45).

Studies report lower body weight, body mass index, or skinfold measures among physically active adults than among their sedentary counterparts (3,5–7,39). Regular physical activity contributes to weight maintenance and/or reduction by increasing caloric expenditure (1,6,46). Research indicates that physical activity does not necessarily produce a compensatory increase in appetite or energy intake (6,47).

As a component of a weight reduction program, physical activity favors the loss of body fat and helps to preserve lean body tissue (6,46,48). Minimizing lean tissue loss helps to protect against a decrease in metabolic rate which can increase the propensity to regain weight (48). Physical activity in conjunction with moderate energy restriction may also enhance dietary compliance (49), help to maintain weight loss (6,7,50,51), and improve maximal oxygen consumption or functional capacity (52).

The 1995 *Dietary Guidelines for Americans* (5) recognizes the importance of physical activity, along with a healthful diet, to maintain a healthy body weight. These guidelines call for 30 minutes or more of moderate physical activity on most, and preferably all, days of the week. Health professional organizations such as The American Dietetic Association support this position (3).

**Diabetes Mellitus.** The goals of managing adult-onset or non-insulin dependent diabetes mellitus (NIDDM) include achieving and maintaining normal blood glucose, lipid, and blood pressure levels (1,53). Although there are few data regarding the effects of combined dietary modification and physical activity on NIDDM, regular physical activity is recommended to help achieve

*"Successful weight management for adults requires a life-long commitment to healthful behaviors emphasizing eating practices and daily physical activity that are sustainable and enjoyable,"* states the American Dietetic Association (3).

and maintain normal blood glucose levels and a reasonable body weight (1,6,53). Epidemiological data indicate a protective effect of physical activity against developing NIDDM (6,54,55). The benefits of physical activity appear to be most pronounced for individuals at high risk for developing NIDDM (1,55).

**Cancer.** Epidemiological studies provide fairly consistent support for a protective effect of regular physical activity against colon cancer, the third most common cancer among adults (6,9). Physical activity may reduce colon cancer risk by stimulating colon peristalsis, thereby speeding up the movement of dietary factors, bile acids, and carcinogens through the gastrointestinal tract. Physical activity may also favorably affect the immune system (9,56), alter prostaglandin synthesis (6), and, in association with a lower body mass, create a metabolic environment less conducive to the growth of cancer (9).

Although less consistent than for colon cancer, epidemiological findings indicate that regular physical activity may reduce the risk of breast cancer, especially in premenopausal or younger women (6,9,57,58). Evidence is too limited or inconsistent to support conclusions regarding the effect of physical activity on other cancers (6,9).

**Osteoporosis.** Throughout life, regular weight-bearing physical activity helps to maintain the normal structure and functional strength of bone (1,6). Increasing peak bone mass reached by age 30 and protecting against bone loss in later years reduces the risk of osteoporosis, a debilitating bone-thinning disease affecting 20 million women and 7 to 12 million men in the U.S. (59).

Numerous studies indicate that regular weight-bearing physical activity, especially throughout life, helps to protect against osteoporosis (6,60–65). However, physical activity alone is insufficient to protect against this disease (66). In addition to physical activity, diet (especially adequate calcium and vitamin D intake), and hormonal status (estrogen) contribute to skeletal health (66).

Increased physical activity and calcium intake have been demonstrated to increase bone density and decrease bone loss at various skeletal sites (61,67–70). A review of 17 trials found that physical activity exerted beneficial effects on bone mineral density at the lumbar spine at high calcium intakes (i.e., >1,000 mg/day), but not at calcium intakes less than 1,000 mg/day (67). Other studies indicate independent effects of physical activity and dietary calcium on bone health (61,69,70). In a recent investigation involving 422 women ages 25 to 65 years in Finland, both high physical activity and high calcium intake (i.e., 1,475 mg/day versus 638 mg/day) were associated with higher total bone mineral content than in participants who were less physically active and consumed lower amounts of calcium (70).

Weight-bearing aerobic activities such as walking, tennis, and low impact aerobics, as well as high-intensity strength training, improve bone density (6,68). When 39 postmenopausal, sedentary women participated in either high-intensity strength training exercises two days a week for one year or remained sedentary, bone density in the exercise group increased by an average of 1.5%, whereas it declined by about 2% in the sedentary women (68). The high-intensity strength training not only helped to preserve bone density, but it also increased muscle strength and balance, all of which can reduce the risk of future osteoporotic fractures (68).

Clearly, regular weight-bearing exercise benefits bone health at all ages. Because the benefits of weight-bearing exercise are site specific, it is best to participate in a variety of physical activities.

## LATER ADULT YEARS

Physical activity is especially important for older adults because of their often low functional status and high incidence of major chronic diseases (6,12,71,72). A recent cross-sectional study involving over 2,000 adults 65 years of age and older associated high intensity physical activity with lower blood insulin, triglyceride, and fibrinogen levels, reduced obesity, higher HDL cholesterol levels, and reduced risk of heart attacks and heart injury (72). Similarly, physical activity in

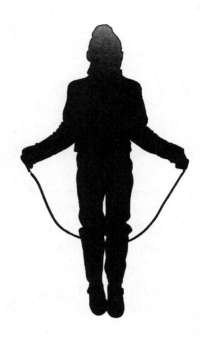

*All Americans, children and adults, are encouraged to participate in about 30 minutes of moderate intensity physical activity on most, and preferably all, days of the week.*

later adult years positively affects multiple risk factors for osteoporotic fractures (i.e., skeletal fragility, muscle weakness, and deteriorating balance) (6,8,68).

Physical activity in later adult years may help improve muscle strength, aerobic endurance, functional capacity, gait, joint flexibility, balance, reaction time, and overall quality of life (6,8,12,13,68). Reduced muscle strength is a major cause of disability among older adults (12). Resistance or strength training has been demonstrated to be beneficial for even frail, institutionalized elderly adults aged 72 to 98 years (13). Also, the increased energy needs resulting from a more physically active lifestyle may allow older adults to improve their overall nutritional intake when energy needs are met by nutrient-dense foods.

## RECOMMENDATIONS FOR A PHYSICALLY ACTIVE LIFESTYLE

There is a general consensus among medical and physical activity experts that all Americans, children and adults, should participate in about 30 minutes of moderate intensity physical activity on most, and preferably all, days of the week (2,5–8). It is now widely recognized that moderate intensity activity equivalent to brisk walking at 3 to 4 mph, and not necessarily a structured, vigorous exercise program, confers health benefits. Resistance or strength exercise at a moderate intensity for two to three days a week is also recommended, especially for older adults (8,13,61,68,73).

Motivating sedentary individuals to become more physically active is a major challenge (35,74). The key to encouraging individuals to lead more physically active lifestyles is to help them identify activities that they enjoy, feel competent and safe doing, and fit into their schedules and budgets (8,35).

Physical activity alone is not the answer to health. Rather, physical activity should be combined with a healthful diet made up of a variety of foods in moderation from the major food groups (3,5). To help the public put food, nutrition, and physical activity messages into action, the Dietary Guidelines Alliance (4) has implemented a campaign called "It's All About You." This campaign provides action tips for the following five supporting messages: "Be Realistic," "Be Adventurous," "Be Flexible," "Be Sensible," and "Be Active" (4). The "Be Active" message encourages the public to think fun and remember that small amounts of physical activity add up over time (4).

## REFERENCES

1. Blair, S.N., E. Horton, A.S. Leon, et. al. Med. Sci. Sports Exerc. 28(3): 335, 1996.

2. Pate, R.R., M. Pratt, S.N. Blair, et. al. JAMA 273: 402, 1995.

3. The American Dietetic Association. J. Am. Diet. Assoc. 97: 71, 1997.

4. The Dietary Guidelines Alliance. Reaching Consumers With Meaningful Health Messages. A Handbook for Nutrition and Health Communicators. A project of the Dietary Guidelines Alliance, 1996.

5. U.S. Department of Agriculture and U.S. Department of Health and Human Services. Nutrition and Your Health: Dietary Guidelines for Americans. 4th edition. Home & Garden Bulletin No. 232. Washington, DC: U.S. Government Printing Office, 1995.

6. U.S. Department of Health and Human Services. Physical Activity and Health: A Report of the Surgeon General. Atlanta, GA: U.S. Department of Health and Human Services, Centers for Disease Control and Prevention, National Center for Chronic Disease Prevention and Health Promotion, 1996.

7. NIH Consensus Development Panel on Physical Activity and Cardiovascular Health. JAMA 276: 241, 1996.

8. Fletcher, G.F., G. Balady, S.N. Blair, et. al. Circulation 94: 857, 1996.

9. World Cancer Research Fund in association with American Institute for Cancer Research. Food, Nutrition and the Prevention of Cancer: a Global Perspective. Washington, DC: American Institute for Cancer Research, 1997.

10. International Life Sciences Institute. Improving Children's Health Through Physical Activity: A New Opportunity. A Survey of Parents and Children About Physical Activity Patterns. July 1997.

11. Telama, R., L. Laakso, X. Yang, et. al. Am. J. Prev. Med. 13: 317, 1997.

12. Evans, W.J., and D. Cyr-Campbell. J. Am. Diet. Assoc. 97: 632, 1997.

13. Fiatarone, M.A., E.F. O'Neill, N.D. Ryan, et. al. N. Engl. J. Med. 330: 1769, 1994.

14. Paffenbarger, R.S., Jr., J.B. Kampert, I.-M. Lee, et. al. Med. Sci. Sports Exerc. 26(7): 857, 1994.

15. Kushi, L.H., R.M. Fee, A.R. Folsom, et. al. JAMA 277: 1287, 1997.

16. Kujala, U.M., J. Kaprio, S. Sarna, et. al. JAMA 279: 440, 1998.

17. The American Dietetic Association. Nutrition Trends Survey 1997. September 1997.

18. Federation of American Societies for Experimental Biology, Life Sciences Research Office. Prepared for the Interagency Board for Nutrition Monitoring and Related Research. Third Report on Nutrition Monitoring in the United States: Executive Summary. Washington, DC: U.S. Government Printing Office, December 1995.

19. National Center for Health Statistics. Healthy People 2000 Review, 1995–96. Hyattsville, MD: Public Health Service, 1996.

20. U.S. Department of Agriculture, Agricultural Research Service. Data tables: results from USDA's 1996 Continuing Survey of Food Intakes by Individuals and 1996 Diet and Health Knowledge Survey, [Online]. ARS Food Surveys Research Group. December, 1997. Available (under "Releases"): <http://www.barc.usda.gov/bhnrc/foodsurvey/home.htm> [February 25, 1998].

21. Centers for Disease Control and Prevention, U.S. Department of Health and Human Services, National Center for Chronic Disease Prevention and Health Promotion. CDC's Guidelines for School and Community Programs to Promote Lifelong Physical Activity Among Young People. March 1997.

22. Division of Health Examination Statistics, National Center for Health Statistics, Division of Nutrition and Physical Activity, National Center for Chronic Disease Prevention and Health Promotion, CDC. MMWR 46(9) (March 7): 199, 1997.

23. Bar-Or, O., J. Foreyt, C. Bouchard, et. al. Med. Sci. Sports Exerc. 30: 2, 1998.

24. Ogden, C.L., R.P. Troiano, R.R. Briefel, et. al. Pediatrics 99(4): e1, 1997.

25. Mei, Z., K.S. Scanlon, L.M. Grummer-Strawn, et. al. Pediatrics 101(1): e12, 1997.

26. Dietz, W.H. J. Nutr. 128: 411s, 1998.

27. Christoffel, K.K., and A. Ariza. Pediatrics 101: 103, 1998.

28. Vuori, I. Nutr. Rev. 54(4): 11s, 1996.

29. Dyson, K., C.J.R. Blimkie, K.S. Davison, et. al. Med. Sci. Sports Exerc. 29(4): 443, 1997.

30. Gunnes, M., and E.H. Lehmann. Acta Paediatr. 85: 19, 1996.

31. Teegarden, D., W.R. Proulx, M. Kern, et. al. Med. Sci. Sports Exerc. 28: 105, 1996.

32. Raitakari, O.T., S. Taimela, K.V.K. Porkka, et. al. Med. Sci. Sports Exerc. 29(8): 1055, 1997.

33. Johnson-Down, L., J. O'Loughlin, K.G. Koski, et. al. J. Nutr. 127: 2310, 1997.

34. Blair, S.N., J.B. Kampert, H.W. Kohl, III, et. al. JAMA 276: 205, 1996.

35. Clark, K.L., In: Cardiovascular Nutrition. Strategies and Tools for Disease Management and Prevention. P. Kris-Etherton and J.H. Burns (Eds). Chicago, IL: The American Dietetic Association, 1998, p. 27.

36. Marragat, J., R. Elosua, M.-I. Covas, et. al. Am. J. Epidemiol. 143: 562, 1996.

37. Leaf, D.A., D.L. Parker, and D. Schaad. Med. Sci. Sports Exerc. 29(9): 1152, 1997.

38. Koenig, W., M. Sund, A. Doring, et. al. Circulation 95: 335, 1997.

39. Pols, M.A., P.H.M. Peeters, J.W.R. Twisk, et. al. Am. J. Epidemiol. 146: 322, 1997.

40. Folsom, A.R., D.K. Arnett, R.G. Hutchinson, et. al. Med. Sci. Sports Exerc. 29(7): 901, 1997.

41. Mensink, G.B.M., D.W. Heerstrass, S.E. Neppelenbroek, et. al. Med. Sci. Sports Exerc. 29(9): 1192, 1997.

42. Niebauer, J., R. Hambrecht, T. Velich, et. al. Circulation 96: 2534, 1997.

43. The Sixth Report of the Joint National Committee on Prevention, Detection, Evaluation, and Treatment of High Blood Pressure. Arch. Intern. Med. 157: 2413, 1997.

44. Kuczmarski, R., K.M. Flegal, S.M. Campbell, et. al. JAMA 272: 205, 1994.

45. National Institute of Diabetes and Digestive and Kidney Diseases, National Institutes of Health. Physical Activity and Weight Control. NIH Publ. No. 96-4031, April 1996.

46. Hill, J.O., and R. Commerford. Int. J. Sports Nutr. 6: 80, 1996.

47. King, N.A., A. Tremblay, and J.E. Blundell. Med. Sci. Sports Exerc. 29: 1076, 1997.

48. Pritchard, J.E., C.A. Nowson, and J.D. Wark. J. Am. Diet. Assoc. 97: 37, 1997.

49. Racette, S.B., D.A. Schoeller, R.F. Kushner, et. al. Am. J. Clin. Nutr. 62: 345, 1995.

50. Grodstein, F., R. Levine, L. Troy, et. al. Arch. Intern. Med. 156: 1302, 1996.

51. Schoeller, D.A., K. Shay, and R.F. Kushner. Am. J. Clin. Nutr. 66: 551, 1997.

52. Kraemer, W.J., J.S. Volek, K.L. Clark, et. al. J. Appl. Physiol. 83(1): 270, 1997.

53. American Diabetes Association. Diabetes Care 21(suppl.1): 32, 1998.

54. Burchfiel, C.M., D.S. Sharp, J.D. Curb, et. al. Am. J. Epidemiol. 141: 360, 1995.

55. Lynch, J., S.P. Helmrich, T.A. Lakka, et. al. Arch. Intern. Med. 156: 1307, 1996.

56. Hoffman-Goetz, L. Nutr. Rev. 56(s): 126, 1998.

57. Thune, I., T. Brenn, E. Lund, et. al. N. Engl. J. Med. 336(18): 1269, 1997.

58. Gammon, M.D., E.M. John, and J.A. Britton. J. Natl. Cancer Inst. 90: 100, 1998.

59. Looker, A.C., E.S. Orwoll, C.C. Johnston, Jr., et. al. J. Bone Miner. Res. 12(11): 1761, 1997.

60. American College of Sports Medicine. Med. Sci. Sports Exerc. 27(4): i, 1995.

61. Nelson, M.E., E.C. Fisher, F.A. Dilmanian, et. al. Am. J. Clin. Nutr. 53: 1304, 1991.

62. Etherington, J., P.A. Harris, D. Nandra, et. al. J. Bone Miner. Res. 11(9): 1333, 1996.

63. Alekel, L., J.L. Clasey, P.C. Fehling, et. al. Med. Sci. Sports Exerc. 27(11): 1477, 1996.

64. Taffe, D.R., T.L. Robinson, C.M. Snow, et. al. J. Bone Miner. Res. 12(2): 255, 1997.

65. Dook, J.E., C. James, N.K. Henderson, et. al. Med. Sci. Sports Exerc. 29(3): 291, 1997.

66. Heaney, R.P. Nutr. Rev. 54(4): 3s, 1996.

67. Specker, B.L. J. Bone Miner. Res. 11(10): 1539, 1996.

68. Nelson, M.E., M.A. Fiatarone, C.M. Morganti, et. al. JAMA 272: 1909, 1994.

69. Suleiman, S., M. Nelson, F. Li, et. al. Am. J. Clin. Nutr. 66: 937, 1997.

70. Uusi-rasi, K., H. Sievanen, I. Vuori, et. al. J. Bone Miner. Res. 13(1): 133, 1998.

71. Evans, W.J. Nutr. Rev. 54(1): 35s, 1996.

72. Siscovick, D.S., L. Fried, M. Mittelmark, et. al. Am. J. Epidemiol. 145(11): 977, 1997.

73. Nelson, M.E., and S. Wernick. Strong Women Stay Young. New York: Bantam Books, 1997.

74. Andersen, R.E., S.N. Blair, L.J. Cheskin, et. al. Ann. Intern. Med. 127: 395, 1997.

## ACKNOWLEDGMENTS

National Dairy Council® assumes the responsibility for this publication. However, we would like to acknowledge the help and suggestions of the following reviewers in its preparation:

■ Kristine L. Clark, Ph.D., R.D.
Director, Sports Nutrition Program
Assistant Professor of Nutrition
Center for Sports Medicine
Pennsylvania State University
University Park, PA

■ Miriam E. Nelson, Ph.D.
Associate Chief, Human Physiology
Laboratory at the Jean Mayer USDA
Human Nutrition Research Center on Aging
Tufts University
Boston, MA

The Dairy Council Digest® is written and edited by Lois D. McBean, M.S., R.D.

# Alcohol and Health

## THE STORY

*Fountain of youth: A drink a day can help you live longer —* Boston Herald, Dec. 11, 1997

*Studies confirm relationship of alcohol to breast cancer —* New York Times, Feb. 18, 1998

Which of these is the truth: Is alcohol a life-extending elixir or a soothing poison? It's actually a combination of these, depending on how much you drink, your general health, and personal risk factors for a host of health problems, including heart and liver disease, many cancers, and alcoholism.

In the United States, public health campaigns have traditionally urged people to avoid alcohol or cut back on their drinking. And rightly so — heavy drinking is the second leading cause of preventable death in the US, right behind cigarette smoking. Alcohol is implicated in up to half of all fatal traffic accidents. Heavy drinking clearly contributes to liver disease, a variety of cancers, a weakening of the heart muscle, high blood pressure, strokes, and depression, and can take a terrible toll on families and relationships. Even moderate drinking interferes with a host of medications or magnifies their negative side effects.

A new countermovement, though, is touting the apparent benefits of a drink a day on the heart and circulatory system. These recommendations are spurred by studies from around the world showing that alcohol offers some protection against heart disease, the leading cause of death in the US and other developed countries.

The latest, and largest, of these was published in the December 11, 1997 *New England Journal of Medicine*. Researchers from the American Cancer Society, the World Health Organization, and Oxford University looked at causes of death and death rates in half a million men and women, all of whom had answered a questionnaire in 1982 about their drinking, smoking, and other habits. Over the following 10 years, moderate drinkers — those who had a drink a day — were 20 percent less likely to die than people who didn't drink at all, thanks to substantial reductions in death from heart disease.

The overall picture masks some important trends. Even though moderate drinking was associated with an overall lower death rate from heart disease, alcohol's protective effect was relatively small among those at low risk for heart disease and more powerful among those at high risk for it. As expected, deaths from alcoholism; cirrhosis of the liver; cancers of the liver, mouth, throat, larynx, or esophagus; and injuries or accidents were highest among the heaviest drinkers. And when the researchers looked at causes of

death for women, they found a greater risk of dying from breast cancer among women who reported having at least one drink a day compared with nondrinkers.

Other researchers found a similar connection between drinking and breast cancer in an analysis of six long-term studies that included more than 300,000 women, published in the February 18 *Journal of the American Medical Association*. Among women who averaged one or fewer drinks a day, the breast cancer risk was 9 percent higher than it was among nondrinkers. (This doesn't mean that 9 percent of women who have a drink a day will develop breast cancer. Rather, it's the difference between 11 of every 10,000 women developing breast cancer — the current US risk — and 12 of every 10,000 developing the disease.) Among those who reported having two to five drinks a day, breast cancer rates rose by 41 percent.

A study of more than 5,000 Italian women, published in the March 4 *Journal of the National Cancer Institute*, also found a connection between increasing amounts of alcohol and breast cancer. The researchers calculated that more than 20 grams of alcohol (slightly more than one drink) a day and little physical activity accounted for about 20 percent of breast cancers; and

Reprinted with permission from *Health News*, March 31, 1998, pp. 1-2. © 1998 by the Massachusetts Medical Society. All rights reserved.

more than 40 percent among premenopausal women.

Parallel lines of research are showing that we can't view alcohol as all bad or all good. Finding your own balance of benefits and risks may be challenging, but it's well worth the effort.

— *The Editors*

## THE PHYSICIAN'S PERSPECTIVE

*Charles H. Hennekens, MD*
*Associate Editor*

Given the way medical science works, and the way the media interact with scientists, you will probably see more conflicting headlines about alcohol and health in the months to come. Most studies, and the news reports that follow them, examine a single connection — alcohol and heart disease, alcohol and breast cancer, alcohol and mortality. While such narrowly focused studies clearly advance what we know about the impact of alcohol on the body, they don't reflect the broader reality. The alcohol you consume in a glass of wine, beer, or spirits alters mood and metabolism, and influences a variety of organs, including your brain, stomach, intestines, liver, and many glands. The complexity of alcohol's effects make it difficult to untangle its benefits from its risks.

Small amounts of alcohol offer some people subtle physical benefits. A drink before a meal can improve one's appetite and aid digestion, and may also keep bowel movements regular. Furthermore, many people look forward to having a drink at the end of a long, stressful day or enjoy the occasional drink with friends — emotional or psychic benefits that may improve health and well-being.

The scientific jury is still out on the degree to which light to

moderate amounts of alcohol may benefit the heart, despite what the headlines may claim. A number of large, carefully constructed studies support the hypothesis that drinking small to moderate amounts of alcohol helps prevent the development of coronary heart disease. We think that alcohol itself is playing this role by raising levels of protective HDL cholesterol or by preventing the formation of small clots that can block blood vessels in the heart. It may, however, be something about people who drink in moderation that is the real cause. For example, according to a large national survey on American eating habits, moderate drinkers are more likely than nondrinkers or heavy drinkers to exercise, watch their diets, and get adequate sleep, each of which may have an independent and beneficial impact on heart disease.

Moderate drinking carries risks as well as benefits. It may interrupt sleep, or degrade the quality of sleep. It is notorious for impairing judgment. And even modest amounts of alcohol can interact with medications in harmful ways. Some antidepressants, sedatives, painkillers, and anticonvulsants can amplify the effects of alcohol, causing inebriation at lower intakes. Alcohol can also amplify the harmful side effects of some medications. Finally, research has consistently shown that moderate drinking increases the likelihood of dying

from liver disease, strokes caused by bleeding inside the brain, breast cancer, and suicide and accidental deaths.

One thing is clear: Assumptions that the average person should begin to have a drink a day are premature, or even misguided. None of us is the mythical average person. Each of us has a unique personal and family history, as well as habits that predispose us to or protect us from diseases. So alcohol offers each of us different risks and benefits.

Alcohol offers abundant risk and no net benefit for pregnant women, recovering alcoholics, people with a family history of alcohol abuse, anyone with liver disease or a weakening of the heart muscle (cardiomyopathy), and anyone taking medications that may interact with alcohol.

Assuming that you don't fall into any of those categories, the

balance between risk and benefit is harder to calculate. Let me give several examples. A 23-year-old man reaps no net benefit from a drink or two a day, because he is at very low risk for developing heart disease and is at high risk for accidental, often alcohol-related, injury or death. Furthermore, there's no getting an early start since any possible "heart benefits" of alcohol aren't stored up for the future. A 55-year-old man who has high cholesterol levels and whose mother died of a heart attack may benefit from a drink a day, assuming he doesn't fall into any of the categories mentioned above. For a 55-year-old woman with high cholesterol and a family history of breast cancer, the risk-benefit calculation is more complicated. Heart disease kills five to six times more women each year than breast cancer, 236,000 compared with 44,000. And the increase in breast cancer associated with a drink a day or less is small. So on the face of it, the occasional drink may offer a net benefit. But a woman who is more afraid of developing breast cancer than heart disease may want to choose to avoid alcohol.

**The health benefits of an alcoholic drink a day are substantially smaller than those offered by exercise and eating right. So a healthy lifestyle offers you the best chance of avoiding disease and living longer. You can best determine whether or not the occasional drink should be part of that healthy lifestyle by talking with your physician and taking an inventory of your health and health risks.**

**If you decide that it should, the key word must be moderation. Given the complexity of alcohol's physiological, metabolic, and psychological effects, the difference between a little bit of alcohol and a lot may be the difference between preventing disease and premature death, and causing it.**

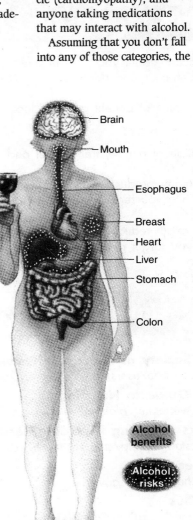

Brain
Mouth
Esophagus
Breast
Heart
Liver
Stomach
Colon
Alcohol benefits
Alcohol risks

## Unit Selections

## Key Points to Consider

❖ How does concern about your weight affect your life and that of your friends? Analyze your attitudes and behavior and describe what, if any, changes are appropriate.

❖ What are the issues of benefit and risk that one should consider before deciding to go on a diet?

❖ Find a description of a new, trendy diet and evaluate it for effectiveness and safety.

❖ Which of the many products with fat and sugar substitutes do you like? What is your purpose in using them? Do you reduce total calories by using these products?

❖ Do you think weight reduction should be a national goal? Why or why not? What population groups would you target and what strategies would you use?

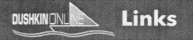 **Links**  **www.dushkin.com/online/**

These sites are annotated on pages 4 and 5.

*If you wish to grow thinner, diminish your dinner, And take to light claret instead of pale ale; Look down with an utter contempt upon butter, And never touch bread till it's toasted—or stale.*
—H.S. Leigh, A Day for Wishing

There have been times and places in history when being fat was considered beautiful. Harry Golden, writing in *Only in America* (Cleveland, Ohio: The World Publishing Company, 1958), tells how it was on the Lower East Side of New York when he was a boy. For 2 cents and accompanied by lots of fanfare, the salesman would guess a person's weight and weigh him or her in public. It was a big social event on Saturday night in a society where women bragged about gaining 5 pounds and practiced ways of simulating double chins.

Most of today's society, however, does not view fat pounds with pride. Thin is in. It is the willowy person who is seen as beautiful, socially acceptable, and appealing to the opposite sex. Many of us with bulges and bumps will knead and pound, use saunas, and starve ourselves—anything to lose a pound. In spite of ourselves, however, we are doing some things right. Fewer people are dieting, and more people realize the necessity for a permanent lifestyle change if lower weights are to be achieved and maintained. Seventy percent of the population claims to be eating more healthily than they did three years ago.

Inevitably, a discussion of weight turns to definitions. When is a person overweight? How much can one weigh and still be healthy? There is considerable scientific support for a causative connection between obesity and increased risks of numerous degenerative diseases such as diabetes, hypertension, and gallstones. However, a candid observer might argue that nobody agrees on appropriate weights and that recommendations bounce up and down like a yo-yo. There is truth in this observation. Most recently, as the first brief article in this unit notes, the federal government's first clinical definition defines obesity as a body mass index (BMI) of 25 or greater. But through the years there also has been evidence of less correlation between higher weights and health risks as people get into their seventies, even support for somewhat higher weights as people age. An additional article in this unit specifically addresses the issue of mortality rates in relation to body mass index and differences between men and women.

In despair, many of us on the plus side of accepted weight guidelines have asked, "What is a body to do?" We briefly hoped that the discovery of the protein leptin would provide a real breakthrough, but such is not yet the case, as an article on obesity and the brain indicates. Three articles attempt to provide answers, however, by identifying what has worked for successful weight losers and by challenging a number of very popular myths about weight loss. In the first of these articles we learn that losing weight is hard work but possible—even if we've failed before. Then we face some of the myths regarding exercise. Finally, several smaller meals as opposed to fewer large ones is suggested, especially for people approaching and reaching the golden years.

Simple answers as to why people gain weight would be a cause for celebration. If there is a magic word used with weight loss, it is exercise, and its significance can hardly be overstated. The one simple thing about weight gain is that it represents an energy unbalance, an intake of more calories than the body uses. One solution, then, is to increase activity. Indeed, a study at Johns Hopkins University showed that children who watch at least 4 hours of television daily are fatter than those who watch less and are presumably more active. Two-thirds of teenagers get minimum amounts of exercise, and a fifth of girls get no exercise at all. Even larger numbers of adults are inactive. We might ask what happened to physical education in the schools. Only Illinois still requires daily physical education in all grades. Although not specifically included in this unit, an article on exercise and nutrition does appear in unit 3.

For a long time we have believed that reducing fat intake would result in lower weight. According to surveys, people *are* eating lighter versions of favorite foods, a topic treated in unit 1. Furthermore, it would seem that we're making progress toward the recommended 30 percent of calories or less from fat, for the percentage of calories attributed to fat is now between 33 percent and 34 percent, down from 40 percent a decade ago and 45 percent around 1965. Some of this reduction is merely an illusion. Because we have simultaneously kept total fat the same *and* increased the number of calories consumed, the percentage of fat calories automatically has declined. But weights continue to go up. In fact, it is generally conceded that, in affluent nations, obesity has become an epidemic.

Surveys indicate that 54 million Americans, or 27% of the population, will go on a diet this year. As many as half of adult women and a quarter of adult men are dieting at any given time. Even more dramatic is the high number of grade school and adolescent girls who have reported weight loss attempts, often at the behest of their mothers. Dieters will try different methods, often joining a locally available weight-loss program such as Weight Watchers or Nutri/System. In a critical review, *Environmental Nutrition* looks at the various components of nine popular programs and identifies the pros and cons of each. A related article explores the effectiveness of dieting techniques.

Although drugs have been available to treat obesity for nearly 50 years, it is only in the last decade that they have become widely used. A combination drug known as "fen-phen" was extremely popular but has been withdrawn due to a possible link to heart valve problems. An article on "natural" therapeutics explores the advisability of using alternative chemical aids.

Two articles on eating disorders conclude this unit. It is ironic, in a country with the highest prevalence of obesity, that we are simultaneously very concerned about the millions who are starving themselves. Eating disorders, with their high morbidity and mortality rates, often are not diagnosed because the behaviors seem culturally normal. It may be no surprise that anorexia nervosa is seven times more common in strict ballet schools as compared to the rest of the population, and that half of these young women are amenorrheic. Almost 20 percent of high school wrestlers exhibit eating-disordered behaviors during wrestling season as well. And, unlike the stereotype of the upper-class, suburban white girl, eating disorders are also common among inner-city African Americans and new armed forces female recruits.

**Prevention**

# Guidelines Call More Americans Overweight

In early June, the American Heart Association added obesity to its list of major, controllable risk factors for heart disease, calling it a "chronic disease" and a "dangerous epidemic." Later that month, the federal government issued its first clinical guidelines on obesity. Under the new definition, people are considered overweight if their body mass index (BMI) is 25; previous recommendations put the mark at about 27. This means that 97 million people or 55% of American adults are now considered too fat for their own good.

In developing the guidelines, a panel of 24 experts, convened by the National Heart, Lung, and Blood Institute (NHLBI), conducted an extensive review of the scientific literature on obesity to date. They concluded that being overweight increases the risk of heart disease, stroke, hypertension, lipid disorders, Type 2 diabetes, certain cancers, osteoarthritis, and other chronic conditions. The panel also noted that obesity is second only to smoking as the largest cause of preventable death in the United States.

To calculate BMI, multiply your weight in pounds by 703 and divide that figure by your height in inches squared. A man or a woman (BMIs are for both sexes) who is 5 feet 7 inches tall and weighs 159 pounds would previously have been in the "healthy" range, with a BMI of 25. That person is now considered overweight. But to achieve a BMI of 24, he or she would need to lose only 6 pounds.

Studies have repeatedly demonstrated that modest weight losses — of less than 10 pounds — can significantly lower blood pressure and harmful low-density lipoprotein (LDL) cholesterol. Some experts say that BMIs of 21 or 22 are best, but that anything between 18.5 and 25 is generally healthy. (The BMI is a reasonable measure for most people, but the formula may not apply to very muscular individuals.)

In addition to BMI, the guidelines call for doctors to measure patients' waist circumference because excess abdominal fat may increase the risk for diabetes and cardiovascular disease. A waist measurement of more than 40 inches in men and over 35 inches in women is considered a marker for risk in those with a BMI of 25 to 34.9.

The guidelines emphasize that there are no "new" or "magic" cures for weight loss and that the most successful strategy is the tried and true one: eat less and exercise more. The recommendations also note that people should attempt lifestyle modifications for at least 6 months before trying such weight loss drugs as phentermine or sibutramine.

Even when medication is called for, treatment should not last for more than one year because the safety and efficacy of these drugs have not been established beyond that point. The full NHLBI guidelines can be found on the Internet at www.nhlbi.nih.gov/nhlbi/.

From the *Harvard Health Letter*, August 1998, p. 7. © 1998 by the President and Fellows of Harvard College. Reprinted by permission.

# Body Mass Index and Mortality: Differences Between Men and Women

The relationship between body mass index (BMI = weight in kilograms divided by the square of the height in meters) and mortality has been used to examine the effect of obesity on mortality rates and causes for mortality. Several recent studies highlight inconsistencies in the conclusions drawn from such research.

In a large prospective, longitudinal cohort study of a sample of U.S. adults older than 70 at entry in the study, 7260 people (2769 men, 4491 women) were followed for a six-year period. (See Allison DB et al., *International J Obesity*, 1997; 21:424.) The minimum mortality occurred at a BMI of approximately 31.7 for women and 28.8 for men. The results were essentially unchanged, if analyses were weighted, if various disease states were controlled for and unhealthy subjects were excluded. Smoking status was not assessed. Numerous other studies cited in the article found that the relationship between BMI and mortality is not markedly different when controlling for smoking. Income and education were used to control for socioeconomic status, as this may reflect access to health care and living conditions. Indicators of pre-existing health problems significantly affected the relation to mortality. There appears to be a wide range of BMI that is well tolerated by older adults.

Mortality rates in relation to BMI were examined in a larger prospective cohort group of 48,287 younger Dutch men and women (30–54 years of age) over a six-year period. (See Seidell JC et al., *Arch Intern Med*, 1996; 156:958.) All-cause mortality was significantly increased in obese men (BMI > 30) and in underweight men (BMI < 18.5), but not in women. Lung cancer in smokers contributed to the deaths in the underweight men. Underweight men had increased mortality from all causes and from noncancer or noncardiovascular diseases. Coronary heart disease mortality was threefold higher among obese men and women. About 70% of the individuals in this study were between 35 and 45 years of age. Therefore, the effect of the aging process on the relationship

between obesity and mortality could not be addressed as various disease processes that develop late in life due to obesity would not have been identified yet.

In a study of more than 12 years' duration of 62,116 men and 262,019 women (nonsmokers > 30 years old at baseline), greater BMI was associated with higher mortality from all causes and from cardiovascular disease in men and women up to 75 years of age. (See Stevens J et al., *N Engl J Med*, 1998; 338:1.) The relative risk associated with greater BMI declined with age.

Individuals were excluded who may have had weight loss due to illness at the time of baseline measurements. In this study, BMI was estimated only once for each subject. Therefore, the effect of weight change over time could not be addressed.

In a longer follow-up period of 29 years, a smaller group (611 men and 687 women; 20–96 years old) showed a significant linear association between BMI and all-cause mortality in men less than age 65 years at baseline. (See Dorn JM et al., *Am J Epidemiol*, 1997; 146:919.) Body mass index was most strongly related to cardiovascular and coronary mortality in women and younger men. However, this association was not found in older men. Body mass index was not related to an increased risk of death from noncardiovascular disease or cancer in men or women. It is difficult to compare the relationship between mortality and BMI across the studies due to variance in study methodology, such as controlling or not controlling for smoking; failure to adjust for clinical or subclinical illness present at baseline and intermediate risk factors (such as hypertension, hyperlipidemia, and diabetes); difference in cut-off points for categories of BMI; unmeasured characteristics of study subjects; failure to control for weight loss; length of study; and lack of adjustment for baseline age.

However, these recent studies confirm the results of many previous studies that show that increased BMI (obesity) is associated with increased mortality, especially in younger subjects.

From *Nutrition & the M.D.*, May 1998, pp. 6-7. © 1998 by Lippincott, Williams & Wilkins. Reprinted by permission.

# OBESITY AND THE BRAIN

## BY ELIZABETH LASLEY

The fitness marketplace abounds with books and videos promising to turn various flabby body parts to steel. Certainly, trotting along with a svelte celebrity can put paid to those five or ten extra pounds. But the aerobics mavens have no solution for obesity. To find a treatment for this very serious condition, researchers are looking not to the abdomen or derriere, but to the brain.

The brain keeps itself informed as to how much stored energy, in the form of body fat, is available for use. If energy supplies run low, the brain activates stomach rumblings, salivation, thoughts of a nice thick steak—in other words, hunger. From an evolutionary standpoint, it's no bad thing to carry a modest surplus in the energy storehouse (read: tummy and hips); these bulges, though considered unsightly in our culture, mean that energy will be available to ensure survival when the food runs short.

Normally, the brain keeps energy stores in balance. But when body fat accumulates to the point where it becomes a health threat, it signals a disturbance in the brain's energy-information network. And in the present-day United States, when food shortage is

among the least of our problems, it behooves us to find out what is going awry in the intricate system that coordinates hunger and eating. According to the most recent National Health and Nutrition Examination Survey, more than half of Americans over age 20 are now overweight, nearly one quarter being clinically obese. The latter are at risk for potentially fatal diseases such as heart disease, diabetes, and cancer. And, alarmingly, the numbers are increasing.

But the prospects for treating obesity are brightening. In just the last several years, scientists have begun to unravel the mystery of energy regulation in the brain. Not only might this research yield successful weight-loss medications, but it might provide clues about other disorders that occur when the balance of energy is disrupted, such as eating disorders, diabetes, and reproductive disorders.

"There's been tremendous progress in this area," says Cliff Saper of Beth Israel Deaconess Hospital and Harvard Medical School, Boston. "We're beginning to understand the web of chemical signals involved in the body's use of energy—and where their pathways are in the brain."

### Sizing up fat reserves

As early as the 1970s, long before scientific evidence was forthcoming, researchers suspected that fat cells made an unknown factor that told the brain how much fat was in stock. When supplies reached the optimal level, this mysterious informant would advise the brain to decrease food intake. Now, scientists have identified at least two dozen such messengers (hormones and brain chemicals called neurotransmitters), some that suppress appetite, some that stimulate it. The hope is that medications yet to come can adjust the levels of these neurotransmitters, bring energy regulation back into balance, and help people lose weight and keep it off.

So far, the most promising candidate as a fat fighter is a hormone variously called OB protein (after the gene that produces it) or leptin (from the Greek word meaning thin). Though discovered only in 1994, leptin is the very "X factor" predicted by researchers more than 20 years ago. At that time, Douglas Coleman of Jackson Laboratory, Bar Harbor, Maine, surgically connected the circulatory systems of an obese mouse and a normal mouse. Lo and behold, the

From *Brain Work*, July/August 1998, pp. 1-3, 8. © 1998 by the Charles A. Dana Foundation. Reprinted by permission.

obese mouse began to approach normal weight. Coleman surmised that it was missing some weight-reducer that it could borrow from its normal partner. But he could not determine what the agent might be.

The agent was found in 1994, by Jeffrey Friedman, molecular biologist at the Howard Hughes Medical Institute at Rockefeller, New York. Using DNA technology that wasn't around in Coleman's day, Friedman and his colleagues at Rockefeller discovered the hormone, and the gene that produced it. Produced by fat cells when they reach a certain size, leptin circulates in the blood and enters the brain through a major processing center called the hypothalamus. The hypothalamus then adjusts the body's thermostat, boosting metabolism and quelling the brain mechanisms that produce the drive to eat.

The fat mice in Coleman's study were described as *ob/ob* because they carried a mutated version of the gene in question (OB). It is thought that obese people may have mutations in the corresponding human gene, or in the gene that produces the nerve cells' surface molecule, or receptor, that receives the leptin signal. But even before these mutations have been tracked down, giving additional leptin is showing promise as a weight-loss remedy both in mice and in humans.

The first clinical trial of leptin treatment in humans concluded this June. "Obese participants receiving leptin injections lost between one and 15 pounds, the latter receiving the highest dose and losing six or seven percent of body weight," says Andrew Greenberg, director of the Program in Obesity and Metabolism, Tufts University, and leader of the study.

This result is comparable to the weight loss one can expect from drugs currently approved to treat obesity, Greenberg notes, and the dose-response effect is an important confirmation of leptin's effectiveness biologically. All participants were on a weight-loss diet calculated to provide 500 calories less than they needed. However, those on a diet receiving no leptin lost only three or four pounds.

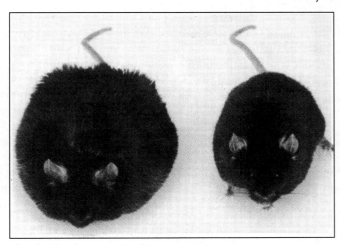

(Left) Mouse with defective ob *gene lacks the* OB *protein (leptin), which regulates the body, signaling the amount of fat stored. (Right) Mouse treated with leptin shed 40 percent of its body weight.*

No major side effects were reported, the most common being a slight swelling at the injection site.

Exactly how leptin brings about weight loss is not known. To confound the matter, unlike the test mice, obese humans are not leptin deficient. In fact, as weight goes up, the levels of circulating leptin increase. But if leptin is not in short supply, why does giving more help?

"It may be that, even though obese humans have high levels of leptin, it still might not be enough, based on their weight, to reset the body thermostat," says Greenberg. "Or they may not be sufficiently sensitive to their own leptin. There's a precedent for this in mature-onset diabetes. These patients have plenty of insulin, but for some reason their bodies don't respond to it properly. Yet they can be treated with insulin injections."

It may be that leptin receptors in the brain are not picking up the signal or are too few in number. "Our study has established, however, that some obese people can respond to extra leptin by losing weight, and that makes leptin a likely candidate for further study."

Friedman finds the study encouraging, though the trial involved only a small group (47 obese patients and 50 lean subjects finished). "The final

word on leptin's usefulness in weight reduction will come when it's tested in large numbers of people," he says. Larger multicenter trials have already begun with about 500 people.

One feature of leptin, however, is likely to limit widespread use: it is not absorbed when taken by mouth and can be given to people only by injection.

### The appetite network

Researchers suspect that leptin plays a more complex role than mere obesity prevention. After all, being too fat was probably not something evolving animals needed to worry about. "It was more plausible for leptin to regulate the body's response to starvation," says Jeffrey Flier, an endocrinologist at Beth Israel Deaconess.

It turns out that, when leptin levels fall too low, other neurotransmitters that stimulate the appetite are activated. Scientists are now studying whether the receptors for these neurotransmitters can be blocked to keep down hunger and weight. One, dubbed NPY, got off to a promising start as a hunger producer; when injected into the brains of rats, it triggered ravenous feeding. But the work of Richard Palmiter and colleagues at the Howard Hughes Institute at the University of Washington, Seattle, casts doubt on NPY's exclusive status in the "feeding center." Palmiter engineered mice that were missing either the NPY gene or the receptor, reasoning that if NPY is what causes eating, mice born without it should have no feeding urge, rendering them thin and puny. But, "they looked perfectly normal to us," Palmiter says. He concludes that though NPY may play a role in feeding, it isn't a solo performer. Members of the supporting cast—and potential targets for fat-busting drugs—include two proteins that are elevated in *ob/ob* mice; they are called, exotically, agouti-related peptide and melanocyte-concentrating hormone. The newest candidates, not yet much explored, are in the so-called "orexin" group.

### Other areas of exploration

Leptin weaves in and out of other conditions besides obesity. Using leptin to bring down weight may have a beneficial effect on diabetes, in which the body does not make enough insulin or fails to respond to it properly. Without insulin, blood sugar cannot enter and nourish the body's cells. Since obesity is thought to be a trigger for diabetes, anything that promotes weight loss can help fend off the disease. In addition, researchers at the Indiana University School of Medicine have reported findings from laboratory studies that suggest leptin may play a regulatory role in glucose metabolism directly within human fat tissue.

Insufficient leptin will throw off the body's mechanisms of growth and reproduction. "The brain uses fat supplies to gauge whether there's enough energy to do what needs to be done. If the amount of leptin suggests there isn't, the brain begins to shut off the luxuries—such as growing, reaching puberty, and having babies—in favor of sheer survival," says Saper.

Lack of leptin is also seen in the extreme thinness that results from anorexia, although here, for some reason, the low levels of the hormone do not touch off the customary hunger response. Low leptin also activates the hormones called glucocorticoids, involved in both the body's reaction to stress and in the working of the immune system. "Leptin clearly can influence the stress response," notes Jeffrey Flier.

Although leptin's role in anorexia, stress, and the immune response is unclear, teasing apart its pathways of communication may open up new ways to study these areas as well as what happens when they go awry. "The neural circuitry activated by leptin is highly complex," says Friedman. "To truly understand it, the challenge is to find the complete set of neurotransmitters and receptors and figure out what they do."

*Elizabeth Lasley is Assistant Editor of* BRAIN Work *.*

# What It Takes to Take Off Weight (And *Keep* It Off)

JUST 2 SHORT MONTHS after Fen-Phen, the popular weight-loss drug combination, was pulled from the market because of its link to a life-threatening heart disorder, the Food and Drug Administration approved another weight-loss medication, Meridia. But if the experience of successful weight losers is any indication, the new drug won't be the solution for shedding pounds either.

After surveying almost 800 people who have kept off at least 30 pounds for at least 1 year, researchers compiling a National Weight Control Registry found that only 4 percent of them used pills. Anne Fletcher, a registered dietitian, has had a similar finding. When she located more than 200 people who kept off at least 20 pounds for at least 3 years, she discovered that while many had tried weight-loss drugs at one time or another, pills helped virtually none of them with the final effort—the one that led to long-term success.

Ms. Fletcher, a former executive editor of the Tufts *Letter* who wrote about her findings in 2 books, *Thin for Life* and *Eating Thin for Life*, (Chapters/Houghton Mifflin Co., Boston), also came across several other facts about successful weight losers that dovetailed with those compiled at the National Weight Control Registry. A number of them turn common notions about weight loss on their ear.

For instance, in both groups, **many had been obese since childhood, undercutting the belief that if you've been carrying around extra fat for decades, it's next to impossible to shed it.** In addition, many had 1—or 2—overweight parents, proving that it is quite possible to "stifle" one's genetic legacy, as Ms. Fletcher puts it.

Then, too, **many lost weight once they were middle-aged or older, belying the idea that after a certain age, it's not worth trying to attain a healthier body.** The average age of people in the Weight Control Registry so far is 45. In Ms. Fletcher's books, a number of those she calls "masters at weight control" are in their 60s, 70s, and 80s. One 85-year-old man has kept off 47 pounds for 11 years; a 72-year-old woman, 97 pounds for 3 years.

Which points to another myth about weight loss—that it can only work for people who need to shed on the order of 20 to 30 pounds. The average weight loss of the people in Ms. Fletcher's books was 64 pounds. **Thirty people she tracked kept off 100 pounds—for 5 or more years.** Those in the Weight Control Registry lost, on average, 29 percent of their weight, sending the group's average size from obese to normal.

The weight losers come from all walks of life. Ms. Fletcher mentions a former show girl who took off 97 pounds, a chocolate scientist who melted away 25 pounds, and a state senator who trimmed 35 pounds. They also lost weight—and maintained their losses—in many different ways. Some joined formal programs such as Weight Watchers while others went solo. Some counted fat grams; others, calories. Still others simply kept tight control over portion sizes.

While the different success stories show that there is no one right way to handle food in order to lose weight, certain patterns did emerge, many involving shifts in *attitude*. The following pointers are culled from those patterns of success seen both in Ms. Fletcher's books and the National Weight Control Registry, which is maintained by researchers at the University of Pittsburgh School of Medicine and the University of Colorado Health Sciences Center.

**1.** **Don't view past failures as a sign that you can't succeed.** More than 90 percent of the people in the Weight Control Registry tried to lose weight previously. In fact, they had each lost—and regained—an average of 270 pounds. Nearly 60 percent of those in Ms. Fletcher's books tried to lose weight at least 5 times before they successfully took it off and kept it off.

The trick is to look at previous weight-loss attempts not as failures but, in the words of 2 psychologists, as "a rich library of what worked and what did not." For instance, if eating 3 fruits a day proved helpful last time but trying never to eat ice cream only made you go on ice cream binges, you might go back to eating the fruits and having a small, pre-set serving of ice cream 2 or 3 times a week.

**2.** **No pain, no loss.** It is the rare person who is able to lose weight without feeling a moment's deprivation. "You need to be able to endure some discomfort," Ms.

---

**Did you know...** All lettering on a food package must be at least 1/16 of an inch high, unless the package is extremely small. The letters also can't be more than 3 times as high as they are wide. And promotional words and phrases, including health claims, can't be more than twice the size of the food's name.

From *Tufts University Health & Nutrition Letter,* January 1998, pp. 4-5. © 1998 by Tufts University Diet & Nutrition Letter. Reprinted by permission.

Fletcher says, explaining that not everyone she interviewed "experienced a mystical attitude shift before losing weight that made the process easy."

The Weight Control Registry re-searchers point out that when registry members were asked to compare their successful weight-loss experience with previous attempts, they said they "used more intensive approaches...on the successful attempt." More than 60 percent incorporated a stricter dietary approach, while more than 80 percent noted that they exercised more.

Successful weight losers also appear to devote a great deal of psychological energy to staying with the program, sometimes to the point of seeming obsessive or neurotic—or at least a little loopy. Almost half of those in the Weight Control Registry, for instance, weigh themselves once a day—or more than once a day. In Ms. Fletcher's group, some people plan meals up to a week in advance, while others write down every single thing they eat as a way of monitoring themselves.

The payoffs, however, mean more to them than the freedoms of eating whatever they want whenever they want. The majority of Weight Control Registry members report improvements in all the following areas: quality of life, level of energy, mobility, general mood, self-confidence, physical health, interactions with others, and job performance. As someone in one of Ms. Fletcher's books sums it up, "It's not easy. But it beats the alternative."

**3.** **Break down your weight-loss goal into several smaller lifestyle goals.** A target weight, while motivating, can also be overwhelming and can make your weight-loss attempt seem like an all-or-nothing proposition. After all, if you place all of your energy on reaching that goal weight, then not getting there—or not getting there fast enough—makes it seem as if you've failed and therefore pushes you toward giving up.

But if you break down your efforts into many small lifestyle steps, it's easier to stick to the overall game plan. Let's say, for instance, that you make a pact with yourself to eat at least a half cup of green vegetables everyday; to increase the amount of time you spend exercising every other day by 5 minutes; and to switch from 2 percent fat milk in your coffee to 1 percent fat milk. Then, if you go off track by eating 2 slices of pie after dinner or overeating at a party, you won't end up feeling that your efforts to get down to goal weight have been ruined. You'll be able to count up all your successes, which outnumber the one lapse, and move on without further backsliding. That is, you won't continue to eat even more pie because you won't end up feeling that you've "blown it anyway."

It's called replacing "I will be" goals with "I will do" goals. You can't, in the short run, *be* a certain weight. But you can *do* all kinds of helpful things that will get you closer to that weight and that you can tally as successful lifestyle improvements as you go along. The more specific the goals (rather than vowing to eat fewer sweets, promise yourself not to eat more than a certain number of sweets a week), the easier it will be to add them up.

Small, doable goals will also allow you to be happier with your more healthful lifestyle if you don't ever reach goal weight—or if you reach it and then gain back some of the weight. That's because success will be defined as more than a number on the scale.

**4.** **Plan Indulgences.** "Never," "always," and "everyday" goals are recipes for disaster, Ms. Fletcher says. What, after all, are the odds that you'll never eat a piece of chocolate cake again? With such a plan, her book notes, "you are leaving yourself no room for *gradual* improvement. You are constantly living *one* mistake away from failure, one error away from defeat." Better to plan extremely carefully for eating those foods you love. You might, for instance, measure out just one scoop of your favorite pudding in a small bowl or cup every other night. Or eat 2 squares of a chocolate bar, or a slice of cake or pie as wide as a finger.

That's very hard for some people. Once they taste their favorite food, they simply can't stop. But if you purpose build a pre-set amount of that food int your weight-loss program, you mig have an easier time sticking to just th small portion you allot yourself ar really savoring every bite.

Such an approach makes it easier go from weight loss to weight maint nance. That's because you won't going "off" the diet once you reach go weight. The "diet" will have include foods that you'll want to enjoy at inte vals for the rest of your life.

**5.** **Exercise.** The men in th Weight Control Registry r ported burning more tha 3,500 calories a week through exe cise; the women, almost 2,700 cal ries. That's the equivalent of walki about 4 miles a day. Similarly, most those profiled in Ms. Fletcher's boo exercised 3 to 7 times a week. In oth words, most people who lose weig and keep it off engage in much mo physical activity than Americans typ cally do.

**6.** **Do what you want to make work.** If the icing on a cupca is what you're *really* after, the eat just the icing and throw the re out. You've thrown out food befor Why not throw it out in the service shedding excess pounds?

You also don't have to finish a ca or a bag of candy just because i there. The world won't come to an e if you let the food go stale.

Likewise, don't feel funny abo driving waiters crazy to make sure yo restaurant food is low in fat; or abo pushing half a gargantuan portion o to a second plate. And never feel ob gated to take seconds—or even firsts for fear of offending a host. If someo is insulted because you don't want eat a particular amount or a particul dish he or she prepared, let the proble remain the cook's, not yours.

Doing what you want goes beyor making your own food choices. M Fletcher says the successful weig losers she found also devoted bett attention to themselves in general doing more of what they *wante* instead of what they *should*.

# The skinny on weight loss

*The truth behind these common myths can help you lose weight when you need to—and stop worrying when you don't.*

*Slimming Insoles* help you lose weight "with every step you take." The *Svelt-Patch* "melts away body fat" even "while you sleep." *Absorbit-ALL Plus* supplements will "zap 3 inches from your thighs." Those and numerous other dubious claims exploit the most enduring of all weight-loss myths: There must be some way—short of taking possibly harmful drugs—to slim down quickly and easily. That myth can lead you to neglect the more demanding steps that really can help you lose weight.

Other weight-loss myths are less obvious but no less harmful. They can lead to needless or fruitless efforts to lose weight. Some may even be damaging to your health.

❶ **Myth: You can tell whether or not you need to lose weight by your appearance or by the size of your clothing.**

**Truth:** Many Americans, brainwashed by all the emaciated models they see, have a distorted image of a healthy physique. That's particularly true of those with a wide, big-boned frame, who couldn't possibly slim down to the supposedly ideal waiflike proportions. The decision to lose weight should be based primarily on whether your weight poses any health risk, not on whether you look as thin as you think you should.

Start by calculating your body-mass index (BMI); that measures how fat you are—a primary determinant of risk—by correlating weight to height. To figure your BMI, multiply your weight in pounds by 705, divide by your height in inches, then divide by your height again. In general, the risk of disease—notably coronary heart disease, diabetes, and several common cancers—is lowest for BMIs between 21 and 25; then it increases slightly between 25 and 27, substantially between 27 and 30, and dramatically for scores over 30. (A BMI below 21 is also linked with increased risk—but only because skinniness sometimes results from underlying health problems, not because it's intrinsically unhealthy.)

But you need to check more than just your BMI. For one thing, your BMI does not distinguish between muscle and fat, the real culprit. Further, body fat poses a substantially greater risk in people who have or are susceptible to such illnesses as coronary heart disease, stroke, and diabetes than it does in other people. And regardless of your current BMI, the risk of disease generally starts to rise if you've gained more than about 10 pounds as an adult.

Where the weight sits on your body also affects your health. Fat on the belly is linked with increased blood-cholesterol levels, hypertension, diabetes, and possibly breast cancer, regardless of your overall weight. So even if you have a desirable BMI, a chubby belly increases your risk of disease more than plump hips or thighs do. Women are at increased risk if the ratio of their waist to hip measurements exceeds 0.8, men if the ratio exceeds 1.0. To calculate your ratio, measure your waist at its narrowest point and your hips at their widest; then divide the waist measurement by the hip measurement.

❷ **Myth: Most overweight people could slim down if they just used a little self-control.**

**Truth:** Losing weight is hard. For one thing, your genes have determined the range of possible weights you could reasonably expect to sustain; even if you forced yourself below that range, your body would almost inevitably swing back. In addition, weight loss, particularly rapid loss from diet alone, slows the body's metabolic rate—its basic rate of burning calories. So a person who slims down to 150 pounds, for example, generally must consume fewer calories to maintain that weight than another 150-pound person who has never been overweight.

The good news is that losing just a little weight can substantially reduce your risk of disease. And improving your diet and exercise habits will improve your health even if you don't lose any weight at all.

❸ **Myth: Strength training won't help you lose weight, since it adds pounds of muscle and burns few calories.**

**Truth:** A typical strength-training session—with machines, free weights, or flexible bands—uses up calories at least as fast as moderately paced walking does. More important, muscle tissue burns calories faster than fat tissue, even when you're resting. So building muscle can increase the number of calories you burn throughout the day; that can help you not only lose weight but keep it off. And muscle is denser than fat, so even if you merely lost fat and added muscle, without losing any weight overall, you'd still become trimmer—and healthier.

❹ **Myth: Vigorous exercise promotes weight loss better than moderate exercise.**

**Truth:** A vigorous workout does burn more calories than a milder workout of the same duration. But a long, moderately intense workout burns more calories than a brief, strenuous one. And most people can

Reprinted with permission from *Consumer Reports on Health*, February 1998, pp. 1, 3-4. © 1998 by Consumers Union of U.S., Inc., Yonkers, NY 10703-1057.

# The fen-phen fiasco

Last September, the U.S. Food and Drug Administration persuaded the maker of two weight-loss drugs—dexfenfluramine (*Redux*) and fenfluramine (*Pondimin*)—to pull them off the market. The FDA acted after learning that up to 30 percent of users developed leaky heart valves. Fenfluramine and, to a lesser extent, dexfenfluramine, had recently become popular as part of "fen-phen," a prescription "cocktail" for weight loss that paired either drug with the appetite-curbing stimulant phentermine (*Ionamin*). Here's what to do if you've taken one of the withdrawn drugs—and what you should know about the alternatives.

## The dangerous drugs

For unknown reasons, both drugs seem to damage the heart valves in the same way they curb appetite—by boosting production of the brain chemical serotonin. None of the carefully controlled studies originally submitted to the FDA had even hinted at that problem. But then none of the studies had used the drugs the way many doctors prescribed them in real life: for long periods of time, in combination with other drugs, and in people who were not truly obese.

All former users of fenfluramine or dexfenfluramine should be checked for heart-valve leakage. In particular, those with possible indications of leaky valves—chest pain, fainting, palpitations, or a recently diagnosed heart murmur—should undergo an ultrasound imaging test of the heart called an echocardiogram.

A number of invasive medical or dental procedures—including deep cleaning of the teeth—can cause bacterial endocarditis, a potentially deadly heart infection, in people who have valve disease. So even former users who have no symptoms of the disease should ask their doctor whether they need an echocardiogram if they're about to undergo an invasive procedure. Antibiotics would have to be given before treatment if the test revealed significant leakage.

## New drugs and herbs

Despite the recent debacle, the FDA has approved a new weight-loss drug, sibutramine (*Meridia*), and will probably soon approve another, orlistat (*Xenical*). Both drugs are about as effective as the withdrawn drugs, helping a substantial minority of obese people reduce their weight by an average of 10 percent.

Unlike the withdrawn drugs, sibutramine does not increase secretion of serotonin. But all three drugs make serotonin work more effectively. (Sibutramine is also a stimulant, which further reduces appetite.) Despite the related mechanism, sibutramine does not seem to harm the heart valves. But it can cause other problems, notably increased blood pressure. While that rise is usually small, all sibutramine users must have their blood pressure monitored carefully; people with poorly controlled hypertension should avoid it entirely.

Orlistat fights obesity by inactivating certain intestinal enzymes needed to absorb dietary fat. That can produce bloating, gas, and loose stools if you consume lots of fat. It may also block absorption of fat-soluble vitamins, including vitamins A, D, and E, so users should take a multivitamin supplement. (Early concerns about a possible breast-cancer risk are apparently unfounded.)

The safety of the new drugs won't be clearly established until they've been used extensively. So consider them only if you're truly obese—with a BMI over 30 or a BMI over 27 plus multiple risk factors for obesity (see story)—and have really tried and failed to lose weight without drugs.

## Herbal fens

In the wake of the FDA ban, supplement makers have been flooding health-food stores with concoctions such as *Herbal Phen-Fen*, *PhenTrim*, and *Phen-Cal*. Those names clearly imply that the products offer the weight-loss power of fen-phen without the risk. But there's no good evidence that any of them can help people lose weight. Further, most of them contain ephedra, or ma huang, which has been linked with numerous problems, including nervousness, insomnia, headache, high blood pressure, irregular heart rate, even heart attack and stroke. And some contain chromium, which isolated reports have linked with anemia, kidney failure, and mental impairment.

exercise at a moderate pace for much longer than they can exercise strenuously.

For the average person, building up to sessions lasting at least 45 to 60 minutes, four to five times a week, is generally the most effective exercise regimen for weight loss. Two or preferably three times a week, you should devote some of those minutes to strength training. You could devote the rest to exercises like brisk walking, hiking, bicycling, cross-country skiing, or energetic dancing: They're vigorous enough to burn calories at a reasonable clip, yet sufficiently moderate, interesting, and easy on the joints that the average person could do them for a fairly long time.

❺ **Myth: The best weight-loss diet is a strict, very low calorie regimen.**

**Truth:** Extreme diets rarely work in the long run.

The sharp drop in your metabolic rate after rapid weight loss makes you likely to put the pounds back on. In addition, extreme diets increase the risk of gallstones. And some low-calorie diets—especially those that limit you to only a few foods, such as the popular grapefruit or cabbage-soup diets—might harm your health by depriving you of needed nutrients.

Instead of crash-dieting, try to make changes you can live with. The most healthful approach is to replace high-calorie fatty or sugary foods with more nutritious, lower-calorie foods like whole grains, beans, fruits, and vegetables. If you're already eating a healthful diet—or want to try a more aggressive approach—you could also reduce the size of your portions, particularly of any higher-calorie foods.

❺ **Myth: A low-fat diet will definitely help you lose weight.**

**Truth:** While the typical American diet has become less fatty, the typical American has become fatter, in part because the average intake of calories has actually gone up (see illustration). When people adopt a low-fat diet, they often compensate by eating

## Less fat, but fatter

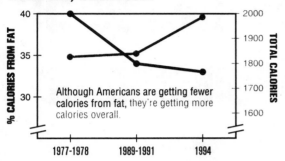

Although Americans are getting fewer calories from fat, they're getting more calories overall.

more than they did before. And many of the new foods manufactured to be low in fat have nearly as many calories as the regular versions, since manufacturers adjust for the loss of palate-pleasing fat by adding extra carbohydrates or protein. So if you want to lose weight, you need to watch the calories, not just the fat.

**❼ Myth: Cream, butter, lard, and other animal fats are more fattening than vegetable oils like canola and olive.**

**Truth:** Animal fats—as well as certain tropical oils, such as coconut and palm oil—are indeed worse for you than vegetable oils. But that's not because they're more fattening; rather, it's because they're high in saturated fat, which raises blood-cholesterol levels and the risk of coronary disease as well as possibly raising the risk of certain cancers. All fats, regardless of the source, provide the same number of calories, and thus pose the same potential for weight gain.

**❽ Myth: Carbohydrates make you gain weight, while protein helps you lose it.**

**Truth:** Several popular diet books have resurrected the antiquated notion that substituting protein for carbohydrates can melt away fat. But both of those dietary components contain four calories per gram, and the body socks away unused calories from both sources equally efficiently. Further, there's little evidence for the claim that protein helps curb the appetite.

Some diet gurus claim that carbohydrates raise blood levels of the hormone insulin, which in turn increases appetite and also helps convert carbohydrates to body fat. But carbohydrates may boost insulin only in people with insulin resistance, a metabolic disorder that prevents efficient use of the hormone. And there's no evidence that carbohydrates lead to weight gain even in those people. On the contrary, high-carbohydrate foods such as rice, pasta, and bread—preferably whole-grain versions—should be the mainstay of a healthful diet, though you need to go easy on the adornments, like butter and sauce. High-carbo foods are low in calories and fat, high in certain minerals and B vitamins and, if whole grain, high in fiber.

## Summing up

Judge the need to lose weight by your BMI, your body type, and the size of your waist and hips—not by your appearance. If you do need to lose:

■ Do lengthy workouts at the fastest pace that you can comfortably sustain—generally a moderate one. Spend some of that time strength training.

■ Instead of going on a crash diet, replace high-calorie foods with lower-calorie, healthier fare, such as produce and whole grains. If necessary, you can cut the portion sizes as well.

■ Watch your calorie intake even if you're already watching your fat intake.

■ Don't avoid carbohydrates; in fact, eat plenty of them—but go easy on the toppings.

# Several Small Meals Keep Off Body Fat Better Than One or Two Large Ones

As people reach their 50s and 60s, they remain able to burn fat from small meals just as efficiently as younger people. But they become much less able to burn the fat from large meals, according to a preliminary study conducted at Tufts. And that could contribute to the accumulation of body fat commonly seen in older adults.

The Tufts researchers made the finding when they compared the fat-burning ability of two groups of women, one in their 20s and another that was postmenopausal. Each group was given a 250-calorie snack, a 500-calorie meal, and a 1,000-calorie meal. All snacks and meals consisted of various amounts of peanut butter and jelly sandwiches with milk, and all of them had 35 percent of calories from fat.

The result: the older women were able to burn as much fat as the younger women after eating the 250- and 500-calorie portions. But they burned about 30 percent less fat after eating the 1,000-calorie meal, which is more or less the size of a big meal at a restaurant. Specifically, they burned only 187 of the fat calories present, while the younger women burned 246 fat calories. That could add up to a significant difference in body fat stores over time.

If future research confirms the findings, yet another piece of the puzzle about why older people are vulnerable to fat deposition will have been put into place. In the meantime, postmenopausal women and older men may want to hedge their bets by distributing their calories among three or four similar-size meals rather than eating most of their food at lunch or dinner. Women in their 60s and 70s consume, on average, 1,400 to 1,500 calories a day, so for them, that means eating a few 400-

## The younger women burned 246 fat calories from a 1,000-calorie meal; the older women, just 187 fat calories.

to 500-calorie meals rather than a single 750-calorie meal and two very small ones.

Men and women should also engage in strength-training exercises for about 45 minutes twice a week. That builds up muscle, which burns more fat than other body tissues—even when the body is at rest.

From *Tufts University Health & Nutrition Letter,* February 1998, p. 1. © 1998 by Tufts University Diet & Nutrition Letter. Reprinted by permission.

# Winnowing Weight-Loss Programs To Find A Match For You

If you're ringing in the New Year with a resolution to drop those excess pounds, you may be considering joining a weight-loss program. You're not alone. Eight million Americans opted for the likes of Diet Center, Optifast and Weight Watchers in 1996.

In this report, *EN* revisits nine weight-loss methods we reported on in 1994. Though some are remarkably unchanged, all are now cyber-savvy with Internet Web sites. Most have simplified plans and a few offer weight-loss medications. What hasn't changed: You must do your homework before you join.

The current trend among programs is to be user-friendly. For example, Weight Watchers has forsaken its strict portion control exchange system for *1-2-3 Success*, a program that assigns members a daily point allowance, with few limitations on how to spend it. Jenny Craig provides weekly menus based on *Jenny Craig's Cuisine* and even provides a shopping list for the few supermarket foods needed.

Until their recent withdrawal from the market amid charges of heart valve damage (see *EN*, October 1997), *Redux* and fenfluramine (one-half of the un-approved combination known as "fen-phen") were offered by several programs in addition to diet plans. Yet Diet Center, Optifast, Health Management Resources and Nutri/System continue to prescribe phentermine (the other half of fen-phen), despite a recent Food and Drug Administration (FDA) requirement that labels must warn users of possible heart damage.

More vexing is Nutri/System's promotion of *Herbal Phen-Fen* as a natural alternative. Its main ingredient is ephedra (ma huang), a powerful stimulant that can cause high blood pressure, heart attacks, even death. It remains to be seen if any of the programs will offer the newly approved weight-loss drug *Meridia*.

**Weighing the Options.** Finding out the facts can be difficult. Consumer groups have petitioned the Federal Trade Commission to make programs disclose up front their costs, health risks, staff qualifications and past success rates. But for now, you're on your own. Use our quick check list, below. If you can answer yes to most of these questions, you have a better chance for success.

- **Are you ready to lose weight and keep it off** *for better health*? If so, your odds for success are greater.

- **Do you understand the program's format?** Group meetings or individual counseling? Prepackaged fare or supermarket foods? Get the particulars.

- **Does the diet include all the food groups, every day?** If it doesn't, it's not healthful.

- **If the program includes prepackaged food, is it tasty?** Sample it first. If that's not allowed, don't join.

- **Does the program fit your lifestyle?** If you travel or socialize a lot, take that into consideration.

- **Do you know the total cost of the program?** Shedding 25 pounds could cost more than $1,000 at Nutri/System; at TOPS, it runs about $38.

- **Will the plan help you make positive behavior changes?** A good program teaches how to live a healthier lifestyle and provides on-going support for maintaining weight loss.

- **Does the program encourage a safe, personalized exercise program?** Regular physical activity is key to keeping the weight off.

*–Elizabeth M. Ward, M.S., R.D.*

Reprinted with permission from *Environmental Nutrition*, January 1998, pp. 1, 4-5. © 1998 by Environmental Nutrition, Inc., 52 Riverside Drive, Suite 15-A, New York, NY 10024.

| Program* | Environmental Nutrition's<br>Overall Approach |
|---|---|
| **Diet Center**<br>(Akron, OH )<br>(800) 333-2581<br>www.dietcenterworldwide.com | Personalized diet and exercise program, emphasizing healthy body composition. *Exclusively You* option based on supermarket foods; prepackaged cuisine optional. Minimum daily calorie level: 1,200. Vitamin and fiber supplements provided during reducing phase. *Concept 1000* option provides 1,000 daily calories from three meal replacements (shakes or bars) and one regular meal. Some locations offer phentermine. Body composition analysis at the start and every 4 to 6 weeks. |
| **Health Management Resources**<br>(Boston)<br>(617) 357-9876<br>www.yourbetterhealth.com | Makes use of a very-low-calorie diet (VLCD) consisting of fortified, high-protein liquid meal replacements (520-800 calories/day) under medical supervision. *Healthy Solutions* plan (1,000-1,600 calories/day) combines meal replacements with regular foods, including optional prepackaged HMR entrees and five servings of fruits and vegetables daily. Mandatory weekly 90-minute group meetings (60 minutes during maintenance). Dieters assigned personal coaches for weekly meetings or calls. Receive health risk appraisal. VLCD requires written approval from an M.D. for patients with certain medical conditions, such as diabetes. Phentermine available. |
| **Jenny Craig**<br>(La Jolla, CA)<br>(619) 812-7000<br>www.jennycraig.com | *ABC (About Better Choices)* program relies on *Jenny Craig's Cuisine* plus additional supermarket foods. 1,000 to 2,600 calories daily. Optional, weekly *Options Lifestyle* classes and one-to-one counseling. After losing half of goal weight, clients given option to transition to regular foods. |
| **Nutri/System**<br>(Horsham, PA)<br>(215) 442-5300<br>www.nutrisystem.com | Diet based mostly on Nutri/System's prepackaged foods. Reducing diet averages minimum of 1,200 calories/day for women; 1,500 for men. Maintenance diet based on optional purchase of prepackaged fare. Nutri/System's multivitamin/mineral supplement recommended for all dieters, but not included in price. Mostly one-to-one weekly counseling with weigh-in; some centers offer group classes. *Herbal Phen-Fen* and phentermine offered at some centers. |
| **Optifast**<br>(Minneapolis)<br>(800) 662-2540<br>www.optifast.com | Medically supervised program of fortified liquid meal replacements or prepackaged foods, eventually including regular foods. Dieters assigned one of three plans: 800, 950 or 1,200 calories daily. Mandatory weekly sessions promote positive eating behaviors. One-to-one counseling available. Some sites offer phentermine. |
| **Overeaters Anonymous**<br>(Rio Rancho, NM)<br>(505) 891-2664<br>www.overeatersanonymous.org | Nonprofit support group whose members are admitted compulsive eaters. Patterned after the 12-step Alcoholics Anonymous program. Addresses physical, emotional and spiritual aspects of overeating. Members encouraged to seek separate professional help for diet plan and dealing with emotional problems. |
| **Registered Dietitian Consultation**<br>(800) 366-1655 for free referral to local R.D.<br>www.eatright.org | Provides a personalized approach to weight control that takes into consideration your individual needs, including medical history, family situation, eating and exercise habits and preferences, travel and dining-out routines and budget. |
| **TOPS**<br>(Take Off Pounds Sensibly)<br>(Milwaukee)<br>(800) 932-8677<br>www.tops.org | Nonprofit organization whose members meet weekly in groups. Requires members to submit weight goals and diets in written form from health professionals. Provides peer support. Holds periodic contests and recognition programs for weight loss. |
| **Weight Watchers**<br>(Woodbury, NY)<br>(800) 651-6000<br>www.weight-watchers.com | Emphasizes calorie-controlled, high-fiber eating and healthful lifestyle habits. *1-2-3 Success* program assigns members daily food point allotment, which averages 1,250-1,500 calories/day for women. Weekly group meetings with mandatory weigh-in. Need to lose at least five pounds to join. |

\* Listed alphabetically

*Chart compiled by Elizabeth M. Ward, M.S., R.D.*

# Critique of Popular Weight-Loss Programs

| Healthful Lifestyle Components | Staffing | Cost / Results | *EN* Analysis |
|---|---|---|---|
| *Exclusively Me* behavior management program used in conjunction with one-to-one counseling sessions. | Weekly consults with nonprofessional counselors, typically Diet Center graduates. Staff R.D., M.D. and board of health professionals design programs at corporate level. | Fees average $30-$50/week, plus additional $17.50 a day for food for *Concept 1000* option. Maintenance averages $100/year. Expected weight loss: no more than two pounds weekly. Length of reducing phase varies; one-year maintenance program recommended. | **Pros:** Emphasizes body composition, not pounds, as a measure of health. Choice of two diet plans; only *Concept 1000* requires Diet Center foods. **Cons:** Expensive. No professional guidance. No group support. |
| Recommends burning minimum of 2,000 calories/week in physical activity. Addresses lifestyle issues in weekly classes and personal counseling. | Program developed by M.D.'s, R.D.'s, R.N.'s and psychologists. Each location has at least one M.D. and health educator. Dieters on VLCD see M.D. or R.N. weekly. | VLCD averages $150/week, but may be covered by insurance. *Healthy Solutions* averages $20/week plus cost of products. Maintenance averages $80/month. Expected weight loss: one to five pounds weekly. Reducing phase typically lasts 12-20 weeks; refeeding phase lasts 8. Maintenance recommended for up to 18 months. | **Pros:** Few eating decisions. Emphasizes exercise. Supervised by health professionals. **Cons:** Expensive if not covered by insurance. Requires prepackaged food and strong commitment to exercise. May be difficult to transition to regular foods. Side effects of VLCD include intolerance to cold, constipation, dizziness, dry skin and headaches. |
| Emphasizes increased physical activity, changing ingrained habits and balanced eating. | Program developed by R.D.'s and psychologists. M.D.'s, R.D.'s and Ph.D.'s consult on program design. Nonprofessional staff counsels clients. | Costs $99 to $299 to join (latter includes unlimited maintenance). *Jenny Craig's Cuisine* averages additional $70/week. Expected weight loss: up to two pounds weekly. Program length varies, depending on weight goal. Maintenance option of one year or unlimited. | **Pros:** Little food preparation required. Plans available for vegetarians, people with diabetes, breastfeeding moms and those on kosher diets. **Cons:** Must rely on prepackaged foods, making dining out and socializing difficult. Lacks professional guidance at client level. Limited maintenance options. |
| Clients determine weekly goals with consultants, often focusing on exercise. Brochures on health topics available with three-month and 12-month programs. Exercise video and audio tapes available at extra cost. | R.D.'s and health educators develop program. Ph.D. and M.D. consult on program design. L.P.N., R.N. or diet technician acts as personal consultant, providing guidance once a week for 15-20 minutes. | One-month costs about $99; three months about $269; 12 months about $500. Food costs an additional $49-$69/week. Vitamin/mineral supplements also extra. Expected weight loss: no more than two pounds weekly. Program length varies according to weight-loss goals. | **Pros:** Few eating decisions. **Cons:** Expensive. *Herbal Phen-Fen* can be dangerous. Weak on lifestyle education component. Little contact with health professionals. |
| Emphasizes changes in behavior and diet planning for "real" foods in group and counseling sessions. Exercise physiologist available to help design personal exercise plan. | Clients assigned a case manager who coordinates care. Dieters seen regularly by M.D., R.N., R.D. and psychologists; consulting exercise physiologist available. Group meeting leaders are psychologists or R.D.'s. | Costs $1,500 to $3,000 depending on diet and and desired weight loss. Price includes maintenance at some centers. Insurance may cover part of cost. Expected weight loss: no more than 2% of body weight weekly. Reducing phase lasts about 13 weeks; transition phase lasts about six. Maintenance begins at week 20 with no time limit. | **Pros:** Close contact with health professionals. Beneficial for people with serious health problems, who need low calorie level to promote quick weight loss. Few eating decisions. **Cons:** Expensive if not covered by insurance. Must rely on Optifast products during much of reducing phase. May be difficult to transition from liquid diet to regular food. |
| Makes no recommendations for exercise or behavior change. | Nonprofessional group members lead meetings and conduct activities. | Makes no weight-loss claims. Unlimited length. Self-supporting with member contributions. Optional monthly journal, *Lifeline*, costs $12.99/year in U.S. | **Pros:** Inexpensive method of group support. No need to follow a specific diet plan. No weigh-ins. **Cons:** Lacks professional guidance. OA stopped giving out diets in 1987, but some members still advocate unhealthy eating practices, including avoiding carbohydrates. |
| Exercise strongly encouraged as part of sensible weight control. R.D.'s help clients identify barriers to weight loss and maintenance and provide healthy lifestyle education. | R.D.'s have degrees in human nutrition or closely related area, plus practical experience, typically a hospital internship. Often have advanced degrees. Must pass accreditation exam and participate in continuing education. | Costs $35 to $150 per hour; weight-control groups usually substantially less. Insurance may pay for visits. Expected weight loss: usually no more than two pounds/week. | **Pros:** Eating prescription adapted to your lifestyle and medical history. Appropriate for any age group and entire families. **Cons:** Expensive if not covered by insurance. |
| Makes no specific lifestyle or exercise recommendations. | Led by elected volunteer nonhealth professional who directs and organizes activities for one year. Health professionals may be invited to speak at weekly meetings. | First visit free. $20 annual fee, which includes monthly *TOPS News*. Local weekly dues set by each chapter—about $5/month. No claims made for weight loss. Unlimited length. | **Pros:** Inexpensive form of group support. No purchases required. Has potential for long-term participation. **Cons:** Focuses on weight loss as chief measure of success. Must weigh in weekly. Groups vary widely in approach. Program lacks professional guidance. |
| Emphasizes positive lifestyle changes, such as regular exercise. Encourages daily physical activity. *Tools For Living* helps members deal with personal beliefs about being overweight. | M.D. and R.D.'s design and direct program. Group leaders are nonhealth professional program graduates. | Costs $17-$20 to join, plus $10-$14 weekly, which entitles members to unlimited meetings for that week. Meetings free if you maintain goal weight within two pounds for six weeks. Expected weight loss: up to two pounds weekly. | **Pros:** Flexible, easy-to-use program offering group support. Plans available for vegetarians, teens and breastfeeding moms. **Cons:** Lacks professional guidance at client level. No personalized counseling. Weekly weigh-ins. |

© Copyright, 1998 by Environmental Nutrition, Inc., 52 Riverside Drive, New York, NY 10024

# "Natural" Therapeutics for Weight Loss: Garden of Slender Delights or Dangerous Alchemy?

By **David B. Allison, PhD**, and **Steven B. Heymsfield, MD,** Obesity Research Center at St. Luke's-Roosevelt Hospital, New York, NY

## Prescription Drugs in Obesity Treatment

We are one of the fattest nations in the world and are in the fattest time of our nation, even though prescription drugs have been available to treat obesity since the 1950s. The use of these agents was largely frowned upon both by the medical community and the general public until the early 1990s. At that point, for a variety of reasons, attitudes changed dramatically. Behavioral management was shown over the years to be largely ineffective for maintaining long-term weight loss. By 1991, many individuals had regained weight following very-low-calorie formula diet attempts. Shortly after 1992, following the publication of a study by Michael Weintraub, MD, and colleagues describing the combined use of phentermine and fenfluramine, the use of drug treatment for obesity exploded, and in particular, the long-term combined use of phentermine and fenfluramine (known as "fen-phen") became extremely popular. (See Weintraub et al., 1992.)

It is difficult to obtain accurate statistics regarding the number and types of people who received these drugs, because much of this information is generated by pharmaceutical companies and others who consider it proprietary and do not publish it. Nevertheless, it appears that an enormous number of individuals were prescribed these appetite suppressants. Many of these individuals were not obese and received only minimal evaluation and follow-up by qualified physicians. Given this extraordinarily widespread off-label use of these two compounds, it is, in retrospect, perhaps not surprising that negative consequences arose. Recent evidence suggests that the use of fenfluramine and the closely related compound dexfenfluramine produces a form of cardiac valvular disorder in approximately 30% of patients taking these drugs. Although the scientific jury is still out on whether the data convincingly show that these drugs caused the anomalies and whether or not the anomalies are reversible when the drugs are withdrawn, the data were troubling enough that the drugs were voluntarily withdrawn

From *Nutrition & the M.D.*, January 1998, pp. 1-3. © 1998 by Lippincott, Williams & Wilkins. Reprinted by permission.

from the market by the manufacturers at the request of the Food and Drug Administration (FDA).

Although there are still prescription drugs available for the treatment of obesity, the climate has clearly changed for many individuals. Many physicians and patients alike are now concerned about using the currently available drugs, especially long term.

In the wake of this withdrawal, many practitioners and patients are seeking alternatives. Where can they go? There are at least three alternatives they can pursue. The first is to simply abandon their attempts at losing weight either temporarily or permanently. The second is to return to more "traditional" approaches to weight loss, namely volitional attempts at decreasing food intake and increasing physical activity. Third, they can turn to "alternative" therapies, which primarily fall into the realm of herbal and mineral supplements. As of this writing, we are aware of no data to indicate the extent to which patients and practitioners are falling back on one of these strategies versus another. However, our subjective sense and reports from individuals working in each of these areas suggest that the use of alternative therapies is receiving enormous attention.

## Alternative Therapies

The variety of alternative therapies is seemingly endless. We will comment here on three of the most common and try to briefly report what we know about the safety and efficacy of each. However, as will become apparent, in most cases we know very little.

**Ma-Huang**—This is the Chinese name of *Ephedra sinica*, an acrid-tasting stimulant herb. Legend has it that the body guards of Genghis Khan, threatened with beheading if they fell asleep at their post, sipped ephedra tea. Ephedrine, an ephedra extract, was first synthesized in 1927 and is still widely used today as a decongestant. Ma-Huang is primarily used today as an ingredient in herbal weight loss products and presumably acts to lower appetite and potentially increase components of energy expenditure through sympathomimetic mechanisms. Although ephedrine, particularly in combination with caffeine, is an effective short-term weight loss agent, we are not aware of any major randomized double-blind Ma-Huang trials. A crucial concern is the potentially fatal stimulant side effects of ephedra. As a result of this concern, the FDA is considering limiting use to relatively low daily amounts.

**St. John Garcinia Cambogia** (St. John's Wort)—This fruit, with the active ingredient hydroxycitric acid (HCA), is the size of an orange but appears like a small pumpkin as it dangles from the large south Asian Garcinia Cambogia tree. The fruit has been used in southern Asia for its culinary and health promoting benefits for centuries.

**HCA Chromium Piccolinate**—The only non-herbal compound on our brief list, chromium is an essential trace element required for normal protein, fat, and carbohydrate metabolism. Clinical chromium deficiency is exceedingly rare, and blood levels are difficult to measure accurately and interpret. There are two forms of chromium, inorganic and organic. The most popular commercial form of chromium is organic chromium piccolinate. Introduced in 1988, chromium piccolinate gained popularity stemming from reports that it increased lean body mass in male athletes. Currently marketed as promoting muscle mass and lowering body fat, most controlled studies in reputable centers show little or no weight loss or body composition effect. Larger scale, carefully controlled studies using appropriate methodology are needed to finally establish whether or not this widely used weight loss ingredient has any worthwhile properties.

## The "Take-Home" Message

What have, or might, we learn from all this? One lesson we can clearly learn, or be reminded of, from the fen-phen fiasco is that no drug, no matter how long it has been used, comes with absolute assurance of complete safety. Every drug has side effects. Some of these are known, but we can never be sure that we know all the possible side effects. This does not mean that drugs should never be used because they can potentially have unknown risks, but it does cause one to take the risk-benefit analysis quite seriously.

Before prescribing, recommending, or taking a pharmacologically active drug, we should have a fair degree of confidence that the benefits outweigh the risks. For the benefits to outweigh the risks, we need to have a fair degree of confidence that indeed there are benefits. It is quite difficult to argue that individuals with body mass indices much below 28 kg/m$^2$ are sufficiently likely to benefit from weight loss that it outweighs the known and unknown risks of pharmacologic treatment.

The second take-home message stems directly from the first. If we acknowledge that every compound having some pharmacologic action is also very likely to have some side effects, then any herbal- or mineral-based product must either be inert or be open to question with respect to safety.

Therefore, the real question about these "alternative" therapies is not whether they are from eastern or western medicine, from a chemistry lab in a pharmaceutical plant, an exotic plant from a tropical rain forest, or labeled "artificial" or "natural," but rather whether there are sufficient data available from controlled scientific studies to give one confidence that the compound is safe and effective.

We are frequently asked by reporters writing for the general public what to make of the latest product or service being marketed for weight loss. In fact, new products and services are marketed with such rapidity that it is not uncommon for us not to have heard of a particular product when the reporter asks. In these cases, we have a stock question that we suggest reporters ask themselves and any individual suggesting the value of a new weight loss product or service. That question is, "Are there any double-blind, placebo-controlled, randomized clinical trials demonstrating a statistically significant weight loss induced by the product or service and demonstrating side effects within the tolerable range?" If the answer to this question is yes, then we suggest that the reporter examine these studies in detail or we examine them ourselves. If the answer is no, then we suggest that there is no need to pursue the conversation further. The compound may well be safe and effective, but without adequate scientific data, the only reasonable response is to go and collect those data and forestall clinical use until those data are collected.

We believe that this is every bit as true of "herbal," "natural," and "alternative" therapies as it is for manufactured pharmaceuticals. We have begun trying to help generate data on some of these products and hope that others will begin collecting such data, particularly those companies that market these products. In the interim, caution is the order of the day, and we must remember Hippocrates.

## Reference

Weintraub M, Sundareson PR, Schuster B et al., Long-term weight control study I-VII, *Clin Pharmacol Ther*, 1992; 51:581.

# The history of dieting and its effectiveness

*by Wayne C. Miller, PhD*

How effective have diets and dieting programs been in producing weight loss? Throughout the years, dietitians and nutritionists have advocated moderate consistent weight loss through a balanced, energy controlled diet in conjunction with lifestyle changes. Although this may be the healthiest way to lose weight, it is not necessarily the way the public attempts to lose weight.

In the late 1950s and early 1960s, total fasting was used to reduce weight in the massively obese. Weight loss through fasting amounted to 1.0 kg per day the first month followed by 0.5 kg a day thereafter.[1] Although the desired outcome, weight loss, was achieved through fasting, serious side effects such as loss of lean body mass, depleted electrolytes, and death caused fasting to quickly wane in popularity.[1,2,3]

Next on the scene came the high-protein, low-carbohydrate diets of the 1960s and early 1970s. The theory of this epic, which still lingers today, was that carbohydrates (particularly starch) make you fat. Popular diets of that time (e.g. Stillman, Atkins) provided 1,200 to 2,000+ calories per day, with only 5 to 10 percent coming from carbohydrates.[4] On the other hand, 50 to 70 percent of the energy intake on these diets came from fat. The justification of this diet composition was that the high protein content prevented the loss of lean tissue, while the high fat content produced ketosis with its associated appetite suppression. Weight loss on these diets was rapid because of depleted glycogen stores and diuresis, but side effects included nausea, hyperuricemia, fatigue, and refeeding edema.[5]

## VLCD liquids

During the mid 1970s very low calorie liquid diets became commercially available. These diets were known as protein-sparing-modified fasts or liquid protein diets. Their extremely low caloric content (300-400 calories per day) caused rapid weight loss. However, in spite of medical supervision, high quality protein, and potassium supplementation, several deaths due to ventricular arrhythmia occurred with prolonged use. These liquid protein diets were subsequently banned until research studies could assure their safety.[6]

A second generation of very low calorie formula diets became popular in the 1980s. These commercial formula products, such as Optifast and Health Management Resources, became part of a medical approach including patient counseling and support. Diets of 400 to 500 calories per day were offered as well as the option of an 800-calorie plan. At the same time, franchises like Nutri/System and Jenny Craig offered clients pre-packaged foods along with exercise and nutrition counseling. This second generation of very low calorie formula diets and pre-packaged foods has evolved to where many of these commercial programs now offer individualized approaches that emphasize exercise and behavior change.[7] These programs can cost up to $3,000 and/or $70 to $90 per week for food products.[7] Another problem is that these programs have not been well researched for safety and may be as detrimental to health as any other rapid weight loss regimen.[8]

## Lowfat diets

Research related to the health risks of dietary fat in the 1970s and 1980s has spawned a fat-phobic society. Thus, the newest trend in the dieting realm is non-fat or low-fat diets. Fat-free and low-fat versions of foods have become popular while the Pritikin diet, which was first used in the 1970s to combat the risks of degenerative diseases, has been resurrected as a weight-loss diet. Other low-fat programs, like the T-Factor diet, promote counting fat grams rather than calories for weight control. Average weight loss due to reducing dietary fat alone is only 0.1 to 0.2 kg per week.[9,10] Moreover, there is some concern that the abundance of low-fat fat-free calorie-rich snack foods on the market will encourage overconsumption by would-be dieters who concern themselves only with dietary fat.

## Diets challenged

Obesity researchers have been fighting an uphill battle ever since

> ❝ Long term weight loss following any type of intervention was limited to only a small minority of the obese people studied ❞
> — NIH

Reprinted with permission from *Healthy Weight Journal*, March/April 1997, pp. 28-29. © 1997 by Healthy Weight Journal, Research, News and Commentary Across the Weight Spectrum, 402 South 14th Street, Hettinger, ND 58639.

Stunkard and McLaren-Hume concluded that dieting was ineffective for 95 percent of those in a hospital nutrition clinic.[11] Since that time, the use of diets for weight control has been challenged by the public, a growing number of health care professionals, as well as some obesity researchers themselves.[8]

Hence, the National Institutes of Health (NIH) recently convened a Technology Assessment Conference to evaluate the effectiveness of voluntary methods for weight loss and control.

The report for very low calorie diets (VLCDs) revealed that weight loss following a 12-week VLCD totaled 20 kg, with a 35 to 50 percent weight regain after one year.[12,13] Furthermore, dropout rates in some VLCD programs can reach 80 percent. The less restrictive low calorie diets (LCDs) are even less effective. Following a 20-week LCD program, average weight loss is 8.5 kg, with a 33 percent regain after one year, and a 100 percent regain after five years.[14,15]

Nutrition education and behavior modification programs have become popular because they are supposedly self-empowering. However, success on these programs isn't any better than on VLCDs or LCDs. An 18-week behavior modification program will bring about a 10 kg weight loss, with a 95 percent relapse after two years.[15] Similarly discouraging is the finding that community programs, worksite interventions, and home correspondence programs show negligible success after one to three years.[16]

## Weak data advanced

Data to support the effectiveness claims of commercial weight-loss programs was requested by the NIH and FDA at the time of the Technology Assessment Conference. Material was received from only five companies, three representing nonphysician-directed programs and two representing physician-directed programs. For the nonphysician-directed programs, one company submitted one research study and several abstracts. The study demonstrated reduced cardiovascular disease risk following short-term use of the program; the abstracts were judged scientifically inadequate. The second company representing nonphysician-directed programs submitted four research studies, but later withdrew the studies from the NIH review. The third company data was judged inadequate to evaluate.

For the physician-directed programs, one company submitted three research articles and several abstracts. Data from this company was evaluated as inconclusive. The other company representing a physician-directed program was the only company in the industry that submitted data that was scientifically sound. Although this company submitted 55 quality research reports, the NIH committee determined that long-term weight loss following this program was questionable.[17]

## Odd conclusion

Surprisingly enough, even though only one commercial program in the whole industry provided data that could be seen as adequate, and that data provided no evidence for long-term success for weight control, the NIH assessment team concluded: *"Regardless of products used, successful weight loss and control is limited to and requires individualized programs consisting of restricted caloric intake, behavior modification and exercise.[17] "*

It is puzzling how the NIH could come to any effectiveness conclusion based on the paucity of data they received which they themselves judged to be inadequate, questionable, and inconclusive.[17] Only two conclusions seem possible to have been drawn, either 1) no conclusion can be made because there is no data upon which to base a conclusion, or 2) no commercial program is effective at producing long-term weight loss because no company could provide data to show otherwise.

It seems the NIH conclusion for commercial program effectiveness was based on an assumption or hope of what should be effective, not on the data evaluated.

The overall conclusion from NIH as to the effectiveness of any type of method for voluntary weight loss and control was more true to the facts than their conclusion for the commercial industry. The universal consensus of the conference was:

*"Long term weight loss following any type of intervention was limited to only a small minority of the obese people studied.[18] "*

Thus, it seems apparent that there is not enough data to support the claim that diet programs are effective in long-term weight control for a majority of the obese.

The question that is most relevant now is, *what intervention strategies should be used to promote health in the obese, if intervention is deemed appropriate at all?* This question will be addressed in the next issue of *Healthy Weight Journal.*

*Wayne C. Miller, PhD, is Professor of Exercise Science and Nutrition at George Washington University Medical Center, Washington, DC.*

REFERENCES
1. J Am Med Assoc 1964;187:100-106
2. J Am Diet Assoc 1990;90:722-726
3. J Nutr 1986;116:918-919
4. J Am Diet Assoc 1985;85:450-454
5. Clinical Nutrition and Dietetics. New York: Macmillan Publishing Co.; 1991.
6. Am. J. Clin Nutr 1981;34:453-461
7. Environmental Nutr 1994;17:1,3
8. Health Risks of Weight Loss. Hettinger, ND: Healthy Weight Journal; 1995
9. Am J Clin Nutr 1991;53:1124-1129
10. Am J Clin Nutr 1991;54:821-828
11. J Am Diet Assoc 1991;91:1248-1251
12. Ann Int Med 1993;119:688-693
13. Ann Int Med 1993;119:764-770
14. Behav Ther 1987;18:353-374
15. Int J Obesity 1989;13:123-136
16. Ann Int Med 1993;119:719-721
17. Ann Int Med 1993;119:681-687
18. Ann Int Med 1993;119:764-770

# Congress Asked to Take Eating Disorders Seriously

## by Frances M. Berg, MS

Eating disorders are an urgent health and policy issue that demand national attention, said leading experts at a United States Congressional briefing, on July 10, 1997.

Eating disorders are important in terms of sheer numbers—they affect women all along the continuum from serious dieting to severe disorders, reported Ruth Striegel-Moore, PhD, an eating disorder specialist from Wesleyan University. Yet she added, they are trivialized and misunderstood.

"Congress can and must do something to halt this destructive epidemic. In investigating this issue, I learned there are few or no good sources of reliable, scientific information for families and individuals struggling with eating disorders," said Representative Louise M. Slaughter (D-NY).

> "In our culture, women define themselves, in part, through their appearance. Women and girls are at high risk to internalize certain assumptions and ideals such as the thin beauty ideal."

Representatives Slaughter and Nita Lowey (D-NY) held the briefing to introduce their new legislation, the Eating Disorders Information and Education Act. They worked closely with the Labor Health and Human Services Education Appropriations Subcommittee and included eating disorder language in the upcoming appropriations report. Lead sponsors of the briefing, The Prevention of Eating Disorders and the Role of Federal Policy, moderated by Jeanine Cogan, PhD, were the American Psychological Association and the Society for the Psychological Study of Social Issues.

"What's amazing to me is that there is really no federal effort to educate the public," said Representative Lowey. "It is so shocking that even though eating disorders are curable, the majority of people with them suffer for years, and too often suffer alone.... Eating disorders is a women's health issue that demands national attention. I believe that it's our responsibility to educate at the federal level."

### How widespread and serious is the problem?

An estimated 8 to 10 million people suffer from eating disorders, reported David Herzog, MD, Harvard Eating Disorders Center. According to Dr. Herzog, they often affect the most gifted, women at a critical stage of career and family development, having a devastating impact on their reproductive and general health as well as their psychological well being. Eating disorders are associated with high infant death rate, infertility, heart problems, depression, death, and osteoporosis.

"In the early 1980s, we started seeing young women with fractures. And it didn't matter whether they were 40 or 18 or 19. In fact, some of the lowest bone densities were for 19- and 20-year-old women who had the bones of 75- and 80-year-old women... This is a serious problem and we have to intervene early," claims Dr. Herzog.

Herzog said about half of eating disorder patients recover, 30 percent get better, and 20 to 30 percent remain chronically ill. The death rate in his research with 250 young women is 5.6 percent per decade.

Even subclinical forms have serious health consequences, reported Striegel-Moore. "Often the symptoms start early. Ten-year-old girls trying to lose weight already show differences in micronutrient intake for vitamin A and calcium. Already at that age the diets of these girls are not as good as the diets of girls not trying to lose weight."

Diagnosis is typically delayed. Herzog cited two studies showing the difficulties physicians have in recognizing eating disorder symptoms and women have in talking about them. The first study showed doctors were not aware of symptoms in 50 percent of their patients who were found to have eating disorders. The second, in a fertility clinic, identified eating disorders in 58 percent of women who had irregular or no menstrual periods, yet none had been diagnosed by their gynecologists.

Routine screening would help, he said. "In colleges we see high rates of eating disorders. The Harvard Eating Disorders Center was the scientific arm for the first eating disorders screening program, which was held at 600 colleges across the country. A very high percentage, 75 percent (of 9,000 participants), were found to have clinically significant symptoms. That means frequent purging or binging, being obsessed with their food or weight, and an association with social and academic impairment... Of particular concern was that the more seriously affected ethnic minority groups, in this sample, the Native Americans and the Latinos, were the least likely groups to receive a referral for further evaluation and care."

### Social and cultural factors

"Our culture is very important in the development of eating disorders," said Striegel-Moore, "cultural attitudes about the body, the thin ideal for women, and the cultural definition of femininity. In our culture, women

Reprinted with permission from *Healthy Weight Journal*, May/June 1998, pp. 41-43. © 1998 by Healthy Weight Journal, Research, News and Commentary Across the Weight Spectrum, 402 South 14th Street, Hettinger, ND 58639.

define themselves, in part, through their appearance. Women and girls are at high risk to internalize certain assumptions and ideals such as 'the thin beauty ideal.'"

She pointed out that the link between thinness and smoking is being exploited by the tobacco industry. "Cigarettes are being marketed to young girls as a way of staying thin."

Naomi Wolf, author of the best selling book, *The Beauty Myth*, further addressed cultural issues and why girls are at particular risk for developing eating disorders. She charged that, as women have moved into the workplace, the pressures to be thin have intensified and ideals of beauty become more rigid, as a way to undermine their strength and confidence.

"It is time to shift the focus from weight to wellness with a positive emphasis on maximizing health for people of all sizes," said Lisa Berzins, PhD, a psychotherapist and founder of the educational organization, Vitality. "Dieting is clearly a risk factor for the development of an eating disorder among those who are more vulnerable, and is associated with dysfunctional eating patterns, preoccupation with shape, weight, and food, increased irritability, and risk for depression."

## Need for federal consumer protection

The speakers repeatedly asked Congress for greater protection from unsafe and ineffective diet products.

Wolf noted the deaths caused by phen/fen, "American women deserve consumer attention paid to the industry that preys on their insecurities." She charged Congress with making sure the diet industry is not defrauding women and not exploiting them to follow dangerous and extreme calorie-restricted diets.

"It is the role of the FDA to make sure that the products sold in this country are safe and effective," said Zuckerman. "The FTC regulates advertising, but could certainly do a lot more."

Berzins explained the recent legislation that regulates diet advertising in Connecticut, which she helped initiate. "Connecticut is the first state in the country to enact legislation that requires the diet industry to disclose accurate information regarding average amounts of weight loss maintained, based on scientific data drawn from representative samples. And if they don't do that, they have to have a statement that for many dieters weight loss is temporary. We had a signing ceremony for a second law requiring full disclosure of cost, estimated duration of services, the credentials of program staff, and a 3-day cancellation period without liability. We would very much like to see this happen on a federal level."

## What is the role of government?

Herzog called on Congress to develop a national campaign to increase public awareness about eating disorders. Another urgent priority is educating doctors and giving them effective clinical assessment tools to increase reporting. A curriculum needs to be developed for professional training of primary care physicians and mental health professionals.

Wolf advocated cultural changes, including regulating the modeling industry. "They use 14-year-old girls and tart them up to look 35 and it's common knowledge in the modeling industry that models have to keep their weight down through drug abuse, through smoking, and through anorexia. If you have doctors making sure that these employment conditions are safe, meaning that women and girls did not have to maintain their weight at starvation levels in order to work, and to make sure, for instance, that models were still menstruating, that they were not starving so much that they were sub-menstrual, then you go a long way to making sure an industry that influences American girls is not using teenage girls in a punitive or abusive way."

An awareness campaign that enlists teen icons such as rock stars, Jewel and Alanis Morrisette, would help get the message out that "looking like Kate Moss is not worth dying for... Girls are getting their cues about what's socially acceptable from the authority of culture."

Wolf also called for enforcing employment laws, saying that beauty and thinness are being used as job qualifications for women, but not men. "A bona fide occupational qualification to be thin and conventionally attractive, is a differential expectation for women as opposed to men. And that is an illegal employment issue."

---

Tell our daughters you are too precious
for us to let you starve yourselves to death or
blight your bodies in this way.

---

"Congress can affect these issues in many different ways," said Diana Zuckerman, PhD, director of research and policy analysis at the Institute for Women's Policy Research. She said it is the responsibility of government to provide accurate information about health issues.

She called for Congress and federal policy through the Department of Health and Human Services to address eating disorder issues in the following ways:

1. Increase funding for research on the prevention and treatment of eating disorders.
2. Hold consensus conferences to examine these issues. She suggested a conference on how to regulate diet drugs and diet products, and another on the dangers of yo-yo dieting and why long-term weight loss is so rare. "Congressional hearings can bring a lot of visibility to an issue not considered in a serious way before."
3. Launch an awareness and public education campaign.
4. Improve the regulation of diet products through the FDA and FTC.

"This is a very big problem and very complex, and we're not going to change society this week... (but) you are in a position where much is possible on many different levels," she concluded.

Wolf believes that using the authority of Congress to address eating disorders would have great impact. "Then you go a long way not only in stemming this epidemic but giving our women, and most importantly our daughters, the message that they are too precious to waste themselves in the pursuit of this unhealthy, and I would say, this anti-woman ideal.

"If Congress says, 'We take this seriously; let's make this an awareness campaign that treats this as seriously as a drug addiction issue and tell our daughters that you are too precious for us to let you starve yourselves to death or blight your bodies in this way,' that gives girls a sense that an authority in the culture, the highest authority, says we want you to stay healthy, we want you to eat, we want to help you."

Inquiries are referred to the organizer of this briefing, Jeanine C. Cogan PhD. Full transcripts may be accessed at the APA website *www.apa.org/ppo/brfweb2.html.*

# Survival of the 'Best and Brightest'

## by Naomi Wolf

First let me say what an historic occasion I think this is. This briefing attests to the changes in this institution in the last few years as more and more women have assumed leadership. The fact that we're talking about eating disorders in a place like this is a change from 5 years ago, when it was considered virtually unAmerican to question the ideal of thinness in public, let alone to treat it as a matter of serious policy discussion. So this is a truly great day for the health issues of all Americans.

As a young woman coming of age, I began to notice at Yale, where I was an undergraduate, that the best and brightest young women of my generation could barely get through the survival issues of their day, they could barely stay on top of schoolwork, and barely stay on top of social relations, because so many of them were starving themselves half to death or spending a lot of time vomiting compulsively behind closed doors struggling with eating disorders. I began to take a closer look at what this ideal was that so many women were trying to live up to. It turns out that it's profoundly unnatural. Twenty years ago the average fashion model weighed eight percent less than the average woman; today (she) weighs twenty-three percent less.

It's my argument that what I call the beauty myth, the huge cultural pressure for girls and women to live up to these increasingly anorexic norms, supplanted the feminist mystique that Betty Friedan described so eloquently in her book. As women began to move into the workplace, as feminism began to transform the landscape, and women asked for more power, the ideals of beauty became more and more rigid as a way to undermine women's new-found confidence and authority.

While many things cause anorexia, so does calorie-restricted dieting. In our culture, it is normative for women to be living on starvation diets. Dieting centers put women on diets ranging from 500 to 900 calories a day (for) up to 6 months at a time. It's clearly a cultural imperative that is weighing down on women and not on men. That is sick, that is a distortion...

There's something that reinforces women having to live up to these norms, that has to do with the work force. Even if you think you are free to be at your own weight or your own size, very often there's what I have called the PBQ or the Professional Beauty Quotient. In retail, in sales, not to mention the media, and television work, many women find this PBQ operating. Flight attendants have protested about this. Many women find they are expected to fit a rigidly thin ideal in order to stay employed. For many women, their appearance is a criteria by which their workplace abilities are measured. A woman in sales told me that she followed my advice in *The Beauty Myth*, let herself go to her natural healthy weight and she couldn't get work anymore. This is illegal.

I want to ask you to consider the political fallout of this—why it is important for you to treat this as a political issue. Anorexia and bulimia, as an epidemic, are working as a sort of political sedative on our daughters' generation, young women coming of age, young women of college level.

This generation should be the future leaders of America. Instead of being strong and creative and full of resilience, so many young women I speak to on college campuses, again the best and the brightest, are barely making it through at a level of survival, because they're exhausted. They're exhausted because they're starving or vomiting compulsively. This generation's voice is diminished, their reasoning powers are blunted. And this is America's future leadership.

Testimony by Naomi Wolf, author of *The Beauty Myth*, at the Congressional briefing, July 10, 1997.

# BINGE *Eating*

## The Newest Eating Disorder

**JOYCE D. NASH, PH.D.**

"I'm okay until mid-afternoon. Then I start eating, and I eat all evening long. I can't seem to stop. It's not that I'm hungry. I feel full, but I keep on eating. Usually, I'm bored and I don't know what to do with myself."

"In the middle of the night, I get up and raid the refrigerator. I'll eat anything I can get my hands on—a whole carton of Cool Whip plus a bag of cookies, maybe some leftovers from dinner the night before, a whole box of cereal. It's disgusting. If anyone were to walk in on me while I'm doing this, I think I'd die."

CCORDING TO A RECENT REPORT FROM THE CENTERS FOR DISEASE CONTROL and Prevention, 35 percent of adult Americans are overweight and a significant minority are seriously obese. At any given time, tens of millions of people are dieting, even if they aren't overweight. A quarter of all adult men and nearly half of all adult women are currently trying to lose weight. Many of them struggle with binge eating. It has been estimated that 25 to 45 percent of those who seek treatment for obesity and 5 to 8 percent of obese people in the general community are binge eaters. Although not all binge eaters are obese, the more severely obese a person is, the more likely it is that binge eating is a problem.

Most people think of a binge as losing control and eating more than they should or more than they want to and feeling bad as a result. According to the fourth edition of the Diagnostic and Statistical Manual of Mental Disorders (DSM IV), published by the American Psychiatric Association, a "binge" is an episode of eating that is characterized by eating, in a discrete period of time, an amount of food that is definitely larger than most people would eat in a similar period of time under similar circumstances, accompanied by a sense of lack of control or a feeling that one cannot stop eating or control what or how much one is eating.

Binge eating is most commonly associated with bulimia nervosa, an eating disorder that involves binge eating followed by the regular use of compensatory behaviors such as vomiting, excessive exercising, or abuse of laxatives. An eating disorder included for the first time in the DSM IV is binge eating disorder (BED). BED involves persistent and frequent binge eating that is not accompanied by the regular use of the compensatory behaviors that characterize bulimia.

Most people overeat from time to time, and many feel they often eat more than they should. Some people worry about breaking self-imposed eating rules but generally do not eat objectively excessive amounts of food. Gourmands eat large amounts of calories in single sittings and may develop a weight problem, but they enjoy food and suffer little or no distress because of their overeating. Such people do not qualify for a diagnosis of binge eating disorder.

A study (Johnson, Schlundt, Barclay, Carr-Nagle, and Engler, 1995) compared serious binge eaters to "normal" eaters and people who may worry about overeating but do not truly binge eat. They found that all eaters are more likely to overeat if lunch is skipped or if evening snacking occurs. Feeling emotionally distressed can lead to overeating for any person, but people with BED are more likely to binge in response to even moderately negative moods. Serious binge eaters tend

Reprinted with permission from *Healthline,* September 1997, pp. 6-7. © 1997 by Healthline Publishing, Inc., 830 Menlo Avenue, Suite 100, Menlo Park, CA 94025.

to overeat when home alone, while normal eaters tend to overeat in restaurants or in social situations that are associated with positive feelings. Binge eaters eat even if they aren't hungry, and binge eating is often triggered by snacking and eating "junk" foods.

Compared to obese dieters who don't binge, people who meet criteria for BED eat more during regular meals, as well as during episodes of overeating. They diet more frequently and have more weight fluctuations. Serious binge eaters also have higher lifetime rates of psychiatric disorders, including anxiety and mood and personality disorders. They have greater concerns about eating, shape, and weight than do other dieters, and they hold more rigid and extreme dieting attitudes. Binge eaters experience more guilt and self-hatred after a binge, and they are more likely to drop out of treatment and regain more weight after weight loss.

In many ways, people with binge eating disorder are similar to bulimics. Both engage in persistent and frequent binge eating accompanied by loss of control over eating, and both fear weight gain. Bulimics and noncompensating binge eaters are preoccupied with food and body weight and struggle continually to control eating and weight. They both experience intense feelings of body dissatisfaction and frequently have feelings of revulsion toward and loathing of their bodies. Typically, bulimics and people with BED set unrealistically high dieting standards for themselves but lack confidence in their ability to attain their goals. As a result, they alternate between periods of normal eating and periods of bingeing.

However, some important differences distinguish bulimics from people with binge eating disorder. Although people with BED may attempt to compensate to some degree for their binge eating, usually by dieting or occasional purging, they do not demonstrate the regular use of extreme compensatory behaviors that bulimics do. Bulimics usually have overvalued ideas about the importance of thinness, whereas serious binge eaters would be happy to settle for average or even somewhat above average body weight. Bulimics are usually of normal weight and may seek treatment for an eating disorder. People with BED are usually overweight and seek treatment for obesity.

A key difference between bulimics and people with BED has to do with restrictive dieting. Whereas bulimics tend to engage in high levels of dietary restraint—severely restricting caloric intake, possibly accompanied by eating a very restricted selection of foods—people with BED do not engage in much restraint. In bulimics, dieting—or, more specifically, dietary restraint—triggers binge eating. In contrast, dieting does not exacerbate binge eating for most people with BED; in fact, it may help them regain control over eating. However, careful consideration should be given to the pros and cons of undertaking a dieting effort without first seeking treatment for binge eating.

The primary, or overall, goal in treating binge eating is to normalize eating—that is, to help the binge eater say "no" to overeating or chaotic eating and say "yes" to eating that involves healthy choices and moderate consumption of all foods. This is achieved by first adopting a plan of regular eating designed to minimize or eliminate binge episodes. Next, the aim is to achieve overall moderation of food intake without the adoption of rigid rules. Identification and modification of maladaptive thoughts and beliefs that perpetuate the eating problem need to be part of the overall solution. Binge eaters must be helped to cope better with emotions, especially anxiety, loneliness, depression, and anger, and to overcome feelings of shame, inferiority, and fear of criticism. Finally, the issue of acceptance needs to be addressed. This is facilitated by the binge eater learning to change that which can be changed (their thoughts, feelings, and behaviors), to accept that which cannot be changed (certain aspects of their bodies), and to discern the difference between the two.

---

*Dr. Nash is a clinical psychologist in private practice in San Francisco and Palo Alto, and is the author of THE NEW MAXIMIZE YOUR BODY POTENTIAL: LIFETIME SKILLS FOR SUCCESSFUL WEIGHT MANAGEMENT as well as five other books on various behavioral medicine topics.*

# Dysfunctional eating: A new concept

*by Frances M. Berg, MS*

Children are growing up with twisted attitudes toward food, eating and weight because of our cultural fear of fat. They are turning away from normal eating and mealtimes with family to restrained and chaotic eating. Dieting and restricting food often starts as early as age 9, and by age 11 is so common that some researchers have called it the norm.

If abnormal eating is becoming so prevalent, we need to know more about it. What is abnormal, restrictive eating? What are its effects? How can it be measured, and should it be prevented?

Dysfunctional eating is a new, inclusive term to describe the kinds of abnormal, inappropriate eating which are becoming widely prevalent in the developed world, especially among girls and women. It is a disruption of normal eating and, too often, starvation in the midst of plenty.

## What is dysfunctional eating?

Dysfunctional eating is eating which is separated or disjoined from its normal function and normal internal controls.

Normal eating nourishes the body for health, energy and strength, enhancing feelings of well-being, and results in "feeling good." Dysfunctional eating is often focused on eating for thinness, body shaping, or using food for comfort or emotional reasons.

Normal eating is controlled by an internal system that regulates the balance of energy intake with expenditure, through hunger, appetite and satiety signals, so that a person eats when hungry and stops when full and satisfied. Normal eating is flexible and includes eating for pleasure and social reasons. In normal eating a person usually follows regular habits, such as eating three meals and snacks to satisfy hunger.

Dysfunctional eating exists on a continuum between normal eating and eating disorders. It may be of mild, moderate or severe intensity. Individuals may move back and forth across the continuum, returning to normal eating after unsuccessful bouts of dieting, or restricting food so severely they develop debilitating eating disorders from which they cannot recover alone.

Dysfunctional eating includes variations of chaotic eating and chronic dieting as well as both persistent undereating and overeating. There are at least three general patterns: irregular or chaotic eating, consistent undereating, and consistent overeating of much more than the body wants or needs, eating past satiety.

Dysfunctional eating encompasses restrained eating, disordered eating and chronic dieting syndrome. It is also being called disturbed, disruptive, abnormal and emotional eating. The broader focus has the advantage of providing a coherent framework for concerns which have been nebulous and incompletely defined.

Reprinted with permission from *Healthy Weight Journal* (formerly *Obesity & Health*), September/October 1996, pp. 88-92, 99. © 1996 by Healthy Weight Journal, Research, News and Commentary Across the Weight Spectrum, 402 South 14th Street, Hettinger, ND 58639.

In contrast to normal eating, dysfunctional eating most often serves functions other than nourishment, such as to shape the body, improve body image, to seek comfort or pleasure, to numb pain or unhappy memory, or to relieve stress, anxiety, anger, loneliness or boredom.

Dysfunctional eating is regulated by inappropriate external and internal controls, such as "will power," a planned diet, calories or fat grams, or sensory or emotional cues.

Though often the internal function is to relieve stress, it does not do this well. Instead of relieving pain, eating often makes the situation worse, or relief may be fleeting, followed by remorse. It is common to feel guilty, ashamed, uncomfortably full, to regret or berate oneself for having eating or, if unsatisfied, to feel ravenously hungry and fear or anticipate an onrushing eating binge.

Studies suggest that dysfunctional eating is prevalent among girls and women. It appears to be increasing and striking at younger ages as cultural pressures to be thin continue to increase. It may include at times as many as the 50 to 80 percent of girls and women in the U.S., age 11 and up, who report they are trying to lose weight. Increasingly, it includes teenage boys and men, who are re-

---

### A definition

Dysfunctional eating is eating that is separated or disjoined from its normal function and normal regulation.

Normal eating nourishes the body for health, energy and strength, enhancing feelings of well-being, and is regulated by hunger, appetite and satiety. Dysfunctional eating is often focused on eating for thinness, body shaping, or using food to comfort, numb pain, relieve stress, anxiety, anger or loneliness. It is regulated by inappropriate external and internal controls such as "will power," planned diets, or sensory and emotional cues.

Dysfunctional eating includes irregular or chaotic eating, consistent undereating, and consistent overeating of more than the body wants or needs. It exists on a continuum between normal eating and eating disorders, and may be of mild, moderate or severe intensity.

---

sponding to new advertising pressures to reshape their bodies.

Dysfunctional eating is unlikely for infants, small children and others who don't diet or have not learned to interfere with the normal eating process.

## Undereating and overeating

The consistent undereating pattern may have the purpose of shaping the body, or may be because of depression, alcoholism, or other mental or physical factors.

Consistent overeating, which is eating more than the body wants or needs, eating past satiety, is less understood and scarcely researched. Prevalence is unknown.

Overeating patterns may develop for emotional reasons, or from family or peer group habits of eating large amounts of food, or eating more because abundant, good tasting foods are readily available.

In the U.S. today, studies suggest that overeating is being encouraged. People are eating out more, and they favor fast food chains and restaurants where they perceive they are getting more for their money. In response, studies show restaurants are offering larger servings and larger meals.

Body size is not to be taken as an indicator of dysfunctional eating. It cannot be assumed that large persons are eating abnormally, or past the point of satiety. Persons of any size may be eating normally, or they may have eating disorders or dysfunctional eating patterns.

Conditions such as Prader-Willi syndrome, which involves a disruption of hunger, appetite and satiety regulation, may or may not fit into this category.

## Physical effects

The person with dysfunctional eating may often feel tired and lacking in energy, especially when undernourished. There is risk of stunted growth and reduced brain development in children and teens. Bone development may be decreased for youth; for women increased bone demineralization may occur, leading to bone fractures. Puberty may be delayed and sexual interest decreased.

Dysfunctional eating affects weight, yet in its various forms it is associated with a wide range of weights as genetic potential interacts with environmental lifestyle factors. Associated with chaotic eating and dieting, weight often cycles up and down in "yo-yo" fashion. Consistent undereating can be expected to result in a weight lower than normal for that person. Overeating will likely result in a higher weight than might be normal for that individual, perhaps increasing year by year.

## Mental focus

One of the most dramatic effects of dysfunctional eating may be its impact on the thinking process.

As dysfunctional eating becomes more severe, the individual often loses mental focus, mental alertness and the ability to concentrate. Her interests may narrow, turning inward, and she loses ambition. As interest in food heightens the individual tends to lose interest in school work, career, family and friends, and pulls back from social activities.

This increase in food preoccupation is clear in the wartime Minnesota Human Starvation study, and more recently has been researched by Dan Reiff, MPH, RD, and Kim Lampson Reiff, PhD, of Mercer Island, Wash.[4]

# Dysfunctional eating: a description

Contrasted and compared with normal eating and eating disorders

| | Normal eating | Dysfunctional eating _mild_ _moderate_ _severe_ | | Eating disorders |
|---|---|---|---|---|
| **Eating pattern** | Regular eating habits and patterns. Typical pattern in U.S. is to eat three regular meals and snacks to satisfy hunger. | Irregular, chaotic eating — often overeat or undereat, skip meals, fast, binge, diet. Or usual pattern is of overeating or undereating much more or much less than body wants or needs. | | Patterns typical of anorexia nervosa, bulimia nervosa, binge eating disorder, other eating disorders. |
| **Function, purpose of eating** | Eat for nourishment, health, energy. Also for pleasure and social reasons. Eating enhances feelings of well-being makes one "feel good." | Eating often for reasons other than nourishment: to shape body, improve body image, seek comfort or pleasure, numb pain, relieve stress, anxiety, anger, loneliness or boredom. May feel uncomfortable after eating, or have feelings of remorse, guilt, shame. | | Eating almost entirely for purposes other than nourishment or energy, as for body shaping to numb pain, relieve stress. |
| **Use of hunger, appetite and satiety to regulate eating** | Eating regulated by internal signals of hunger, appetite and satiety. Eat when hungry, stop when full and satisfied; usually hungry at mealtime. | Eating often separated from normal controls of hunger, appetite and satiety. May be regulated by "will power," a planned diet, calories or fat grams, emotional or sensory cues, such as sight or smell of food. | | Eating regulated predominantly by external and internal controls other than hunger and satiety. |
| **Prevalence** | Infants, small children, persons who don't diet or interfere with normal eating. At this time, higher rates among males, fewer among females. | Chaotic eating and undereating affect many girls and women in U.S., perhaps at times as many as the 50 to 80 percent age 11 and over who say they are trying to lose weight; also increasing numbers of boys and men. Consistent overeating may occur for both genders. | | Estimated prevalence is 10% of high school and college students; 90-95% female, 5-10% male. |

Reprinted from _Children and Teens in Weight Crisis_, by Frances M. Berg. Copyright 1996. All rights reserved. Publisher's written permission required for reproduction. Published by Healthy Weight Journal, 402 South 14th Street, Hettinger, ND 58639 (701-567-2646; Fax 701-567-2602).

# Dysfunctional eating: effects and relationships

| | Normal eating | Dysfunctional eating (mild, moderate, severe) | Eating disorders |
|---|---|---|---|
| **Physical** | Promotes health, energy, strength, and the healthy growth and development of children and youth. | May typically feel tired, apathetic, lacking in energy, chilled. Increased risk of stunted growth and reduced brain development with undernutrition. Decreased bone development or bone demineralization and higher risk of fractures. Delayed puberty, decrease in sexual interest. | Physical effects may be severe. Mortality reportedly as high as 18% for anorexia nervosa and bulimia nervosa. |
| | WEIGHT: Normal weight for the individual, expressing genetic and environmental factors. Any weight within wide range; usually stable. | WEIGHT: Any weight within wide range depending on genetic potential. Eating pattern may cause weight to decrease, cycle up and down, remain stable, or increase. | WEIGHT: Any weight within wide range, depending on genetic potential and the disorder and its expression. |
| **Mental focus** | Promotes clear thinking ability to concentrate. | Risk of decreased mental alertness and ability to concentrate, narrowing of interests, loss of ambition, and a turning inward. | Diminished capacity to think, memory loss, extreme narrowing of interests. |
| | FOOD THOUGHTS: low key, usually at mealtime. For women, 10-15% of time awake may be spent thinking of food, hunger, weight. | FOOD THOUGHTS: Increased preoccupation with food. Thoughts often focused on eating weight, planning when and what to eat, counting calories or fat grams. Thoughts of food, hunger, weight may occupy 20-65% of time. | FOOD THOUGHTS: Thoughts focused most of time on food, hunger, weight. For untreated anorexia about 90-110%, bulimia 70-90% of time awake (extra 10% includes dreaming). |
| **Emotional** | Promotes mood stability. | Potentially greater mood instability — highs and lows. May be easily upset, irritable, anxious, have lowered self-esteem. Increasing preoccupation and concern with body image. Increased risk of eating disorders. | Greater risk of mood instability and functional depression. |
| **Social** | Social integration; promotes healthy relationships with family, peers and community. | Less social integration, more risk of feeling isolated, self-absorbed and self-focused, stigmatized, disconnected from society, lonely. May have less interest in values of generosity, sharing volunteer activities; less sense of community. | Social withdrawal, isolated from family and friends, avoidance of and by peers, alienation, often eating alone; worsening family relations. |

Reprinted from *Children and Teens in Weight Crisis*, by Frances M. Berg. Copyright 1996. All rights reserved. Publisher's written permission required for reproduction. Published by Healthy Weight Journal, 402 South 14th Street, Hettinger, ND 58639 (701-567-2646; Fax 701-567-2602).

In their book, *Eating Disorders: Nutrition Therapy in the Recovery Process*, the Reiffs provide a food preoccupation scale. Individuals are asked to indicate total conscious time spent thinking about food, weight and hunger at three times in their lives: currently, at its highest, and at its lowest, and to give their age and weight for each. This includes time spent in shopping, preparing food, eating, thinking about eating or food cravings, purging, weighing, reading diet books, suppressing feelings of hunger, using strategies such as smoking or chewing gum to distract from hunger, and thinking about or discussing weight.

The researchers tested more than 500 eating disordered patients on this scale. They found that for untreated anorexia nervosa patients, 90 to 110 percent of waking time is spent thinking about food, weight and hunger. The extra 10 percent comes from dreams of food or weight, or having their sleep disturbed by hunger. Bulimic patients report about 70 to 90 percent.

From the testing he has done, Dan Reiff suggests that for women with normal eating, who are buying and preparing food for the family, the amount of time spent thinking about food, weight and hunger may be about 10 to 15 percent of waking time. In dysfunctional eating, this may occupy about 20 to 65 percent of waking hours, he reports.

In his studies, preoccupation with food is directly related to body weight and the degree and duration of semistarvation. In the Minnesota study, it appeared to be most closely related to the drop in body weight, as the men consumed a fairly adequate diet of 1,500 to 1,700 calories for six months, but lost one-fourth of their weight.

Dysfunctional eating can have severe physical and emotional effects. The individual may become moody, easily upset, irritable, anxious, apathetic and increasingly concerned about body image. She is often self-absorbed and self-focused. Self-esteem may be low, or focused on appearance.

The girl with dysfunctional eating may isolate herself socially, feeling lonely, alienated, and disconnected from society. She may focus less than others on the values of generosity, sharing, caring, and participate less in volunteer and community activities.

## Eating disorder risk

A major concern with the current high prevalence of dysfunctional eating is whether it will increase eating disorders.

A recent review reports that several one- and two-year longitudinal studies find that up to 35 percent of normal dieters progress to pathological dieting, and of pathological dieters, 20 to 25 percent progress to partial or full syndrome disorders. The report also says that 15 to 45 percent of those with partial syndrome progress to full syndrome eating disorders within one to four years.[5]

## Survival traits

Can some of these effects and relationships be explained as natural survival traits?

Early humans must have frequently feasted weeks on the carcass of a mammoth or beached whale, followed by a famine of seven months or seven years.

In deprivation, their bodies would have shut down to conserve fuel, not just with slowed heart rate and metabolism, but in every activity. Growth stopped or was severely stunted. Nearly all fat consumed was routed to storage to replace what was lost, instead of being used normally. Sexual activity and fertility shut down; as starvation progressed it was more critical to care for the young than to procreate. Ultimately, even children were abandoned, as Colin Turnbull reports so vividly in "The Mountain People."

At the same time, starvation causes high stress.

There is no peace for starving people. They crave food and focus all attention on this need. A useful survival trait, this kept our ancestors out hunting food despite weakness or danger, instead of lying listless in the cave, awaiting death. Without this complex internal regulation, the human race could hardly have survived.

But this ancient legacy haunts the dysfunctional eater today.

## Research needed

The adverse factors associated with dysfunctional eating and its high prevalence make further study imperative. Much research is needed in these areas.

How can we identify and measure the various patterns of dysfunctional eating? What causes the related adverse effects: is it abnormal eating habits, insufficient calories, iron or other nutrient deficiencies, weight loss, depleted fat cells, or psychological factors?

If dysfunctional eating is unhealthy, how can it be prevented? And how can normal eating be restored for children and adult women?

Normal eating itself needs study. What is normal eating and does it have its own range of patterns? How can it be measured?

A note of caution: The case made here for normal eating is not meant to imply that nutrition is the primary factor in good mental and physical health, but rather, that each person has a baseline of adequate nutrition, and perhaps an upper level, as well, and when this is disrupted there may be severe disruption of normal life and a diminishing of the mind, body and spirit.

Only when food supply is stable can people eat and live normally, as we interpret this today. With adequate nutrition and regular eating habits, they are able to focus on developing their full potential through a wide range of interests. They can afford the luxury of being generous, sharing, caring, and reaching out to others.

# Research basis

The concepts of dysfunctional eating presented here are based on the insights and research of numerous leaders in obesity, eating disorders and size acceptance fields. Among the important resources are: the early work on restrained eating by Janet Polivy and Peter Herman[6]; writings by Susan Wooley[7]; the work of Ellyn Satter on normal eating and "dieting casualties"[8]; Linda Omichinski's nondiet leadership and program development[9]; work on food preoccupation by Dan and Kim Reiff; starvation studies, including the Minnesota Experiment[10], United Nations reports on world malnutrition[11], and Colin Turnbull's description of starvation pressures on the African Ik tribe in "The Mountain People"[12]; national and local studies showing the high prevalence of dieting and disordered eating among children and adolescents[13]; research revealing the mental and physical effects of eating disorders, and their association with dieting[14]; writings on dieting risks and need to treat chronic dieting syndrome[15]; and the No Diet Day movement, led by Mary Evans Young,[16] and Eating Disorder Awareness Week, sponsored by eating disorder organizations.[17]

Most of this information has been reviewed in *Healthy Weight Journal* over the past 11 years, and is discussed extensively and referenced in the journal's special report "Health Risks of Weight Loss."

REFERENCES:

Berg F. Health Risks of Weight Loss, 1995. Chapter 1. General treatment risks, 14-26; Ch 7. Eating disorders, 56-62; Ch 8. Psychological risks, 63-69; Ch 9. Weight cycling, 70-79; Ch 11. Thinness: a cultural obsession, 89-99; Ch 13. To treat or not to treat, 108-113.

1. Niven C, D Carroll. The Health psychology of women. Harwood Academic Publ., Chur, Switzerland. 1993:115.

2. JADA 1992;92;92:7:851-53; Healthy Weight J/O&H 1993;7:3:46.

3. Third report on nutrition monitoring in the US, Life Sciences Research Office, Dec 1995. Interagency Board for Nutrition Monitoring and Related Research, US Gov Printing Office.

4. Reiff D, KK Lampson Reiff, Eating Disorders: Nutrition Therapy in the Recovery Process, 1992. Aspen, Gaithersburg, MD; Personal communication with Dan Reiff, 1996.

5. Estes L, M Crago, C Shisslak. Eating disorders prevention. The Renfrew Perspective, 1996;2:1:3-5.

6. Herman P, J Polivy. Eating and its disorders, edit Stunkard and Steller, 1984, 141-56. Raven Press; Healthy Weight J Mar/Apr 1996;10:2:32-33.

7. Wooley S, W Wooley. Eating and its disorders, edit Stunkard and Steller, 1984. Raven Press.

8. Satter, Ellyn. How to get your kids to eat — but not too much, Bull Publ, Palo Alto, CA; Workshops, "Treating the dieting casualty," Satter Assoc., Madison, WI.

9. Omichinski L. You Count, Calories Don't, 1992; HUGS facilitator programs, HUGS International, Box 102A, Rt3, Portage la Prairie, Manitoba, R1N 3A3, Canada; Teens & Diets — No Weigh, Healthy Weight J 1996;10:3:49-52; Berg F. Nondiet movement gains strength HWJ/Obesity & Health Sep/Oct 1992;6:5:82-90.

10. Keys A, et al. Biology of human starvation, 1950. U of Minn Press, Minneapolis, MN; Berg F, Starvation stages in weight loss patients similar to famine victims, HWJ/Obesity & Health Apr 1989;3:4:27-30.

11. Berg F. World starvation: weight may be best tool to measure malnutrition, Healthy Weight J May/Jun 1995;9:3:47-49; Body Mass Index: FAO, A measure of chronic energy deficiency in adults, 1994, United Nations report.

12. Turnbull, Colin. The Mountain People, 1972. Simon and Schuster, NY.

13. CDC USHHS, Behavioral Risk Survey; Calorie Control Council, 1991 National Survey; Berg F. Who is dieting in the U.S. Healthy Weight J/Obesity & Health 1992;6:3:48-49; Dieting and purging behavior in black and white high school students, JADA 1992;92:3:306-312; Adolescents dieting; JAMA 1991;266:2811-2812; Berg F. Harmful weight loss practices among adolescents, HWJ/O&H Jul/Aug 1992;6:4:69-72.

14. Fallon P, Katzman M, Wooley S. Feminist perspectives on eating disorders 1994, Guilford Press, NY; Baker D, R Sansone, Overview of eating disorders, 1994:1-10, NEDO; Kaplan A, P Garfinkel. Medical issues and the eating disorders, 1993, Brunner/Mazel, NY; Berg F. Eating disorders: physical and mental effects, Healthy Weight J Mar/Apr 1995;9:2:27-30; Smolak L, M Levine. Toward an empirical basis for primary prevention of eating problems with elementary school children, Eat Disorders 1994;2:4:293-307

15. Andersen A. The last word, Eating Disorders 1994;2:1:81-82; Bowers M. The last word. Eating Disorders 1994;2:4:375-377.

16. Young, Mary Evans. Diet Breaking, 1996, Hodder & Stoughton, London.

17. Biely J. Eating Disorder Awareness Week '96, EDAP Matters Winter 1996;2.

## Unit Selections

## Key Points to Consider

❖ Rank-order three issues of food safety that you think are the most important and justify your selection.

❖ What measures would you suggest to counteract misinformation about food safety and the tactics used by activist organizations?

❖ Observe yourself when you handle food. In what ways might you be the vector of foodborne illness?

❖ Read Upton Sinclair's muckraking novel *The Jungle*. Compare conditions and problems described in this book with today's procedures for ensuring a safe food supply.

❖ Watch in the news for reference to Codex and the participation of our government officials. What is their role and what are they trying to accomplish?

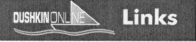 **Links**          **www.dushkin.com/online/**

These sites are annotated on pages 4 and 5.

*The dichotomization of risk distorts the reality that nothing is absolutely safe or absolutely dangerous.*
—Peter Sandman, quoted in "Determining Risk," FDA Consumer, *June 1990.*

In 1906, with the passage of the first Food and Drug Act, the federal government assumed some responsibility for food safety. Increased governmental involvement has been an inevitable trend ever since. With the 1950s came a fear that chemicals in the food supply, especially additives, might be carcinogenic. Congress responded with tighter control on the use and testing of additives. In 1958, the Delaney Clause prevented the use of any additives found to induce cancer in man or experimental animals, and the GRAS (Generally Recognized as Safe) list identified those believed by scientists to be safe for human consumption. This list is periodically revised, and the testing and retesting of additives continues. The Food and Drug Administration (FDA) governs all of these procedures, and books of regulations cover all aspects of food production and service.

Given the complexity of biological interactions, the uniqueness of each human organism, and the multitude of chemicals that potentially could interact, few knowledgeable people would contend that the absolute safety of anything can be ensured. Yet activist groups demand just that and have become experts at escalating a minor or nonexistent issue into a major catastrophe. It has been argued that if it takes programs like *60 Minutes*, or a partisan political group such as the National Resources Defense Council, or a self-appointed watchdog group such as Food and Water, Inc., to create a public issue, then it probably isn't a safety issue at all. Alar—a growth regulator used in apple orchards—is a good example. The scare in 1989 over Alar's safety appears to have been nothing more than media hype, but it seriously hurt the apple industry and shook parents' confidence in apple juice for their children.

The United States' food supply is among the world's safest; yet current surveys indicate that food safety has become a primary issue with consumers. This is hardly surprising, given the media coverage of foodborne illness outbreaks due to cyclospora on raspberries from Guatemala, salmonella at church suppers, and *E. coli* from a variety of products. In fact, one research group discovered that the Hudson Beef recall (25 million pounds) was the third most closely followed news story last year. That bacteria-laden foods do result in significant numbers of ill people cannot be denied. In a recent year, the Council for Agricultural Science and Technology reported 33 million cases and 9 thousand deaths. Other sources suggest that the figures may be even higher. On a yearly basis, total costs of these illnesses are estimated at $3–10 billion.

Some of today's most prevalent foodborne organisms were not public health issues 20 years ago, a sign that conditions and lifestyles have changed. One of these is *E. coli* 0157:H7, which is infamous for causing a 1991 outbreak of food poisoning in Washington State from undercooked hamburger. After repeated outbreaks, it has become clear that this type of contamination is truly serious, sometimes resulting in hemolytic uremic syndrome and kidney failure. *E. coli* accounts for thousands of cases of food poisoning yearly and approximately 250 deaths. It is known that *E. coli* can be carried not just by undercooked hamburger but by raw vegetables, unpasteurized cider, mayonnaise, and other food products as well. Reports indicate that this organism must be aggressively controlled in both the processing industry and the kitchen. Pasteurization and irradiation are two powerful measures currently used commercially, and other methods are being tested.

Many people blame the food industry or the government's food inspection procedures for the presence of illness-producing organisms in the food supply. And, indeed, government agencies are responding to the challenge. A new, state-of-the-art surveillance system permits scientists to determine the cause of an illness outbreak within 24 hours by entering the DNA fingerprinting of a pathogen in a national database. This speeds up intervention strategies to stop outbreaks with only a few illnesses. New tests are available to detect the presence of salmonella and *E. coli* on foods. The FDA has adopted HACCP (Hazard Analysis and Critical Control Points) rules to improve safety control and monitoring in the food production of meat, poultry, and seafood.

While many people assume that foodborne illness is contracted primarily in restaurants, it is revealing to discover that each of us is his or her own worst enemy. Surveys have shown that people fail to follow appropriate sanitation techniques in their own kitchens over 99 percent of the time, but food properly handled in home kitchens could reduce the incidence of disease significantly.

Food irradiation, addressed in an article by John Henkel, has been both a food safety issue and a political issue. Activist groups, such as Food and Water, Inc., effectively used aggressive scare tactics to delay irradiation in this country for a long time. Although it was approved previously in the United States for poultry, fresh produce, spices, and the food eaten by astronauts, only at the end of 1997 was irradiation finally approved for use with red meat. However, it has been recommended by the World Health Organization (WHO) for years and is used in over 20 countries to destroy pathogenic bacteria and to maintain high quality produce over a prolonged shelf life.

Two articles in this unit have international implications. A discussion of mad cow disease is included because of wide media coverage of a new variant of Creutzfeldt-Jakob Disease (CJD) found in Europe. First discovered in the 1920s, CJD is a rare neurological disease which affects about a million people per year worldwide. It has been found, for example, among Midwesterners who consider squirrel brains a delicacy. So far, the new variant is not a safety issue in America. However, more than 20 cases have occurred in Europe, most of them in the United Kingdom. A second article describes Codex, an international set of food standards, which is especially significant when we realize that nearly 40 percent of the fruits and 12 percent of the vegetables in our markets are imported.

The fallacy of the common consumer belief that the word "natural" is a guarantee of safety can be illustrated easily by pointing out the risks associated with snake venom or amanita mushrooms growing on the lawn or in the woods. Some toxins, including carcinogens, occur naturally in food.

Problems arising over the safety of food supplies can be documented throughout history. Sometimes there is disagreement on the extent of the problem and on how to solve it. As consumers, we must accept personal responsibility for safe food handling. We must also continue to expect our regulatory agencies to do their best.

# FOODBORNE ILLNESS:
## ROLE OF HOME FOOD HANDLING PRACTICES

The Principal author of this Scientific Status Summary was S. J. Knable, Ph.D., The Pennsylvania State University

Outbreaks of foodborne illness, such as the highly publicized outbreaks of *Escherichia coli* O157:H7 in the western United States in early 1993 that led to the tragic deaths of four children (CDC, 1993), remind us that under certain circumstances, familiar foods can lead to serious consequences, even death. Despite progress in improving the overall quality and safety of foods produced in the U.S., significant foodborne illness and death due to microbial pathogens still occur....

## FACTORS CONTRIBUTING TO NEW MICROBIOLOGICAL CHALLENGES

Several interrelated factors contribute to new microbiological challenges and risks throughout the food system.

**Demographics and lifestyles.** Demography and lifestyle of U.S. consumers have changed dramatically during the past two decades. The U.S. population has increased and family size has decreased. There are more families with both parents working outside the home and more single-parent households than previously. More children are shopping for and preparing their own food because no parent is home during the day (Goldman, 1990). In addition, the proportion of elderly individuals in the population has also increased and the number of people at increased risk for foodborne illness has grown.

Preference for quick methods of food preparation, convenience foods, fresh and "fresh-like foods," minimally processed foods, and foods that meet specific health/dietary needs has increased. To meet these preferences and the needs of a growing population, new processing, preservation, and packaging techniques have been incorporated into the manufacturing of food products. Distribution networks have become large, centralized, and complex. Changes such as these affect the epidemiology of foodborne illnesses and present new microbiological risks.

Minimally processed foods, for example, are designed for convenience, "fresh-like" state, and extended shelf life. Minimally processed foods present concerns to food manufacturers in maintaining product safety. These foods may receive a lower heat treatment than required for commercial sterility. They may be vacuum packaged or packaged in atmospheres modified by the addition of nitrogen and/or carbon dioxide. Such processing and packaging conditions alter the microbial ecology of foods. The heat treatment may destroy some microorganisms but not others, e.g., bacterial spores. The modified atmospheres may inhibit the growth of some microorganisms surviving the heat treatment, but may enhance the growth of others, even at refrigeration temperatures. The extension of shelf life may allow time for growth of undesirable, harmful microorganisms. This is of particular concern in ready-to-eat products not requiring cooking before consumption....

Several microorganisms that were not previously recognized as important foodborne pathogens have emerged during the past two decades, adding to our microbiological challenges. These pathogens include Norwalk virus, *Campylobacter jejuni*, *E. coli* O157:H7, *Listeria monocytogenes*, *Vibrio vulnificus*, *Vibrio cholera*, and *Yersinia enterocolitica* (IOM, 1992; Doyle, 1991; Doyle, 1985). Some of these microorganisms, *Campylobacter*, for example, may have come to our attention through investigative surveillance and ability of laboratories to identify them (Hedberg et al., 1994). *E. coli* O157:H7 appears to be a new pathogen that acquired genetic determinants for new virulence factors (Whittam et al., 1993; Griffin and Tauxe, 1991). *E.coli* O157:H7 was first recognized as a foodborne pathogen in 1982 and is now known as an important cause of the diarrheal form of hemorrhagic colitis (painful bloody diarrhea) and renal failure in humans (Padhye and Doyle, 1992; Griffin and Tauxe, 1991; Doyle, 1985). In its report on a small outbreak in California, the CDC noted that many unrecognized sporadic cases and small outbreaks of *E. coli* O157:H7 due to

From *Food Technology: Scientific Status Summary*, April 1995, pp. 119-131. Reprinted by permission of *Food Technology: Scientific Status Summary*, a publication of the Institute of Food Technologists' Expert Panel on Food Safety and Nutrition.

## Table 1—Common Foodborne Diseases Caused by Bacteria. *From Cliver (1993)*

| Disease (causative agent) | Latency Period (duration) | Principal Symptoms | Typical Foods | Mode of Contamination | Prevention of Disease |
|---|---|---|---|---|---|
| (*Bacillus cereus*) food poisoning, diarrheal | 8–16 hr (12–24 hr) | Diarrhea, cramps, occasional vomiting | Meat products, soups sauces, vegetables | From soil or dust | Thorough heating and rapid cooling of foods |
| (*Bacillus cereus*) food poisoning, emetic | 1–5 hr (6–24 hr) | Nausea, vomiting, sometimes diarrhea and cramps | Cooked rice and pasta | From soil or dust | Thorough heating and rapid cooling of foods |
| Botulism; food poisoning (heat-labile toxin of *Clostridium botulinum*) | 12–36 hr (months) | Fatigue, weakness, double vision, slurred speech, respiratory failure, sometimes death | Types A&B: vegetables; fruits; meat, fish, and poultry products; condiments; Type E: fish and fish products | Types A&B: from soil or dust; Type E: water and sediments | Thorough heating and rapid cooling of foods |
| Botulism; food poisoning infant infection | Unknown | Constipation, weakness, respiratory failure, sometimes death | Honey, soil | Ingested spores from soil or dust or honey colonize intestine | Do not feed honey to infants —will not prevent all |
| Campylobacteriosis (*Camplyobacter jejuni*) | 3–5 days (2–10 days) | Diarrhea, abdominal pain, fever, nausea, vomiting | Infected food-source animals | Chicken, raw milk | Cook chicken thoroughly; avoid cross-contamination; irradiate chickens; pasteurize milk |
| Cholera (*Vibrio cholerae*) | 2–3 days hours to days | Profuse, watery stools; sometimes vomiting, dehydration; often fatal if untreated | Raw or undercooked seafood | Human feces in marine environment | Cook seafood thoroughly; general sanitation |
| (*Clostridium perfringens*) food poisoning | 8–22 hr (12–24 hr) | Diarrhea, cramps, rarely nausea and vomiting | Cooked meat and poultry | Soil, raw foods | Thorough heating and rapid cooling of foods |
| (*Escherichia coli*) foodborne infections enterohemorrhagic | 12–60 hr (2–9 days) | Watery, bloody diarrhea | Raw or undercooked beef, raw milk | Infected cattle | Cook beef thoroughly pasteurize milk |
| (*Escherichia coli*) foodborne infections entroinvasive | at least 18 hr (uncertain) | Cramps, diarrhea, fever, dysentery | Raw foods | Human fecal contamination, direct or via water | Cook foods thoroughly; general sanitation |
| (*Escherichia coli*) foodborne infection enterotoxigenic | 10–72 hr (3–5 days) | Profuse watery diarrhea; sometimes cramps, vomiting | Raw foods | Human fecal contamination, direct or via water | Cook foods thoroughly; general sanitation |
| Listeriosis (*Listeria monocytogenes*) | 3–70 days | Meningoencephalitis; stillbirths; septicemia or meningitis in newborns | Raw milk, cheese and vegetables | Soil or infected animals, directly or via manure | Pasteurization of milk; cooking |
| Salmonellosis (*Salmonella* species) | 5–72 hr (1–4 days) | Diarrhea, abdominal pain, chills, fever, vomiting, dehydration | Raw, undercooked eggs; raw milk, meat and poultry | Infected food-source animals; human feces | Cook eggs, meat and poultry thoroughly; pasteurize milk; irradiate chickens |
| Shigellosis (*Shigella* species) | 12–96 hr (4–7 days) | Diarrhea, fever, nausea; sometimes vomiting, cramps | Raw foods | Human fecal contamination, direct or via water | General sanitation; cook foods thoroughly |
| Staphylococcal food poisoning (heat-stable enterotoxin of *Staphylococcus aureus*) | 1–6 hr (6–24 hr) | Nausea, vomiting, diarrhea, cramps | Ham, meat, poultry products, cream-filled pastries, whipped butter, cheese | Handlers with colds, sore throats or infected cuts, food slicers | Thorough heating and rapid cooling of foods |
| Streptococcal foodborne infection (*Streptococcus pyogenes*) | 1–3 days (varies) | Various, including sore throat, erysipelas, scarlet fever | Raw milk, deviled eggs | Handlers with sore throats, other "strep" infections | General sanitation, pasteurize milk |
| *Vibrio parahaemolyticus* foodborne infection | 12–24 hr (4–7 days) | Diarrhea, cramps; sometimes nausea, vomiting, fever, headache | Fish and seafoods | Marine coastal environment | Cook fish and seafoods thoroughly |
| *Vibrio vulnificus* foodborne infection | In persons with high serum iron: 1 day | Chills, fever, prostration, often death | Raw oysters and clams | Marine coastal environment | Cook shellfish thoroughly |
| Yersiniosis (*Yersinia enterocolitica*) | 3–7 days (2–3 weeks) | Diarrhea, pains mimicking appendicitis, fever vomiting, etc. | Raw or undercooked pork and beef; tofu packed in spring water | Infected animals especially swine; contaminated water | Cook meats thoroughly, chlorinate water |

Reprinted with permission from the American Council on Science and Health (ACSH), New York, NY

undercooking of hamburger in the home probably occur throughout the U.S. (CDC, 1994a).

*Listeria monocytogenes* has been recognized as a human pathogen for several decades but the importance of food as a vehicle for transmission has only recently been identified (Doyle, 1985). *L. monocytogenes* is widely distributed in the environment and carried in the intestinal tracts of a variety of animals and humans (Doyle, 1985). Of significance to food safety, the microorganism can grow, although slowly, at refrigeration temperatures. *Listeria monocytogenes* causes illness primarily in individuals at increased risk for foodborne illness. Infection with *L. monocytogenes* may result in meningitis, miscarriage, and perinatal septicemia (Doyle, 1985). *S. enteriditis* can contaminate whole shell eggs when infected hens transmit the pathogen to the egg when it is produced. The global incidence of this serotype increased dramatically from 5% of all isolates in the U.S. in the 1970s to 20% of isolates in 1989 (St. Louis et al., 1988).

Emergence of these microbial health threats (diseases and their causative agents) may be due to several factors. These include: emergence of new microorganisms, recognition of existing diseases previously undetected, and changes in the environment that provide an epidemiologic "bridge" (IOM, 1992). The potential for foods to be involved in the emergence or reemergence of microbial threats to humans is great, largely because there are many points in the food system at which food safety can be compromised (IOM, 1992). . . .

## FACTORS CONTRIBUTING TO FOODBORNE ILLNESS IN THE HOME

The extent of the hazards associated with pathogenic microorganisms and the risk of acquiring foodborne illness depend on several factors. These include type of pathogen, number of microorganisms ingested, and the consumers' susceptibility to the pathogen.

**Pathogens.** Pathogenic bacteria, viruses, fungi, parasitic protozoa, other parasites, and marine phytoplankton may cause foodborne illness. One way foodborne illness may arise is from infection by microorganisms and parasites. Infection occurs when pathogens, such as *Campylobacter* or *Salmonella*, in the ingested food, grow in the host's intestine. The infection may involve subsequent growth in other tissues or the production of toxin, in which case the illness is classified as a toxicoinfection. Foodborne illness may also stem from intoxication. Intoxication occurs when pathogens, such as *S. aureus*, produce toxin in a food or when a toxic chemical occurs in food before consumption. Common foodborne diseases caused by pathogenic microorganisms or their toxins are described in Tables 1–4. Depending on host susceptibility, foodborne illness may be mild to severe or lead to serious chronic complications such as arthritis, carditis, Guillain-Barre' syndrome, and hemolytic anemia (CAST, 1994; Smith, 1994; Archer and Young, 1988; Mossel, 1988; Archer 1985) or death. The complications that may be associated with certain foodborne illnesses are listed in Table 5.

Among outbreaks of known etiology reported to the Centers for Disease Control and Prevention (CDC) between 1973 and 1987, bacterial pathogens were responsible for most of the outbreaks (66%) and cases (92%; Bean et al., 1990). . . .

About 60% of the foodborne illnesses reported to CDC from 1973–1987 were of unknown etiology. The inability to determine the etiologic agent in reported outbreaks may be attributable to late or incomplete laboratory investigations, lack of recognition of the pathogen as a disease agent, or inability to identify the pathogen with available laboratory techniques (Bean and Griffin, 1990; Bean et al., 1990). . . .

The ability of several bacterial pathogens to multiply rapidly to dangerous levels in foods allowed to warm up or to remain warm for an extended period is responsible for their frequent implication in foodborne illness. Some pathogens, however, such as *L. monocytogenes*

*"The potential for foods to be involved in the emergence or reemergence of microbial threats to humans is great ... (IOM, 1992)."*

---

**Table 2—Common Foodborne Diseases Caused by Viruses.** *From Cliver (1993)*

| Disease (causative agent) | Onset (duration) | Principal Symptoms | Typical Foods | Mode of Contamination | Prevention of Disease |
|---|---|---|---|---|---|
| Hepatitis A (Hepatitis A virus) | 15–20 days (weeks to months) | Fever, weakness, nausea discomfort; often jaundice | Raw or undercooked shellfish; sandwiches, salads, etc. | Human fecal contamination, via water or direct | Cook shellfish thoroughly; general sanitation |
| Viral gastroenteritis (Norwalk-like viruses) | 1–2 days (1–2 days) | Nausea, vomiting, diarrhea, pains, headache, mild fever | Raw or undercooked shellfish; sandwiches, salads, etc. | Human fecal contamination, via water or direct | Cook shellfish thoroughly, general sanitation |
| Viral gastroenteritis (rotaviruses) | 1–3 days (4–6 days) | Diarrhea, especially in infants and young children | Raw or mishandled foods | Probably human fecal contamination | General sanitation |

*Reprinted with permission from the American Council on Science and Health, New York, NY*

and *Y. enterocolitica*, can grow at refrigeration temperatures and others, such as *E. coli* O157:H7, and viruses, can cause illness at very low levels in foods.

Certain pathogens may be a greater problem in the home than in foodservice establishments or in commercially prepared foods. Approximately 92% of the 231 outbreaks of botulism from 1973–1987 were associated with food prepared in the home, especially home-canned foods (Bean and Griffin, 1990). . . .

**Foods.** A variety of foods are associated with foodborne illnesses, including foods of animal origin, such as fish and shellfish, red meats, poultry, fruits and vegetables, eggs, and dairy products (CAST, 1994; Bean and Griffin, 1990; Bryan, 1988a). In recent years, foodborne illnesses have been associated with novel substrates, such as potatoes, sauteed onions, garlic-in-oil mixtures, cooked rice, and sliced fruits. Vegetables grown in the ground or close to it are likely to be contaminated by

the spore-forming bacteria *C. botulinum*, *C. perfringens*, and *B. cereus* (Bryan 1988a). Outbreaks of botulism have been associated with foil-wrapped baked potatoes left at room temperature, sauteed onions, and garlic-in-oil mixtures. Outbreaks of *B. cereus* food poisoning have been associated with cooked rice held at room temperature.

**Mishandling Factors.** From 1973–1987, 7,458 outbreaks and 237,545 cases of foodborne illness were reported to the CDC. Among the 7,219 outbreaks in which it was reported, the site of preparation of the implicated food was a commercial or institutional establishment in 79% of outbreaks and the home in 21%, with variations for different illness etiologies (Bean and Griffin, 1990). Sporadic cases and small outbreaks in homes, however, are considered far more common than cases constituting recognized outbreaks and comprise most of the foodborne illness cases in the U.S. (Schuchat et al. 1992; Tauxe, 1992, 1991; Bean and

**Table 3—Common Foodborne Diseases Caused by Protozoa and Parasites.** *From Cliver (1993)*

| Disease (causative agent) | Onset (duration) | Principal Symptoms | Typical Foods | Mode of Contamination | Prevention of Disease |
|---|---|---|---|---|---|
| (PROTOZOA) Amebic dysentery (*Entamoeba histolytica*) | 2–4 weeks (varies) | Dysentery, fever, chills; sometimes liver abscess | Raw or mishandled foods | Cysts in human feces | General sanitation; thorough cooking |
| Cryptosporidiosis (*Cryptosporidium parvum*) | 1–12 days (1–30 days) | Diarrhea; sometimes fever, nausea, and vomiting | Mishandled foods | Oocysts in human feces | General sanitation; thorough cooking |
| Giardiasis (*Giardia lamblia*) | 5–25 days (varies) | Diarrhea with greasy stools, cramps, bloat | Mishandled foods | Cysts in human and animal feces, directly or via water | General sanitation; thorough cooking |
| Toxoplasmosis (*Toxoplasma gondii*) | 10–23 days (varies) | Resembles mononucleosis fetal abnormality or death | Raw or undercooked meats; raw milk; mishandled foods | Cysts in pork or mutton, rarely beef; oocysts in cat feces | Cook meat thoroughly; pasteurize milk; general sanitation |
| (ROUNDWORMS, Nematodes) Anisakiasis (*Anisakis simplex, Pseudoterranova decipiens*) | Hours to weeks (varies) | Abdominal cramps, nausea, vomiting | Raw or undercooked marine fish, squid or octopus | Larvae occur naturally in edible parts of seafoods | Cook fish thoroughly or freeze at -4° F for 30 days |
| Ascariasis (*Ascaris lumbricoides*) | 10 days –8 weeks (1–2 years) | Sometimes pneumonitis, bowel obstructions | Raw fruits or vegetables that grow in or near soil | Eggs in soil from human feces | Sanitary disposal of feces; cooking food |
| Trichinosis (*Trichinella spiralis*) | 8–15 days (weeks, months) | Muscle pain, swollen eyelids, fever; sometimes death | Raw or undercooked pork or meat of carnivorous animals (e.g., bears) | Larvae encysted in animal's muscles | Thorough cooking of meat; freezing pork at 5° F for 30 days; irradiation |
| (TAPEWORMS, Cestodes) Beef tapeworm (*Taenia saginata*) | 10–14 weeks (20–30 years) | Worm segments in stool; sometimes digestive disturbances | Raw or undercooked beef | "Cysticerci" in beef muscle | Cook beef thoroughly or freeze below 23°F |
| Fish tapeworm (*Diphyllobothrium latum*) | 3–6 weeks (years) | Limited: sometimes vitamin B-12 deficiency | Raw or undercooked fresh-water fish | "Plerocercoids" in fish muscle | Heat fish 5 minutes at 133°F or freeze 24 hours at 0°F |
| Pork tapeworm (*Taenia solium*) | 8 weeks–10 years (20–30 years) | Worm segments in stool; sometimes "cysticercosis" of muscles, organs, heart, or brain | Raw or undercooked pork; any food mishandled by a *T. solium* carrier | "Cysticerci" in pork muscle; any food —human feces with *T. solium* eggs | Cook pork thoroughly or freeze below 23°F; general sanitiation |

*Reprinted with permission from the American Council on Science and Health, New York, NY*

## Table 4—Common Foodborne Diseases Caused by Toxins in Seafood. *Adapted from Cliver (1993)*

| Disease (causative agent) | Onset (duration) | Principal Symptoms | Typical Foods | Mode of Contamination | Prevention of Disease |
|---|---|---|---|---|---|
| (TOXINS IN FINFISH) Ciguatera poisoning (ciguatoxin, etc.) | 3–4 hr (rapid)<br><br>12–18 hr (days–months) | Diarrhea, nausea, vomiting, abdominal pain<br><br>Numbness & tingling of face; taste & vision aberrations, sometimes convulsions, respiratory arrest, and death (1–24 hrs) | "Reef and island" fish: grouper, surgeon fish, barracuda, pompano, snapper, etc. | (Sporadic); food chain, from algae | Eat only small fish |
| Fugu or pufferfish poisoning (tetrodotoxin, etc.) | 10–45 min to ≥ 3 hr | Nausea, vomiting, tingling lips and tongue, ataxia, dizziness, respiratory distress/arrest, sometimes death | Pufferfish, "fugu" (many species) | Toxin collects in gonads, viscera | Avoid pufferfish (or their gonads) |
| Scombroid or histamine poisoning (histamine, etc.) | minutes to few hours (few hours) | Nausea, vomiting, diarrhea, cramps, flushing, headache, burning in mouth | "Scombroid" fish (tuna, mackerel, etc.); mahimahi, others | Bacterial action | Refrigerate fish immediately when caught |
| (TOXINS IN SHELLFISH) Amnesic shellfish poisoning (domoic acid) | | Vomiting, abdominal cramps, diarrhea, disorientation, memory loss; sometimes death | Mussels, clams | From algae | Heed surveillance warnings |
| Paralytic shellfish poisoning (saxitoxin, etc.) | ≤ 1 hr (≤ 24 hr) | Vomiting, diarrhea, paresthesias of face, sensory and motor disorders; respiratory paralysis, death | Mussels, clams, scallops, oysters | From "red tide" algae | Heed surveillance warnings |

*Reprinted with permission from the American Council on Science and Health, New York, NY*

## Table 5–Medical Complications Associated with Certain Foodborne Infections. *From CAST (1994)*

| Bacterial Infections Transmitted by Foods | Complications/sequelae |
|---|---|
| *Aeromonas hydrophila* enteritis[a] | Bronchopneumonia, cholecystitis |
| Brucellosis | Aortitis, epididymo-orchitis, meningitis, pericarditis, spondylitis |
| Campylobacteriosis | Arthritis, carditis, cholecystitis, colitis, endocarditis, erythema nodosum, Guillain-Barre' syndrome, hemolytic-uremic syndrome, meningitis, pancreatitis, septicemia |
| Escherichia coli (EHEC-types) enteritis | Erythema nodosum, hemolytic uremic syndrome, seronegative arthropathy, thrombotic thrombocytopenic purpura |
| Q-fever | Endocarditis, granulomatous hepatitis |
| Salmonellosis | Aortitis, cholecystitis, colitis, endocarditis, epididymoorchitis, meningitis, myocarditis, osteomyelitis, pancreatitis, Reiter's disease, rheumatoid syndromes, septicemia, splenic abscesses, thyroiditis, septic arthritis (sickle-cell anemic persons) |
| Shigellosis | Erythema nodosum, hemolytic-uremic syndrome, peripheral neuropathy, pneumonia, Reiter's disease, septicemia, splenic abscesses, synovitis |
| *Vibrio parahaemolyticus* enteritis | Septicemia |
| Yersiniosis | Arthritis, cholangitis, erythema nodosum, liver and splenic abscesses, lymphadenitis, pneumonia, pyomyositis, Reiter's disease, septicemia, spondylitis, Still's disease |
| **Parasitic Infections Transmitted by Foods** | **Complications/sequelae** |
| Cryptosporidiosis[b] | Severe diarrhea, prolonged and sometimes fatal |
| Giardiasis[b] | Cholangitis, dystrophy, joint symptoms, lymphoidal hyperplasia |
| Taeniasis | Arthritis, cysticercosis (*T. solium*) |
| Toxoplasmosis | Encephalitis and other central nervous system diseases, pancarditis, polymyositis |
| Trichinosis | Cardiac dysfunction, neurologic sequelae |

[a]Suspected to be foodborne or waterborne.
[b]Waterborne.

Griffin, 1990; Schwartz et al., 1988). Foodborne illness in the home is reported much less frequently than institutional outbreaks because fewer people are typically involved. Additionally, sporadic cases of mild illnesses are less likely than more serious illnesses to result in medical attention, reporting, and investigation.

Bryan (1988b) reviewed the handling errors leading to foodborne illness outbreaks in the U.S. reported to CDC between 1961 and 1982. The top 12 factors contributing to 345 outbreaks resulting from mishandling/mistreatment of foods in the home are listed in Table 6. Use of contaminated foods or raw ingredients, inadequate cooking/canning/heat processing, and obtaining food from an unsafe source were the three leading factors contributing to foodborne illness in the home. Raw animal products may contain low levels of pathogenic microorganisms and cause illness if not properly cooked. For example, poultry may contain various species of *Salmonella* and *Campylobacter*; shell eggs may contain species of *Salmonella,* especially *S. enteritidis;* and ground beef may contain various pathogens, including *E. coli* O157:H7. Shellfish from sewage-polluted waters, raw milk, and wild mushrooms are foods obtained from unsafe sources. Microorganisms associated with these foods may be spread during preparation and may survive inadequate heating. Bacterial spores may be present on soil-grown cereals, vegetables, and fruits and may survive heating that is less severe than heating in a pressure cooker.

The fourth and fifth factors, improper cooling and lapse of time between preparation and eating, are time and temperature violations. The sixth factor is contamination of food by food handlers. People who carry foodborne pathogens in their intestinal tracts or touch fecally contaminated surfaces and fail to completely remove traces of fecal contamination by proper hand washing may contaminate any food they touch.

Bean and Griffin (1990) listed the mishandling factors thought to contribute to 1,678 foodborne illness outbreaks occurring during 1973–1987 with corresponding etiologies. Improper storage or holding temperature was the factor most often reported in *B. cereus* (94%), *C. perfringens* (97%), *Salmonella* (84%), *S. aureus* (98%), and group A *Streptococcus* (100%) outbreaks. Inadequate cooking was the factor most often reported in outbreaks due to *C. botulinum* (91%), *V. parahaemolyticus* (92%), and *Trichinella spiralis* (100%). Food from an unsafe source was the factor most often cited for outbreaks due to *Brucella* (100%), *Campylobacter* (67%), ciguatoxin (83%), mushroom poisoning (98%), and paralytic shellfish poisoning (100%). Personal hygiene was most frequently reported in *Shigella* (91%), Hepatitis A (96%), Norwalk virus

(78%), and *Giardia* (100%) outbreaks. For each year from 1983–1987, Bean et al. (1990) reported that the most common practice that contributed to foodborne disease was improper

**Table 6–Top Twelve Factors Contributing** *to 345 Outbreaks of Foodborne Disease Caused by Mishandling and/or Mistreatment of Foods in Homes in the U.S., 1973-1982. From Bryan (1988b)*

| Rank | Contributing Factor | Percent[a] |
|---|---|---|
| 1. | Contaminated raw food/ ingredient | 42.0 |
| 2. | Inadequate cooking/ canning/heat processing | 31.3 |
| 3. | Obtained food from unsafe source | 28.7 |
| 4. | Improper cooling | 22.3 |
| 5. | Lapse of 12 or more hours between preparing and eating | 12.8 |
| 6. | Colonized person handling implicated food | 9.9 |
| 7. | Mistaken for food | 7.0 |
| 8. | Improper fermentations | 4.6 |
| 9. | Inadequate reheating | 3.5 |
| 10. | Toxic containers | 3.5 |
| 11. | Improper hot holding | 3.2 |
| 12. | Cross-contamination | 3.2 |

[a]Percentage exceeds 100 because multiple factors contribute to single outbreaks.

storage or holding temperature, followed by poor personal hygiene of the food handler.

Usually several sequential factors result in foodborne illness (Bryan, 1988b). These are: (1) a pathogen must reach the food, (2) it must survive there until ingested, (3) in some cases, it must multiply to reach infectious levels or produce toxins, and (4) the person ingesting the food must be susceptible to the levels ingested. For example, in staphylococcal food poisoning, *S. aureus* typically reaches cooked food during handling. With sufficient time at room temperature or during inadequate cooling in too large a container in the refrigerator, the pathogen produces enterotoxin. The first six of the top 12 factors contributing to foodborne illness outbreaks (listed in Table 6) are either contamination and/or time and temperature-related errors. These errors account for the vast majority of foodborne illnesses in the home.

### PREVENTING FOODBORNE ILLNESS IN THE HOME

Everyone in the food system, from those

*"Everyone in the food system, from those who produce food to those who prepare it, has a role in food safety."*

who produce food to those who prepare it, has a role in food safety. People in each segment of the food system need to understand the compelling reasons for proactive control of food safety. These reasons include: (1) microorganisms are ubiquitous in the environment and are found on raw agricultural products, (2) pathogens may survive minimal preservation treatments, (3) humans may introduce pathogens into food products during production, processing, distribution and/or preparation just before consumption, (4) depending on individual susceptibility, foodborne illness can range from mild to severe and life-threatening, with chronic complications.

People need to be aware of the control they have in their own kitchen for foodborne illness. They also need to understand how important food handling practices—acquisition, storage, preparation, serving, and dealing with leftovers—affect food safety. The top four mishandling factors cited in Table 6 are the most critical food handling practices to stress in food safety programs (Bryan, 1988b). Messages to the public about handling practices important in maintaining the safety of new unfamiliar food products may also be useful.

**Messages and Educational Strategies.** The most effective and practical strategy for controlling hazards and assuring food safety throughout the food system is the Hazard Analysis and Critical Control Points (HACCP) concept (Bauman, 1990). Successful application of the HACCP concept requires monitoring the points, processes, or practices that are critical for food safety and then actively controlling them to prevent problems from occurring. The food processing industry has effectively applied HACCP to the control of foodborne pathogens since the 1970s (Bauman, 1990). HACCP is relevant to all stages of the food system, from production to consumption. Education and training of people in each segment of the food system—from producers, retailers, foodservice operators, to preparers—should be an integral part of HACCP. Educational efforts, varying appropriately for different target audiences, should be proactive and messages should be HACCP-based, clear, consistent, and persuasive.

The U.S. Dept. of Agriculture (USDA, 1989) applied the HACCP concept in developing educational material for consumers. The agency identified five "educational critical control points" defined as the points most important in preventing foodborne illness but least understood by consumers. The points identified were: acquisition, storage, preparation, service, and handling leftovers. For example, in "A Quick Consumer Guide to Safe Food Handling" the agency provides the following advice based on the five critical control points:

- When you shop, buy cold food last, get it home fast.
- When you store food, keep it safe, refrigerate.
- When you prepare food, keep everything clean, thaw in refrigerator.
- When you're cooking, cook thoroughly.
- When you serve food, never leave it out over two hours.
- When you handle leftovers, use small, shallow containers for quick cooling.
- When in doubt, throw it out.

Similarly, the agency's safe food handling labels, shown in Fig. 1, required in July 1994 on packages of raw and partially cooked meat and poultry products, provide advice based on critical control points.

Some foodborne pathogens present few risks to most individuals but life-threatening risks to others, e.g., those with immunosuppression due to illness or medications, infants, pregnant women, and elderly individuals. Special educational emphasis should be given to these "at risk" groups. These individuals need to understand that they are more susceptible to foodborne illness even if they consume very low levels of foodborne pathogens, and therefore, must vigilantly use proper food handling practices. They must understand the need to avoid eating raw or undercooked animal foods, such as unpasteurized milk, avoid eating raw or undercooked seafood, particularly molluscan shellfish, and prevent cross-contamination between raw and cooked foods during preparation and storage. Individuals in these "at risk" groups and those who serve them need to understand that they should thoroughly cook raw animal foods to at least 160°F to kill any pathogens that may be present, promptly refrigerate leftovers in small shallow containers, and reheat leftovers to 165°F before consumption. Because outbreaks involving many deaths have occurred in nursing homes as a result of consumption of undercooked eggs or products made from raw eggs, the CDC recommends use of pasteurized eggs for institutions such as nursing homes and hospitals (CDC, 1990). The CDC recommends that, to avoid listeriosis, people at high risk use proper food handling practices and thoroughly wash raw vegetables before eating, avoid eating soft cheeses (e.g., Mexican-style and feta) and reheat ready-to-eat foods (e.g., hot dogs) thoroughly to at least 165°F. The CDC also said that these individuals may choose to avoid foods from delicatessen counters and to thoroughly reheat cold cuts to at least 165°F before eating (CDC, 1992; Schuchat et al., 1992).

Caregivers of infants younger than age one must understand the need for close attention to their use of sanitary containers, potable water (safe drinking water), good personal hygiene

*"Education and training of people in each segment of the food system—from producers, retailers, foodservice operators, to preparers—should be an integral part of HACCP."*

(hand washing), and sanitary practices in the preparation of infant formula. If possible, individuals who change diapers in institutional day care centers should refrain from preparing foods for infants. Because microorganisms may be introduced into the formula from the infant during feeding, leftover infant formula should be discarded after each feeding and a new container should be prepared immediately before the next feeding.

The CDC (1994b) suggested that because messages about behaviors that prevent or foster emerging infections are often most effective before unsafe behaviors develop, educational efforts targeting children and adolescents should be emphasized. Similarly, the National Advisory Committee on Microbiological Criteria for Foods (NACMCF), formed in 1988 by agencies of the U.S. Depts. of Agriculture, Health and Human Services, Commerce, and Defense, recommended the development of a basic food safety curriculum and specific lesson plans with accompanying audiovisual materials for public and private school systems (Rhodes, 1991). The NACMCF also advised that training be provided for teachers of children, initially, in grades 4–6. Further, the committee said that public service announcements were needed to foster the awareness of food safety principles (Rhodes, 1991). Additional strategies for reaching consumers include providing information in leaflets at retail markets, in recipes, in computer programs, and on computer networks. Safe food handling educational programs for national television audiences similar to those targeted at preventing AIDS and automobile injuries would be helpful.

As new innovative foods, such as minimally processed foods, are developed, clear, HACCP-based information about the importance of refrigeration and other handling practices would be useful. The NACMCF recommended the development of a mandatory, uniform logo, to read "*Important* Must Be Kept Refrigerated," for perishable refrigerated items for which temperature is the key element of safety (Rhodes, 1991). Because temperature maintenance can be extremely important, the committee also recommended that manufacturers use time/temperature indicators where possible to show product mishandling. Sherlock et al. (1992) suggested that consumer education may be necessary to ensure the success of time/temperature indicators. Incorporation of food handling information into product labels may be useful to actively and continuously educate consumers about new food products and the necessary safe food handling practices.

**Resources for Consumers and Educators.** A variety of information about food safety, including food handling tips, is available for

### Safe Handling Instructions

This product was prepared from inspected and passed meat and/or poultry. Some food products may contain bacteria that could cause illness if the product is mishandled or cooked improperly. For your protection, follow these safe handling instructions.

Keep refrigerated or frozen. Thaw in refrigerator or microwave.

Keep raw meat and poultry separate from other foods. Wash working surfaces (including cutting boards), utensils, and hands after touching raw meat or poultry.

Cook thoroughly.

Keep hot foods hot. Refrigerate leftovers immediately or discard.

Fig. 1—Label *as described in Code of Federal Regulations, title 9, parts 317 and 381*

consumers and educators from several sources including: federal agencies (Food and Drug Administration, USDA, CDC), food industry trade organizations, scientific societies, food science and nutrition departments at land grant colleges and universities, and other organizations. Information formats include printed materials and videos for educators, other professionals, and the public. Much of the material is free or available for a nominal cost. Some material is written specifically for certain groups of people, such as people at high risk for foodborne disease. Information published by federal agencies may also be available from the local offices of these agencies.

As part of a national campaign to reduce the risk of foodborne illness and to increase knowledge of food-related risks from food production through consumption, the FDA and USDA established in 1994 the Foodborne Illness Education Information Center (Beltsville, MD). The Center is developing an educational database that will be made available to educators, trainers, and organizations producing educational and training materials for food workers and consumers. The database is accessible through a variety of electronic networks such as Internet, the National Agriculture Library electronic bulletin board, and PENpages' International Food and Nutrition Database.

The USDA's Food Safety and Inspection Service also operates a Meat and Poultry Hotline (1-800-535-4555) to answer questions about safe handling of meat and poultry. The number of consumer calls to the Hotline has grown steadily since 1985. Journalists, cookbook authors, and extension agents also use the Hotline for the latest information about food safety (USDA, 1994, 1991a,b). Similarly, the FDA operates a Seafood Hotline (1-800-FDA-4010) to answer questions about seafood safety.

## CONCLUSION

Because microorganisms are ubiquitous in the environment they naturally occur on plants and animals. A small percentage of these microorganisms are pathogenic and, therefore, require control measures. Humans may also introduce pathogens into foods during production, processing, distribution, and/or preparation. Everyone in the food system, from people who produce food to those who prepare it, has a significant role in food safety, including activities broadly defined as food handling.

Surveys have found that some people consider homes the least likely place for food safety problems to occur. In contrast, epidemiologic studies indicate that sporadic cases and small outbreaks in homes comprise most of the foodborne illness cases in the U.S. Botulism, campylobacteriosis, and listeriosis are often caused by mishandling of foods in the home. Additional epidemiologic studies on sporadic cases of *Salmonella* and *E. coli* O157:H7 are urgently needed to help determine the magnitude of problems associated with these pathogens and to determine common causes and sites of preparation of implicated foods.

Several changes in society contribute to microbiological challenges. People have expressed concern about food safety, but some appear to be unaware of the home food handling practices that can affect their risk of acquiring a foodborne illness. Education, with specific programs targeted at individuals at high risk, is the key means for increasing public awareness of foodborne disease risks and preventing foodborne illness. To enable the public to make informed food safety decisions affecting their health, educational efforts must provide compelling reasons for the need for vigilance in proper food handling practices. Information about the means for preventing, controlling, or eliminating microbial hazards must be clear, consistent, and science-based.

## REFERENCES

Archer, D.L. 1985. Enteric microorganisms in rheumatoid diseases: Causative agents and possible mechanisms. J. Food Protect. 48: 538-545.

Archer, D.L. and Kvenberg, J.E. 1985. Incidence and cost of foodborne diarrheal disease in the United States. J. Food Protect. 48: 887-894.

Archer, D.L. and Young, F.E. 1988. Contemporary issues: Diseases with a food vector. Clin. Microbiol. Rev. 1: 377-398.

Bauman, H. 1990. HACCP: Concept, development, and application. Food Technol. 44(5): 156-158.

Bean, N.H. and Griffin, P.M. 1990. Foodborne disease outbreaks in the United States,1973-1987: Pathogens, vehicles, and trends. J. Food Protect. 53: 804-817.

Bean, N.H., Griffin, P.M., Goulding, J.S., and Ivey, C.B. 1990. Foodborne disease outbreaks, 5-year summary, 1983-1987. J. Food Protect. 53(8): 711-728.

Bennett, J.V., Holmberg, S.D., Rogers, M.F., and Solomon, S.L. 1987. Infectious and parasitic diseases. In "Closing the Gap: The Burden of Unnecessary Illness," Oxford University Press, New York.

Bryan, F.L. 1988a. Risks associated with vehicles of foodborne pathogens and toxins. J. Food Protect. 51: 498-508.

Bryan, F.L. 1988b. Risks of practices, procedures and processes that lead to outbreaks of foodborne diseases. J. Food Protect. 51: 663-673.

Buchanan, R.L. and Deroever, C.M. 1993. Limits in assessing microbiological food safety. J. Food Protect. 56(8): 725-729.

CAST. 1994. Foodborne Pathogens: Risks and Consequences. A report of a Task Force of the Council for Agricultural Science and Technology, Ames, Iowa.

CDC. 1990. Update: *Salmonella enteritidis* infections and shell eggs-United States, 1990. Morbid. Mortal. Wkly. Rept. 39: 909-912, Centers for Disease Control and Prevention, Atlanta, Georgia.

CDC. 1992. Update: Foodborne listeriosis—United States, 1988-1990. Morbid. Mortal. Wkly. Rept. 41(15): 251-258, Centers for Disease Control and Prevention, Atlanta, Georgia.

CDC. 1993. Update: Multistate outbreak of *Escherichia coli* O157:H7 infections from hamburgers-Western United States, 1992-1993. Morbid. Mortal. Wkly. Rept. 42: 258-263, Centers for Disease Control and Prevention, Atlanta, Georgia.

CDC. 1994a. *Escherichia coli* O157:H7 outbreak linked to home-cooked hamburger—California, July 1993. Morbid. Mortal. Wkly. Rept. 43: 213-215, Centers for Disease Control and Prevention, Atlanta, Georgia.

CDC. 1994b. Addressing Emerging Health Threats: A Prevention Strategy for the United States. Centers for Disease Control and Prevention, Atlanta, Georgia.

Cliver, D.O. 1990. Organizing a safe food supply system. IV. Consumer's role in food safety. In "Foodborne Diseases," ed. D.O. Cliver, pp. 361-367. Academic Press, New York.

Cliver, D.O. 1993. "Eating Safely: Avoiding Foodborne Illness," ed. A. Golaine, American Council on Science and Health, New York.

Cousin, M.A., Jay, J.M., and Vasavada, P.C. 1992. Psychrotrophic microorganisms. In "Compendium of Methods for the Microbiological Examination of Foods," ed. C. Vanderzant and D.F. Splittstoesser, 3rd ed., pp. 153-168. American Public Health Association, Washington, D.C.

Doyle, M.P. 1985. Food-borne pathogens of recent concern. Ann. Rev. Nutr. 5: 25-41.

Doyle, M.P. 1991. A new generation of foodborne pathogens. Contemp. Nutr. 16(6), General Mills Nutrition Department, General Mills, Stacy, Minn.

FMI. 1994. Trends in the U.S.: Consumer Attitudes and the Supermarket 1994. Food Marketing Inst. Washington, D.C.

Goldman, D. 1990. The new consumer, superbrands 1990. Adv. Weekly Suppl., Sept. 17, pp. 25-32.

Griffin, P.M. and Tauxe, R.V. 1991. The epidemiology of infections caused by *Escherichia coli* O157:H7, other enterohemorrhagic *E. coli*, and the associated hemolytic uremic syndrome. Epidemiol. Rev. 13: 60-98.

Hauschild, A.H.W. and Bryan, F.L. 1980. Estimate of cases of food- and waterborne illness in Canada and the United States. J. Food Protect. 43: 435-440.

Hedberg, C.W., MacDonald, K.L., and Osterholm, M.T. 1994. Changing epidemiology of food-borne disease: A Minnesota perspective. Clin. Infect. Dis. 18: 671-682.

IOM. 1992. "Emerging Infections: Microbial Threats to Health in the United States," ed. J. Lederberg, R.E. Shope, and S.C. Oaks, Jr., Institute of Medicine, National Academy Press, Washington, D.C.

Jay, J.M. 1992a. Microbiological food safety. Crit. Rev. Food Sci. Nutr. 31(3): 177-190.

Jay, J.M. 1992b. "Modern Food Microbiology," 4th ed. Van Nostrand Reinhold, New York.

Jones, J.M. 1992. "Food Safety." Eagan Press, St. Paul, Minn.

Lechowich, R.V. 1988. Microbiological challenges of refrigerated foods. Food Technol. 42(12): 84-89.

Lee, L.A., Gerber, A.R., Lonsway, D.R., Smith, J.D.,

Carter, G.P., Puhr, N.D., Parrish, C.M., Sikes, R.K., Finton, R.J., and Tauxe, R.V. 1990. *Yersinia enterocolitica* O:3 infections in infants and children, associated with the household preparation of chitterlings. N. Engl. J. Med. 14: 984-987.

Ollinger-Snyder, P. and Matthews, E. 1994. Food safety issues: Press reports heighten consumer awareness of microbiological safety. Dairy, Food, Environ. Sanita. 14(10): 580-589.

Mossel, D.A.A. 1988. Impact of foodborne pathogens on today's world, and prospects for management. An. Hum. Health. 1: 13-23.

Padhye, N.V. and Doyle, M.P. 1992. *Escherichia coli* O157:H7: Epidemiology, pathogenesis, and methods for detection in food. J. Food Protect. 55: 555-565.

Penner, K., Kramer, C., and Frantz, G. 1985. Consumer food safety perceptions. MF774. Kansas State Univ. Ext. Service, Manhattan, Kansas.

Potter, J.E. 1994. The role of epidemiology and risk assessment: A CDC perspective. Dairy, Food, Environ. Sanita. 14(12): 738-741.

Rhodes, M.E. 1991. Educating professionals and consumers about extended-shelf-life refrigerated foods. Food Technol. 45(4): 162-164.

Roberts, T. 1993. Cost of foodborne illness and prevention interventions. In "Proceedings of the 1993 Public Health Conference on Records and Statistics. Toward the year 2000 - Refining the Measures," pp. 514-518. U.S. Dept. of Health and Human Services, Washington, D.C.

Schuchat, A., Deaver, K.A., Wenger, J.D., Plikaytis, B.D., Mascola, L., Piner, R.W., Reingold, A.L., and Broome, C.V. 1992. Role of foods in sporadic listeriosis: I. Case-control study of dietary risk factors. J. Am. Med. Assn. 267(15): 2041-2045.

Schwartz, B., Broome C.V., Brown, G.R., Hightower, A.W., Ciesielski, C.A., Gaventa, S., Gellin, B.G., and Mascola, L. 1988. Association of sporadic listeriosis with consumption of uncooked hot dogs and undercooked chicken. Lancet 2: 779-782.

Sherlock, M., Fu. G., Taoukis, P.S., and Labuza, T.P. 1992. Consumer perceptions of consumer type time-temperature indicators for use on refrigerated dairy foods. Dairy, Food, Environ. Sanita. 12: 559-565.

Smith, J.L. 1994. Arthritis and foodborne bacteria. J. Food Protect. 57(10): 935-941.

St. Louis, M.E., Morse, D.L., Potter, M.E., DeMelfi, T.M., Guzewich, J.J., Tauxe, R.V., and Blake, P.A.

1988. The emergence of grade A eggs as a major source of *S. enteritidis* infections: New implications for the control of salmonellosis. J. Am. Med. Assn. 259: 2103-2107.

Tauxe, R.V. 1991. Salmonella: A postmodern pathogen. J. Food Protect. 54: 563-568.

Tauxe, R.V. 1992. Epidemiology of *Campylobacter jejuni* infections in the United States and other industrialized nations. In "*Campylobacter jejuni*—Current Status and Future Trends," eds. I. Nachamkim, M.J. Blaser, L.S. Tompkins, p. 9-19. American Society for Microbiology, Washington, D.C.

Tauxe, R.V. 1995. Personal communication. Centers for Disease Control and Prevention, Atlanta, Georgia.

Todd, E.C.D. 1989. Preliminary estimates of the cost of foodborne disease in the United States. J. Food Protect. 52: 595-601.

USDA. 1989. A margin of safety: The HACCP approach to food safety education. Project Report. U.S. Dept. of Agriculture, U.S. Government Printing Office, Washington, D.C.

USDA. 1991a. The Meat and Poultry Hotline. A retrospective, 1985-1990. U.S. Dept. of Agriculture, U.S. Government Printing Office, Washington, D.C.

USDA. 1991b. USDA's Meat and Poultry Hotline links scientists and consumers. Food News for Consumers 7(4): 4-5. U.S. Dept. of Agriculture, Food Safety and Inspection Service, Washington, D.C.

USDA. 1994. Making the connection: An update - USDA's Meat and Poultry Hotline, 1993. U.S. Dept. of Agriculture, U.S. Government Printing Office, Washington, D.C.

USDA/FDA. 1991. Results of the Food and Drug Administration's 1988 health and diet survey—Food handling practices and food safety knowledge for consumers, U.S. Dept. of Agriculture and Food and Drug Administration, Washington, D.C.

Whittam, T.S., Wolfe, M.L., Wachsmuth, K., Orskov, F., Orskov, I., and Wilson, R.A. 1993. Clonal relationships among *Escherichia coli* strains that cause hemorrhagic colitis and infantile diarrhea. Infect. Immunol. 61(5): 1619-1629.

Williamson, D.M. 1991. Home Food Preparation Practice: Results of a National Consumer Survey. M.S. thesis. Cornell University, Ithaca, New York.

Williamson, D.M., Gravani, R.B., and Lawless, H.T. 1992. Correlating food safety knowledge with home food-preparation practices. Food Technol. 46(5): 94-100.

# New risks in ground beef revealed

It looked as though the government acted effectively. Less than a year after undercooked, bacteria-laden hamburgers led to hundreds of illnesses and four deaths in the infamous Jack-in-the-Box incident of 1993, the U.S. Department of Agriculture declared the offending strain of bacteria—E. coli 0157:H7—an "adulterant." The legal implication: meat containing the bug is not considered fit for sale and is subject to federal seizure.

Nevertheless, illness-producing bacteria have become the leading cause of acute kidney failure among children in the United States, causing some 40,000 illnesses and 250 to 500 deaths each year. According to a team of Tufts University researchers, the government may be missing the forest for the trees by focusing primarily on E. coli 0157:H7. Judging by a new report from the group, as much as 25 percent of ground meat sold in supermarkets may contain other types of bacteria that are just as capable of causing kidney failure and related complications.

For a closer look at the state of the meat supply and some answers on how you can protect yourself and your loved ones, we spoke with the lead researcher of the new study, David W. Acheson, MD, of the Division of Geographic Medicine and Infectious Diseases at the Tufts New England Medical Center.

**Q:** *Ever since the Jack-in-the-Box story hit the media, fingers have been pointed at* E. coli *0157:H7 as the emerging culprit in food-borne illness. Why are you saying it's not the only one that's so lethal?*

**Dr. Acheson:** To answer that, let me roll back a bit. Bacteriologists discovered *E. coli* 0157:H7 back in 1982. It caused two very unusual outbreaks of grossly bloody diarrhea—one in Oregon and the other in Michigan. That was really when it got on the scientific map. By the mid to late '80s, it was determined that *E. coli* 0157 was making a toxin that was essentially identical to a toxin that had been discovered about a hundred years ago, called Shiga toxin.

Over the past ten years it has become very clear that Shiga toxin, not the bacteria themselves, is causing the problems associated with *E. coli* 0157:H7. It has also become clear that many other strains of bacteria are capable of producing Shiga toxin. What's happened is that the toxin genes have been moving around the world. Particles called bacteriophages are able to jump from one strain of bacteria and land in another. The bacteriophages then give the bacteria the genes that enable them to produce Shiga toxin.

**Q:** *So shouldn't the government be looking for Shiga toxin rather than* E. coli *0157:H7?*

**Dr. Acheson:** Yes, that's where the logic is. Look for the toxins, or look for *all* the toxin-producing bacteria and get away from the dogma of just checking for 0157. That's what has led us down this track here at Tufts.

**Q:** *How many types of bacteria can make Shiga toxin?*

**Dr. Acheson:** So far in North America more than 50

From *Tufts University Diet & Nutrition Letter,* June 1996, pp. 3-6. © 1996 by Tufts University Diet & Nutrition Letter. Reprinted by permission.

different types of *E. coli* have been linked to illness caused by Shiga toxin. The same numbers are coming out of Europe, South America, and Australia. In fact, in Australia there's almost no 0157:H7. But in January of last year there was a really nasty outbreak of illness due to an 0111 strain of *E. coli* in sausage. About two dozen people ended up with serious kidney complications, and one child died.

We've been trying to get Australians to realize that they need to move away from 0157. They test for it, even though they don't have it, and what they don't routinely test for is 0111.

Ironically, the United States imports a lot of beef from Australia, and according to my colleagues in Australia, the USDA makes the Australian meat companies test their beef for 0157 before they export it. There's evidence that 0111 is killing people in Australia, and it's in Australian cattle. But do we look for it in our imported Australian meat? No—we test for the bug they *don't* have in Australia. It's like a head-in-the-sand mentality.

**Q:** *It sounds like* E. coli *is the big problem, and we should try to get rid of all strains of it.*

**Dr. Acheson:** Actually, most strains of *E. coli* are "good" bacteria. We've all got millions of them in our guts, and we'd be a mess without them. It's just the toxin-producing strains that are a problem.

In the last couple of years it has also come out that Shiga toxin genes seem to be able to jump into bacteria other than *E. coli*. There was an outbreak in Europe in 1994 linked to a bacterium called *Citrobacter freundii*. It's part of the same general family as *E. coli*, but it's somewhat different. The outbreak occurred among a group of kids who had eaten something known in Germany as green butter, which is regular butter mixed with parsley. It turned out the parsley had been grown with cow manure or hadn't been washed properly. When these kids got sick, the illness was traced to Shiga toxin genes in the *Citrobacter*.

A similar thing was reported in Australia this year. A 5-month-old girl got sick from a strain of bacteria called *Enterobacter cloacae*, which had Shiga toxin genes in it.

**Q:** *Is there a test on the market that labs can use to check for Shiga toxin rather than just 0157?*

**Dr. Acheson:** Yes, we've been working on the Shiga toxin for years, and one of the things we developed was a rapid, accurate test that detects its presence. Following the Jack-in-the-Box outbreak, we decided we should try to do something to get the test out there where it could be useful. So Meridian Diagnostics in Cincinnati took it and made it suitable for use in hospital clinics. This way when a patient presents with diarrhea or bloody diarrhea, you're not just looking

for 0157. You can also use a variation of the test to check for toxins in, say, ground beef.

**Q:** *Are many people using the test?*

**Dr. Acheson:** No, not routinely. Many labs don't even check for 0157 in the stools of potentially affected patients. The Centers for Disease Control and Prevention published a survey this year showing that only about 50 percent of labs are looking for 0157. It's really quite scary how little attention is being paid to this.

**Q:** *What about the meat industry? Why isn't it testing for Shiga toxin or for bacteria other than 0157?*

**Dr. Acheson:** According to our research, 25 percent of ground beef is contaminated. If the results of our study are borne out with larger studies, I can see why the meat industry doesn't want to test for the toxin. It's going to cost them to do the test, and it's going to cost them to deal with the meat that comes up positive for Shiga toxin.

Still, it's only fair that consumers know that it's not just 0157 that's a problem, and the meat they're buying off their supermarket shelves is potentially as deadly as the half-cooked meat served in Jack in the Box in 1993.

**Q:** *What led you to conclude that 25 percent of ground beef may be contaminated with Shiga toxin?*

**Dr. Acheson:** We wanted to see whether the test we had developed to check for Shiga toxin in human stool was able to identify it in ground beef. So we bought ground beef and spiked it with different strains of toxin-producing bacteria. But we found that some of our "controls," non-spiked beef samples used for comparison, were kicking over positive for the toxin.

Of course, that set us all wondering what was going on here. So we mounted a very small scale study in which various members of the lab just went to supermarkets and bought ground beef, both here in Boston and in Cincinnati. We used several different tests and found that 25 percent of the samples contained toxin-producing bacteria. And none of it was *E. coli* 0157:H7.

**Q:** *It's enough to make a person never want to eat another hamburger. Is it safe to eat ground beef?*

**Dr. Acheson:** Yes, so long as it's thoroughly cooked and properly handled. [See box on next page.] You know, I think people have learned to be very careful with chicken because of *Salmonella* bacteria. They've woken up to the fact that if they prepare chicken on the countertop, they get out the bleach and make sure that everything is washed. But they may not do the same with ground beef. And it's fun to play with. The kids will come in and say, "Oh, let's make hamburgers." But in reality beef with toxin-producing bacteria is potentially as deadly, if not more so, than chicken with *Salmonella*.

**Q:** *Why are Shiga toxin-producing bacteria so harmful?*

**Dr. Acheson:** One of the things is that the infectious dosage seems to be really small. From studying the Jack-in-the-Box incident, scientists reckon that some of the hamburgers they rescued from the distributors contained only 100 or 200 toxin-producing bacteria per quarter-pound burger. That's much different than *Salmonella* food poisoning, in which it might take a million bacteria to get sick. This probably explains why person-to-person transmission is such a big deal. In fact, about 20 percent of U.S. outbreaks of 0157:H7 occurred in daycare settings and nursing homes and were caused by relatively few bacteria spread, for example, by not washing hands after changing diapers.

Another reason Shiga-producing bacteria are so harmful is that they are likely to make you much sicker than you would be with *Salmonella*. Roughly 5 to 10 percent of people who get sick enough to seek the attention of a physician end up with hemolytic uremic syndrome (HUS), a serious illness that often leads to kidney failure. Of those who get HUS, about 5 percent die during the acute stages of the disease, and 5 percent suffer major medical complications such as stroke or permanent kidney damage requiring transplant or dialysis. Of the remainder, 2 or 3 years later, probably half of them will still have significant kidney damage. So although it's not a frightfully common problem, it's not just like your regular food poisoning where you spend a couple of days in the bathroom and it's all over.

**Q:** *Most of the media coverage of hemolytic uremic syndrome seems to focus on children as the victims. Can, say, a middle-aged person suffer serious illness from Shiga toxin?*

**Dr. Acheson:** It can hit at any age, but it seems that children and the elderly are the most vulnerable. If you want to put numbers on it, I'd say that consumers under 10 and over 75 are the two populations that are hardest hit. We don't know exactly why, but it's probably related to the immune system. In young children, immunity hasn't fully kicked in yet, and in the elderly it's waning.

**Q:** *How can a parent tell if a child is sick with Shiga toxin?*

---

## Bacteria busters: Tips for keeping food safe

To prevent illness from *E. coli* 0157:H7 and other Shiga toxin-producing bacteria, heed the following advice.

- At the supermarket, make sure meat and poultry are bagged separately from fruits and vegetables or that the meat is wrapped in a small plastic bag. Produce bagged along with meat can become contaminated with bacteria if the meat's juices seep out of the package and onto the fruits and vegetables. And since fruits and many vegetables are not cooked, any toxin-producing bacteria that reach them will not be destroyed.

- Rinse fruits and vegetables thoroughly with cold water before serving. Toxin-producing bacteria reside in animal feces rather than produce. But some outbreaks of illness due to *E. coli* 0157:H7 have been linked to lettuce and other produce that apparently had been exposed to fecal matter during growing or transport to the supermarket. Even cantaloupe and other melons with inedible skins should be rinsed carefully. The knife used to cut the fruit can carry bacteria lurking on the exterior into the fleshy inside of the fruit.

- During cooking, flip steaks with tongs or a spatula rather than a fork. Unlike ground beef, in which bacteria are mixed throughout the meat during the grinding process, steak harbors bacteria only on the surface. Sticking a fork into the meat, however, injects the interior with bacteria from the outside.

- Cook all meat and poultry to 160 degrees Fahrenheit. The meat should not look pink, and the juices should run yellow, with no trace of pink or red.

- Wash with hot soapy water hands, utensils, cutting boards, and countertops that have come into contact with raw meat or poultry. Also wash sponges and dishcloths used to wipe surfaces exposed to raw meat.

- When dining out, order hamburgers and other ground beef items well-done.

- Buy pasteurized apple cider or heat fresh cider to 160 degrees Fahrenheit. In 1991, about two dozen people were infected with *E. coli* 0157:H7 after drinking fresh cider at a mill in Massachusetts. Public health officials suspect that the contaminated cider was made with unwashed apples that had fallen off the tree and come into contact with animal feces on the ground.

- Do not drink raw milk.

- Wash hands thoroughly after changing diapers. If your child is in a daycare setting, make sure the staff does the same.

**Dr. Acheson:** That's one of the big problems, because its initial presentation is like any other illness a kid gets. Symptoms usually start 1 or 2 days after exposure. There isn't much of a fever, and about half the kids have vomiting and generalized abdominal pain, and they just feel bad. Often, they will have non-bloody diarrhea, which may or may not progress to bloody diarrhea.

Then, typically, the gut part of the disease—the abdominal pain, vomiting, and diarrhea—begins to get better. But as the gut part is improving or is even gone altogether, the child re-presents with a stroke, seizure, or kidney failure. One thing we're working on in our lab is figuring out how the toxin gets from the inside of the gut, where the bacteria produce it, across the gut wall and to the brain and kidneys. We don't know whether it is actually getting into the bloodstream or whether something else is going on.

Of course, the important thing for parents is that you're not going to want to run and have a checkup done every time your child gets diarrhea. But if the child has *bloody* diarrhea, unquestionably ask for a Shiga toxin test.

**Q:** *If parents start talking Shiga toxin, won't some pediatricians think they're crazy? Are physicians even aware of this problem?*

**Dr. Acheson:** Probably not as aware as they should be. We've got a real education job to do. There have been multiple cases in the literature of kids going to a doctor with these kinds of symptoms and then having their appendixes taken out or, in adults, having surgery to check for intestinal disease. In the meantime, somebody sends a stool sample off for a test, and then 3 days after the surgery they find toxin-producing bacteria. Some poor kid has gone through an operation and general anesthesia just because people don't think of Shiga toxin.

But consumers can go into the physician's office with an article like this and say, "Look, it may be Shiga toxin."

**Q:** *Once someone is diagnosed with Shiga toxin, what kind of treatment is available?*

**Dr. Acheson:** There is a drug called Synsorb-Pk being tested in Canada that mops up Shiga toxin in the gut. It looks moderately promising, but it's not a panacea. Unfortunately, there isn't a wonder drug.

But for me both as a physician and a parent, I'd want to know if my child had Shiga toxin. I mentioned the two phases: the diarrhea, vomiting, and fever that seem to get better; and the second stage where a child presents with a seizure or stroke. If you know that a child is infected with toxin-producing bacteria, you can at least watch for signs of kidney failure and for the other things we know happen. And you can be in there with supportive therapy. Being aware, watching fluid balance and other vital signs, can help avoid dialysis and may prevent strokes.

# Why You Need A Kitchen Thermometer

YOU'VE GRILLED YOUR hamburger until it looks brown in the middle, so it's safe to eat, right? Wrong, says the U.S. Department of Agriculture's Food Safety and Inspection Service. The government bacteria busters warn that you can't use visual cues like color or texture to judge whether ground meat has been cooked thoroughly enough to kill potentially harmful microbes.

The only way to know for sure whether ground beef—or any meat, poultry, or casserole—has been safely cooked is to use a kitchen thermometer. Unfortunately, in a survey conducted by the USDA, only about half of those questioned said they do. Considering that dangerous pathogens like *E. coli* 0157:H7 can be killed only at high temperatures, that's a lot of people who are putting themselves at unnecessary risk of foodborne illness.

The reason that using your eye to judge a burger's "doneness" won't cut it is that the natural pigment of raw red meat (which can range from purple to red to brown depending on the age of the animal and whether the meat was exposed to air) could change to brown before the meat is fully cooked, according to Bessie Berry, manager of the USDA's Meat and Poultry Hotline. Using marinades can also make a burger appear brown before it has reached a safe internal temperature.

Testing a burger to see whether the juices run clear is an equally faulty method. "What does 'clear' really mean?" challenges Ms. Berry. "Should the juice have no color at all? Or just no evidence of pink? The color you see could change according to the background lighting, the plate you use, and how much juice you squeeze out of the burger."

The meat thermometers that everyone should depend on (instead of their eyes) come in several models, and safe temperatures will differ according to what type of meat,

poultry, or casserole you're cooking. (See charts below.) When checking a meat's temperature, make sure to put t thermometer in the deepest, thickest part of the roast or patty. You may have to turn chops, chicken breasts, or burgers sideways to get an accurate reading. Make sure your thermometer is properly calibrated (you can do this by taking the temperature of boiling water, which should read 212 degrees Fahrenheit), and always wash it in hot, soapy water after each use.

*Note:* While checking temperatures at the grill or stov may sound cumbersome, some types of thermometers tak only 10 seconds or so to get a reading.

## Know When Your Dinner Is *Really* Don

Here are the minimum internal temperatures that different foods must reach to be safe to eat, according to the USDA. These temperatures appl whether the foods are roasted, broiled, grilled, baked, or fried.

| | degrees Fahrenhei |
|---|---|
| Ground beef, veal, lamb, pork | 160 |
| Beef, veal, lamb (steaks, roasts, chops) | 145 |
| Pork (roasts, chops) | 160 |
| Ham | |
| uncooked | 160 |
| precooked | 140 |
| Poultry | |
| ground chicken, turkey | 165 |
| whole chicken, turkey | 180 |
| breasts | 170 |
| thighs, wings | 180 |
| Stuffing (cooked alone or in bird) | 165 |
| Egg dishes, casseroles | 160 |
| Leftovers* | 165 |

\* Reheated soups and gravies should be brought to a rolling boil. All other leftovers should be hot and steaming.

## Finding a Food Thermometer

| Type of Thermometer | What It's Best For* |
|---|---|
| **Liquid-Filled** | Roasts, casseroles, and soups. Thermometer can remain in food while it's cooking. Must be placed at least 2 inches deep; it can't measure temperature in thin foods. Takes 1 or 2 minutes to get a reading. |
| **Bimetal (oven-safe)** | Roasts, turkeys, or other large items. This is the traditional "meat thermometer" that remains in food throughout cooking; it can be read at a glance, but the long probe makes it a poor choice for foods less than 3 inches thick. Also, since the metal stem conducts heat, readings must be taken in two or three different places to avoid getting a false high reading. Takes 1 or 2 minutes to get a reading. |
| **Bimetal (instant-read)** | Roasts, casseroles, and soups. Since it reads temperature in 15 to 20 seconds, it can be used to check foods at the end of cooking time. However, it can't be used in the oven while food is cooking, and it must be inserted sideways into thin foods. |
| **Thermistor (digital)** | Any foods; especially good for thin foods like burgers because it needs to be inserted only 1/2 inch deep. Reads temperature in 10 seconds; digital face is easy to see. However, it can't be used in the oven while food is cooking. |

\* Based on technical information from the USDA Food Safety and Inspection Service

**Did you know...** Unrefrigerated ground beef should be thrown out after 1 hour (not the usual 2) if it is a hot day with the temperature over 90 degrees.

From *Tufts University Health & Nutrition Letter*, June 1998, p. 6. © 1998 by Tufts University Diet & Nutrition Letter. Reprinted by permission.

# For Safety's Sake: Scrub Your Produce

## THE STORY

Any savvy traveller knows the rules: On trips to a developing country, avoid the local fruits and vegetables. If you eat salads, juices, or produce that isn't peeled or cooked, you risk a bout of nasty stomach upset.

Now it seems the same rules apply even to trips to your local supermarket and favorite hometown restaurant. Over and over, Americans are hearing about local outbreaks of gastrointestinal disease traced to raw fruits or vegetables contaminated with dangerous microorganisms.

Several months ago, nearly 200 Michigan schoolchildren developed stomach pains and jaundice and were found to have hepatitis A. Epidemiologists traced their illness to a school treat of strawberry shortcake. The dessert was made from frozen strawberries that had been grown in Mexico, processed in southern California, and contaminated with the hepatitis A virus somewhere in their travels.

Last summer, an outbreak of infectious diarrhea also was caused by imported berries: Raspberries from Guatemala were identified as the vehicle that infected North Americans from New York to Texas to Toronto with an unusual diarrhea-causing parasite called *Cyclospora cayetanensis.* Again this year, cases in five states seem linked to raspberries from Guatemala.

But produce need not be imported to be dangerous. Last fall in the Western US, dozens of cases of bloody diarrhea — and one death — were traced to a batch of organic apple juice made from California apples that had somehow been contaminated with the virulent bacteria *E. coli* 0157:H7.

*E. coli* 0157:H7 is the same microbe that contaminated undercooked hamburger meat in the infamous Jack-in-the-Box outbreak of 1993 that resulted in the deaths of four children. It also caused illness traced to contaminated lettuce in 1995.

What may appear to be an increase in produce-related outbreaks has been ascribed to a number of factors, including far more produce from around the world entering the US, more widespread use of national-brand packaged and processed foods, and scientific techniques that enable better tracking of outbreaks. The outbreaks have concerned not only consumers but also federal officials, who now estimate that up to 33 million cases of food-borne illness occur in the US yearly, resulting in about 9,000 deaths and an annual expense of some $3 billion.

President Clinton recently proposed that $43 million of the 1998 budget be used to improve food safety by expanding surveillance and diagnosis networks. Proposals for reorganizing food-protection agencies are also afoot. Until such steps have an impact on the safety of your supermarket produce section, how can you ensure that you and your family will not become part of the worrisome statistics?

— *The Editors*

## THE PHYSICIAN'S PERSPECTIVE

*Abigail Zuger, MD*

It seems like the ultimate paradox. Just as medical science announces that fruits and vegetables can protect you from everything from cancer to heart disease, you learn that your gastrointestinal health may suffer severely for your efforts.

In fact, it is easy enough to reap the benefits of raw fruits and vegetables while avoiding their risks by taking just a little extra care with your food-buying and preparation habits.

The produce-associated outbreaks described above may appear all quite different — they involved different kinds of organisms (parasites, viruses, bacteria) contaminating different kinds of fruits and vegetables (berries, apples, lettuce) that were grown in different parts of the world and prepared in different ways.

Even so, these incidents have enough in common to easily deduce a set of rules for

Reprinted with permission from *Health News,* June 24, 1997, p. 3. © 1997 by the Massachusetts Medical Society. All rights reserved. For information on subscribing to *HealthNews,* please call (800) 848-9155.

avoiding similar disasters. Plainly speaking, all the outbreaks occurred because of fecal contamination. At some point in the growth and processing of the implicated fruit or vegetable, human or animal feces contaminated its surface. It may have been contaminated water used to irrigate a berry patch in Guatemala, or manure from a California cow infected with *E. coli* 0157:H7 that was spread underneath an apple tree and touched the falling fruit. It may have been the dirty hands of a worker ill with hepatitis A, picking fruit in a Mexican berry patch without adequate bathroom facilities. However it happened, the microbe grew whole colonies on the surface of the fruit or vegetable, which may have traveled thousands of miles and arrived on someone's plate without being washed clean.

Thus the first and most important rule for preventing foodborne disease: Scrub your produce carefully. Then scrub your cutting board with soap and water, and then scrub your hands. Even without soap, a good rinse can rid fruit and vegetable skins of most harmful organisms. It may not completely eliminate the risk of cyclospora in the tiny crevices of berries, but it should decrease the risk. If the skin of a piece of produce is broken, toss it out: Organisms may have crawled into the pulp beyond the reach of your scrubbing. After washing, refrigerate all cut or peeled fruits and vegetables.

What about liquids like the tainted California apple juice? That question perplexed French scientist Louis Pasteur in the 19th century when he was trying to eradicate milk-borne disease. Pasteurization was his solution — and it still is today.

Briefly heating beverages and then rapidly cooling them can kill most feces-associated bacteria and make even contaminated drinks safe. The California juice was unpasteurized: Some raw food aficionados eschew pasteurization, arguing that it detracts from taste and nutritional content. While these issues are certainly debatable, the health benefit of pasteurization is not. Avoid unpasteurized foods. If you feel like buying raw cider at a roadside stand, go right ahead — but if you want to be certain of its safety, boil it before drinking.

Finally, what to do about produce served in a restaurant or at a party or mass-prepared school lunches? These answers are less clear. Any item that is clearly the worse for wear (slimy lettuce or gritty, dirty fruit) should be avoided, as should any item that has been implicated in a current outbreak.

**Fruits and vegetables are essential to a healthy diet and needn't be shunned. But if you want to be absolutely sure to steer clear of produce-associated illness, you might elect to do most of your raw fruit and vegetable eating at home, where you can make sure that thorough washing precedes serving and eating. HN**

------------------------------------

*Abigail Zuger, MD, a specialist in infectious diseases, is an attending physician at Beth Israel Medical Center in New York.*

# Mad cows and Americans

Readers worried about mad cow disease have often asked us whether they ought to stop eating beef in order to avoid the fatal brain disorder known as Creutzfeldt-Jakob disease (CJD). *Eating beef, so far as anyone knows, does not cause CJD.* Mad cow disease does not exist in the U.S., and CJD is very rare (one case per year per million people). No one knows what causes this type of CJD, but it is not transmissible. There is a transmissible type, known an kuru, first observed in New Guinea, where people sometimes consumed human brains. That practice has ceased, and kuru is gone.

Here's the story, in brief, on bovine spongiform encephalopathy (BSE), also called mad cow disease. It showed up in English dairy herds in 1985, causing cows to behave erratically and then die. Hundreds of thousands of animals have been slaughtered as a precaution. There's been intense anxiety about human exposure and a concerted scientific effort to find out what's going on. Dairy and beef cattle require a high-protein diet; in England and elsewhere ground-up remains of sheep and other animals are fed to cattle. (Some people look upon this practice as sensible recycling of scarce resources; others regard it as coerced cannibalism.) In sheep, spongiform encephalopathy is called scrapie. Perhaps the cows got their disease from eating scrapie-afflicted sheep. It's an educated guess, but still only a theory. In any case, the British government has banned the feeding of sheep and other ruminants to cows and has taken many other precautions.

### Mysteries unsolved

The big question is whether BSE shows up in humans as CJD. Some researchers believe the causative agent is a strange inanimate protein particle called a "prion." Prions, whatever else they may do, have made for some of the most hair-raising pop-science reading since the invention of space aliens. One difference between a prion and a virus is that heat can kill a virus, but only reduces the number and/or activity of prions somewhat. Nobody can say prions don't exist and aren't extremely dangerous. Dr. Stanley Prusiner of the University of California at San Francisco won the Nobel Prize in 1997 for his work on prions. But other experts think prions are a red herring and that the culprit is a virus.

Researchers in England have found a very small increase in the number of cases of CJD in humans—21 people have died of it in recent years. They fear that BSE was the source, and it also appears that ten of the cases represent a variant, or new form, of CJD, designated NCJD. While CJD usually occurs in older people, this outbreak occurred mostly in the young, and has caused death quickly. There is no definitive evidence, however, that the new form comes from BSE. The prions from the brains of these victims were not the same as the cow prions. And only two of the victims were connected with the cattle industry. There's also been a small rise in CJD in countries where BSE is unknown. There is little evidence to even suggest that BSE can be transmitted to humans. Horrifying as it is, CJD (and its new variant) is still extremely rare. And since the herds were slaughtered, no new cases have been diagnosed in cattle, or in humans. The epidemic among cattle in England is over, thanks to swift and effective government action there.

### What's going on here

Meanwhile, the Centers for Disease Control and Prevention here has begun surveillance for the new variant of CJD: no cases yet. The USDA is testing cattle for BSE (none in the cow-brain samples so far examined). The U.S. has long had strict regulations against importing any kind of diseased animal or plant. Imports of beef from countries with BSE have been banned since 1989, and cattle imported before then were tracked down and put under surveillance or killed. The safety of gelatin imports (a beef by-product) is under review. The FDA, following recommendations of the World Health Organization, has proposed a ban on feeding ground-up ruminants (cows, sheep, goats) to other ruminants. But the U.S. livestock industry had already voluntarily stopped this practice, which was never as widespread here as it was in England. The use of any kind of animal tissue in cattle feed may also be banned. Other steps have been taken or are under consideration. It's an enormous job for regulatory agencies.

Dr. Prusiner, the Nobelist, told the *San Francisco Chronicle* that he celebrated winning the prize by eating a steak and that he has no fears about U.S. beef.

**No panic:** *You may already have cut down on beef to avoid saturated fat; and if you follow our advice, you don't eat hamburgers rare. Those are sensible decisions. But there's no reason to fear that beef will give you a deadly brain disease.*

Reprinted with permission from *University of California at Berkeley Wellness Letter,* September 1998, p. 4. © 1998 by Health Letter Associates. For information, call (800) 829-9170.

# IRRAD

*by John Henkel*

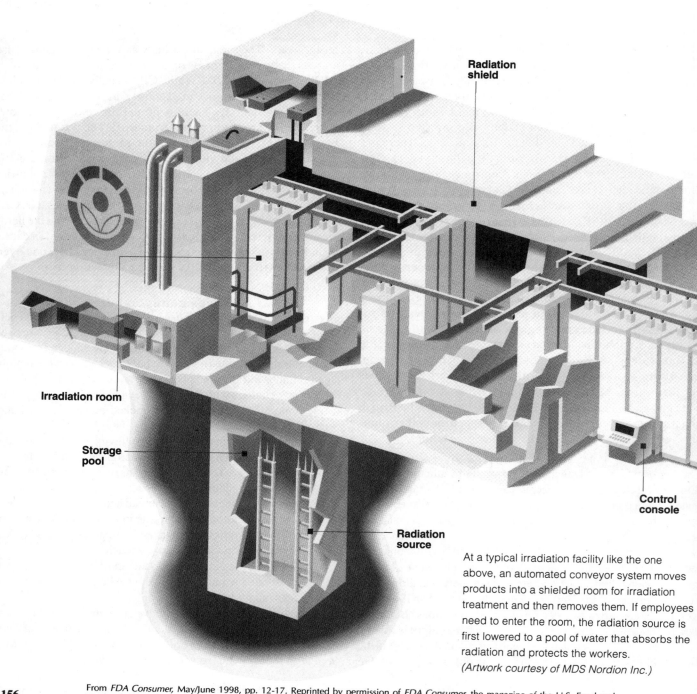

**Radiation shield**

**Irradiation room**

**Storage pool**

**Radiation source**

**Control console**

At a typical irradiation facility like the one above, an automated conveyor system moves products into a shielded room for irradiation treatment and then removes them. If employees need to enter the room, the radiation source is first lowered to a pool of water that absorbs the radiation and protects the workers.
*(Artwork courtesy of MDS Nordion Inc.)*

From *FDA Consumer*, May/June 1998, pp. 12-17. Reprinted by permission of *FDA Consumer*, the magazine of the U.S. Food and Drug Administration.

# ATION

## A Safe Measure For Safer Food

**BEEF** is one of the U.S. food industry's hottest sellers—to the tune of 8 billion pounds a year, according to trade figures. Whether at a fast-food meal, a dinner on the town, or a backyard barbecue, beef is often front and center on America's tables.

But in recent years, beef, especially ground beef, has shown a dark side: It can harbor the bacterium *E. coli* O157:H7, a pathogen that threatens the safety of the domestic food supply. If not properly prepared, beef tainted with *E. coli* O157:H7 can make people ill, and in rare instances, kill them. In 1993, *E. coli* O157:H7-contaminated hamburgers sold by a fast-food chain were linked to the deaths of four children and hundreds of illnesses in the Pacific Northwest.

In 1997, the potential extent of *E. coli* O157:H7 contamination came to light when Arkansas-based Hudson Foods Inc. voluntarily recalled 25 million pounds of hamburger suspected of containing *E. coli* O157:H7. It was the largest recall of meat products in U.S. history.

Nationally, *E. coli* O157:H7 causes about 20,000 illnesses and 500 deaths a year, according to the federal Centers for

Conveyor
system

Unloading
processed
product

Loading
unprocessed
product

INFOGRAPHIC BY SAM WARD

# FDA's approval of red meat irradiation adds to a lengthy list of foods approved for the process, including poultry, fresh fruits and vegetables, and dry spices.

Disease Control and Prevention. Scientists have only known since 1982 that this form of *E. coli* causes human illness.

To help combat this public health problem, the Food and Drug Administration last December approved treating red meat products with a measured dose of radiation. This process, commonly called irradiation, has drawn praise from many food industry and health organizations because it can control *E. coli* O157:H7 and several other disease-causing microorganisms. As with other regulations governing meat and poultry products, irradiation will be authorized when the U.S. Department of Agriculture completes its implementing regulations.

Though irradiation is the latest step toward curbing food-borne illness, the federal government also is implementing other measures, which include developing new technologies and expanding the use of current technologies.

**A Long Safety Record**

FDA's red meat approval added another product category to the already lengthy list of foods the agency has approved for irradiation since 1963. These include poultry, fresh fruits and vegetables, dry spices, seasonings, and enzymes.

As part of its approval, FDA requires that irradiated foods include labeling with either the statement "treated with radiation" or "treated by irradiation" and the international symbol for irradiation, the radura (pictured above). Irradiation labeling requirements apply only to foods sold in stores. For example, irradiated spices or fresh strawberries should be labeled. When used as ingredients in other foods, however, the label of the other food does not need to describe these ingredients as irradiated. Irradiation labeling also does not apply to restaurant foods.

FDA has evaluated irradiation safety

for 40 years and found the process saf and effective for many foods. Before proving red meat irradiation, the agen reviewed numerous scientific studies conducted worldwide. These included research on the chemical effects of ra diation on meat, the impact the proces has on nutrient content, and potential toxicity concerns.

In this most recent review and in pr vious reviews of the irradiation proces FDA scientists concluded that irradiat reduces or eliminates pathogenic bact ria, insects and parasites. It reduces spoilage, and in certain fruits and veg etables, it inhibits sprouting and delay the ripening process. Also, it does not make food radioactive, compromise nut tional quality, or noticeably change foo taste, texture or appearance as long as it applied properly to a suitable product.

Health experts say that in addition t reducing *E. coli* O157:H7 contamina tion, irradiation can help control the p tentially harmful bacteria *Salmonella* and *Campylobacter*, two chief causes food-borne illness. The Centers for Di ease Control and Prevention estimates that *Salmonella*—commonly found in poultry, eggs, meat, and milk— sicke as many as 4 million and kills 1,000 p year nationwide. *Campylobacter*, fou mostly in poultry, is responsible for 6 million illnesses and 75 deaths per yea in the United States. A May 1997 presi dential report, "Food Safety from Farm Table," estimates that "millions" of Ame cans are stricken by food-borne illness each year and some 9,000, mostly the v young and elderly, die as a result.

FDA officials emphasize that thoug irradiation is a useful tool for reducing food-borne disease risk, it complemen but doesn't replace, proper food han dling practices by producers, processo and consumers.

**Limited Success So Far**

Though irradiation would appear to

# Many spices are irradiated, which eliminates the need for chemical fumigation to control pests.

have much going for it, retail outlets have been slow to carry irradiated foods. This, experts say, is partially because many store owners and food producers fear consumers won't buy the products based on misgivings about radiation in general.

But some stores have plunged in anyway—with limited success. Carrot Top, a Chicago-area grocery market, was one of the first to carry irradiated fruits (see "Berry Successful Irradiation"). Owner Jim Corrigan says the products have been selling steadily since 1992. Other stores—mostly small, independent markets—have followed suit, offering irradiated vegetables, fruits and poultry to a modest, but loyal, group of irradiation-savvy customers.

Because irradiated red meat is not yet on the market, it remains to be seen if consumers will buy products such as irradiated ground beef—or if large food processors will even offer it. Irradiated products sold to date have cost slightly more than their untreated counterparts because of the extra step irradiation adds to food processing. But in the future, these costs could be offset by improved shelf life and increased consumer demand, according to food trade groups.

Major food companies such as poultry processors, meat packers, and grocery chains have yet to embrace irradiation, not only because of perceived consumer attitudes, but also due to logistics. Food Technology Service Inc., in Mulberry, Fla., is the only irradiating facility dedicated solely to treating agricultural products. More than 40 other facilities nationwide primarily handle sterilization of medical supplies, though these plants also can irradiate food products. In fact, it was a New Jersey-based medical irradiation company, Isomedix Inc., that petitioned FDA to approve red meat irradiation.

Beyond physical distances and lack of facilities, sheer product volume makes it unlikely that irradiation will be wide-

## Berry Successful Irradiation

The huge sign hanging over the rows of boxed strawberries left little doubt for Chicago-area grocery shoppers that the produce before them was something new and unusual.

Not that the berries looked any different. But the massive poster above them bore a message in mammoth letters that might as well have been neon: "Treated by irradiation for freshness and health." To the store owner's surprise, patrons flocked to the new product, buying nine times more of it than of standard strawberries.

That scene took place in 1992 at Carrot Top, one of the first retail stores to venture into the then-uncharted realm of irradiated foods. The decision to stock radiation-treated berries in the store, however, came slowly. Owner Jim Corrigan spent about a year reading up on the irradiation process and passing details to his regular customers through periodic newsletters. He says informing customers before the store actually stocked the new products helped allay possible fears.

When the Florida-grown strawberries finally arrived, along with irradiated oranges and grapefruits, shoppers were well acquainted with the process and responded with sales.

Today, Corrigan remains enthusiastic. He says irradiation ensures that strawberries will be free of insects and will keep longer—in some cases, up to three weeks, versus three to five days for conventional berries.

"One of our ways of rating the freshness of strawberries is to examine the small hairs that grow by the seed," he says. "If they are standing up and plentiful, the strawberries are still fresh. [With irradiated strawberries] we see a lot of that after three weeks."

The products remain steady sellers, and Corrigan has since added irradiated onions and papayas to his stock. ■

—J.H.

# Irradiating food is similar to passing luggage through an airport scanner.

spread anytime soon. The domestic poultry trade, for instance, processes about 25 billion pounds per year, according to industry figures. Says Kenneth May, spokesman for the National Broiler Council, which represents poultry producers: "We think [irradiation is] a process that will work. But for practical purposes, we just don't see anything happening with it in the near future." He adds, however, that if the public really wants an irradiated product, the poultry industry will find a way to deliver it.

## Will Consumers Accept It?

Before irradiation can really take off, the public must "warm up" to a method associated with nuclear energy, a source that carries its share of negative perceptions. George Pauli, Ph.D., FDA's food irradiation safety coordinator, compares irradiation to milk pasteurization, another decontaminating process that dramatically curbed disease but took decades before achieving public acceptance. "When the public finally sees a need for irradiation and realizes its value, I think people will accept it, maybe even demand it," Pauli says. "But you have to give them time."

A Louis Harris poll released in 1986 found that 76 percent of Americans considered irradiated food a hazard. But later studies have shown that consumer attitudes can be changed through education.

In 1995, researchers at the University of Georgia reported that 87.5 percent of consumers had heard of irradiation but knew little about it. So the university set up a "simulated supermarket setting" and labeled irradiated products, put posters at the point of sale, and developed a slide show explaining irradiation. "Our goal was to see which one of those techniques was most effective in changing people's attitudes," says Kay McWatters, agricultural research scientist and one of the study authors.

The study found that any kind of education helps convey the benefits of irradiation, McWatters says. "But the one that turned out most effective was the

## Approved Uses of Irradiation

FDA approved the first use of irradiation on a food product in 1963 when it allowed radiation-treated wheat and wheat flour to be marketed. In approving a use of radiation, FDA sets the maximum radiation dose the product can be exposed to, measured in units called kiloGray (kGy). The following is a list of all approved uses of radiation on foods to date, the purpose for irradiating them, and the radiation dose allowed.

| Food | Approved Use | Dose |
|---|---|---|
| Spices and dry vegetable seasoning | decontaminates and controls insects and microorganisms | 30 kGy |
| Dry or dehydrated enzyme preparations | controls insects and microorganisms | 10 kGy |
| All foods | controls insects | 1 kGy |
| Fresh foods | delays maturation | 1 kGy |
| Poultry | controls disease-causing microorganisms | 3 kGy |
| Red meat (such as beef, lamb and pork) | controls spoilage and disease-causing microorganisms | 4.5 kGy (fresh) 7 kGy (frozen) |

slide show, because visual images and [narration] are much more attention-getting than just a static label or poster."

After the study's education strategy, about 84 percent of participating consumers said irradiation is "somewhat necessary" or "very necessary." Fifty-eight percent said they would always buy irradiated chicken if available, and 27 percent said they would buy it sometimes.

Another study in 1997 by the Food Marketing Institute had similar results. After receiving education about the process, 60 percent of those in the study said they would buy irradiated foods.

Carrot Top owner Corrigan also discovered this on a small scale after sending his regular customers information about irradiation in periodic newsletters.

## Luggage and Milk

Other studies, however, show that many consumers still question if irradiation is safe. They wonder if the process transfers radiation to the product or if it causes chemical changes in the food that might be hazardous. Even the word "irradiation" is scary to some, carrying images of atomic explosions or nuclear reactor accidents.

**Radiolytic products**, formed when food is irradiated, are similar to those formed by cooking food. FDA has found them to be safe.

But as long as radiation is applied to foods in approved doses, it's safe, says FDA's Pauli. Similar to sending luggage through an airport scanner, the process passes food quickly through a radiation field—typically gamma rays produced from radioactive cobalt-60. That amount of energy is not strong enough to add any radioactive material to the food. The same irradiation process is used to sterilize medical products such as bandages, contact lens solutions, and hospital supplies such as gloves, sutures and gowns. Many spices sold in this country also are irradiated, which eliminates the need for chemical fumigation to control pests. American astronauts have eaten irradiated foods since 1972.

Irradiation is a "cold" process that gives off little heat, so foods can be irradiated within their packaging and remain protected against contamination until opened by users. Because a few bacteria can survive the process in poultry and meats, it's important, Pauli says, to keep products refrigerated and to cook them properly.

Irradiation interferes with bacterial genetics, so the contaminating organism can no longer survive or multiply. Although chemicals called radiolytic products are created when food is irradiated, FDA has found them to pose no health hazard. In fact, the same kinds of products are formed when food is cooked.

**Praises and Protests**

Though irradiation has its share of detractors, many prestigious organizations endorse it, including the World Health Organization, the International Atomic Energy Agency, the American Medical Association, and the American Dietetic Association. Trade groups such as the National Meat Association, the Grocery Manufacturers of America, and the National Food Processors Association also support irradiation.

However, some groups have given irradiation a thumbs down. Consumer activist Jeremy Rifkin, president of the Pure Food Campaign, says more atten-

## Radiation's Positive Side

Scientists first studied radiation as a way to improve food products in the 1930s, but research didn't begin in earnest until just after World War II. At that time, the U.S. Army was seeking a means to lessen dependence on refrigeration and replace K rations and other preserved products that troops used in the field.

In the early 1950s, the Atomic Energy Commission (now part of the U.S. Department of Energy) explored food irradiation as part of President Eisenhower's "Atoms for Peace" program. This research differed from the Army's in that it examined the effects smaller radiation doses had on certain fruits and vegetables. The end result was not a sterile product but one where insects would be killed or sterilized. Because this produce still could spoil, refrigeration was needed. But at least potentially harmful insects would not cross state or national borders.

Such research, augmented by studies from other countries, established that the most important benefit from irradiation could be the control of disease-causing pathogens and that the maximum practical and effective dose depended on the food and the purpose for irradiating. ■

—J.H.

tion should be placed on raising healthier livestock, which he says would reduce pathogens and make irradiation unnecessary. The Center for Science in the Public Interest calls irradiation "expensive" and "an end-of-the-line solution to contamination problems that can and should be addressed earlier."

But with so many influential organizations backing irradiation, along with concerns about rising numbers of disease cases, the stage is set for the pro-

cess to pick up momentum, despite negative sentiments, supporters say. First, however, says FDA's Pauli, the food industry needs to get more irradiated products into the marketplace. "Most people in this country haven't even seen an irradiated food," he says. "When products start appearing, then the public can make up its mind."

*John Henkel is a staff writer for* FDA Consumer.

# Codex: Protecting Consumers' Health and Facilitating International Trade

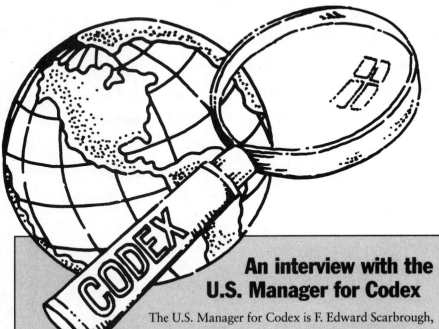

## An interview with the U.S. Manager for Codex

The U.S. Manager for Codex is F. Edward Scarbrough, Ph.D., whose office is part of the United States Department of Agriculture's (USDA) Food Safety and Inspection Service. Dr. Scarbrough coordinates all Codex activity within the United States and works closely with delegates to the various committees, members of Congress and non-governmental organizations. He reports to USDA's Under Secretary for Food Safety, Catherine Woteki, Ph.D., and takes direction from a steering committee chaired by Dr. Woteki and composed of senior government officials.

### Dr. Scarbrough, does adhering to Codex standards mean giving up the sovereignty of our own food safety regulations?

"Not in the least. Codex is a baseline. We can have our higher standard and are not required to adhere to those Codex standards which we feel do not protect consumer safety. We are working within Codex to make sure that baseline is grounded on sound science and is the highest standard possible."

### Who are the Steering Committee Members?

"In addition to officials from the involved agencies—FDA, USDA and EPA—the Steering Committee includes representatives from the State Department and the Office of the U.S. Trade Representative. Although they give a broader perspective to our Codex activities, science and consumer safety are still the main guiding factors."

### What are some top Codex issues?

"Labeling of products made from biotechnology. Our policy is that if the resulting product is the same as a food not produced through biotechnology, there is no need to label it. The Europeans appear to have more concerns about the safety of biotechnology than do consumers in the United States. This may be because consumer education has been under way for a longer period of time in the United States."

Not long ago, winter meant canned fruits and vegetables and root vegetables that could be stored for weeks. Now, thanks to improved relations with other countries in the 1990s and sophisticated transportation and distribution systems, during winter months, consumers in the United States can enjoy fresh grapes and other fruits from Chile, corn and asparagus from Mexico and a wide variety of foods from around the world.

For most consumers, fresh fruits and vegetables in winter are welcome luxuries, and few give the products' sources a second thought. But, are Chilean grapes as safe as California grapes, and is Mexican corn as safe as that from Indiana? Who is watching out for the consumer's welfare in the global food market?

The *Codex Alimentarius* Commission or Codex, is an intergovernmental, United Nations-based organization that establishes international food standards to protect consumers' health and facilitate world trade in food. It was created in 1962 by two United Nations organizations, the Food and Agriculture Organization and the World Health Organization. The nine-volume Codex Alimentarius contains the Codex standards which help guide world food trade. Codex committees establish agreed upon levels of food additives as well as permitted levels of pesticide and veterinary drug residues. It also sets food hygiene, labeling and packaging standards and prescribes methods of analysis and sampling.

Reprinted with permission from *Food Insight*, May/June 1998, pp. 2-3. © 1998 by the International Food Information Council Foundation (IFIC).

Codex standards, guidelines and recommendations are used as references by the World Trade Organization in settling international disputes in food trade as specified in the 1994 General Agreement on Tariffs and Trade (GATT) Uruguay Round Sanitary and Phytosanitary International Trade Agreement. This made Codex one of the pivotal organizations to countries, including the United States, involved in international food trade. There are 158 countries that belong to Codex. If challenged in a trade dispute, a country must prove that it at least meets Codex standards. If its standards are more stringent, then the country must present scientific evidence demonstrating the need for a higher level of protection.

## How Codex Works

The Codex Commission meets every two years and adopts standards. Proposals for work originate from committees composed of government delegates from member countries. The United States' delegates are from the U.S. Department of Agriculture (USDA), the Food and Drug Administration and the Environmental Protection Agency. Industry input comes directly from non-governmental organizations that participate in Codex meetings as observers, and recently, consumer groups were invited to participate.

The adoption process for approving standards is quite formal. For Codex to adopt a new food standard, it must proceed through an eight-step process involving the appropriate

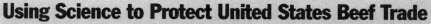

# Using Science to Protect United States Beef Trade

A good example of using Codex to protect against artificial trade barriers is United States beef. In the early 1970s, the Food and Drug Administration (FDA) approved the use of certain hormones to enhance growth and leanness in beef cattle. The FDA saw no significant risk in the use of minuscule amounts of growth promoters, which are administered through an ear patch and are not injected or fed. The European Union (EU), however, refused to import United States beef, claiming it posed a consumer health risk. In 1990, a Codex panel of experts determined that beef raised in the United States that used hormones is safe, but the Codex Commission failed to adopt standards incorporating the use of hormones until 1995. The United States then filed a complaint with the World Trade Organization, which it won. The EU now must either allow importation of such beef from the United States or pay the government almost $100 million in reparations.

committees, government and interested party comments and the Commission. This process provides time for countries and interested parties to comment.

## Standards For the World Food Supply

Ninety-six percent of the world's population live in countries other than the United States. As trade barriers fall, and a portion of the U.S. food supply continues to be imported, it is important that federal government health officials participate in Codex to help achieve standards that are as stringent as those protecting consumers in this country.

For example, a new standard proposed by the European Union would not require the pasteurization of milk used to manufacture certain soft cheeses because the Europeans are of the opinion that pasteurization inhibits flavor and mars texture. The United States opposes this proposal because it believes that without pasteurization, or a similar safety measure, the safety of the cheeses might be compromised, and has indicated it will ban cheese imports made from raw milk. USDA's Manager for Codex, F. Edward Scarbrough, Ph.D., says consumer safety is the guiding principle behind the United States' stance on pasteurization of soft cheeses, and there is no sci-

entifically sound alternative that will offer the same level of consumer protection.

Should Codex adopt a standard allowing certain cheeses to be made with raw milk, the United States does not have to permit imports meeting that standard under current trade agreements. If the United States were to lose a dispute settlement on this issue, it would have to pay reparations to the exporting countries to protect those countries against artificial trade barriers. Nevertheless, the ruling would not force the United States to import the cheeses, and the United States may be able to prove scientifically that a higher level of protection is needed for its consumers.

## Standards Based on Science

Participation in the Codex process is important to U.S. agribusiness. According to Agriculture Secretary Dan Glickman, "Agriculture's future depends on expanded trade...We need foreign markets to continue [increasing] farm prosperity here at home." By participating in the Codex process, the United States can try to assure that standards are based on science and do not become artificial trade barriers.

Codex serves a significant role in watching over the world food supply. The challenge for the United States is to make science-based decisions the norm for Codex.

## Unit Selections

## Key Points to Consider

❖ Why do you think people are so vulnerable to quackery? When have you been a victim?

❖ Identify three current fallacies that you believe are the most dangerous to nutritional health. Why are they fallacies?

❖ Make a list of characteristics you would look for in a *reliable* information source. Use them to evaluate nutrition articles in your local newspaper or a nutrition-oriented talk show.

❖ Decide if there are any herbals you could safely use right now and which ones should wait for scientific testing and judgment. What criteria did you use?

❖ Explore a variety of Web sites for nutrition information and decide if they offer reliable information.

❖ How do you feel about pharmacies promoting supplements, herbals, and homeopathic remedies? What are the issues to consider?

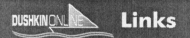 **Links**  **www.dushkin.com/online/**

These sites are annotated on pages 4 and 5.

*Does it contain any experimental reasoning, concerning matter of fact and existence? No. Commit it then to the flames; for it can contain nothing but sophistry and illusion.*
—David Hume, in An Enquiry Concerning Human Understanding, 1748

In ancient Rome, Cato the Elder prescribed cabbages to cure "everything that ails you" and continued to do so even though his wife died from the "fevers." London pharmacists, in 1632, believed that bananas were so important to health that only trained druggists should administer them. Early in the history of this country, Elisha Perkins promoted vinegar as the cure for yellow fever, yet he died of this disease. All were sincere but wrong. Yet, almost any product, device, or regimen that promises the moon and 5 miles more will acquire a following of users and believers.

Quackery is misinformation about health, according to the Food and Drug Administration (FDA). Certain fallacious statements have been made repeatedly by promoters for years, among them: "The American food supply is worthless because it is grown on depleted soil," "Everybody needs vitamin supplements for insurance," "Sugar from honey is healthier than table sugar," and "Natural is better." Such misinformation may be easier to find than facts. For example, popular talk show hosts provide a good promotional forum for misinformation, since their need to capture a large audience draws sensationalism. Nutritionists often have despaired of counteracting the exaggeration and blatantly false information frequently distributed through the popular information media.

This unit begins with 25 indicators that should cause the consumer to suspect quackery. Typically, those who misrepresent the truth warn that today's food supply is deficient, that processing techniques are harmful, and that dire consequences will result if one doesn't use supplements. Of course, these promoters are likely to offer an easy solution through the use of certain products—their products.

The second article "How Quackery Sells" will help us to understand the strategies of promoters who have fine-tuned the art of selling to an exquisitely high level. They know how to influence the emotions of the vulnerable, easily convinced customer so that he or she will buy, even though some small inner voice advises against it.

Since surveys repeatedly have shown the media to be the primary source of nutrition and food-safety information, the accuracy of what is reported is an important issue. Hardly a newspaper or periodical is published without mention of a new study that has produced "important" information about a health issue. Often these reports predict dreadful consequences from something we commonly do or consume. "Yet Another Study—Should You Pay Attention?" suggests a set of guidelines to assist the consumer in deciding what to ignore and when to take a study seriously.

Many of us rely more and more on the Internet for answers to our questions. Here, too we must be watchful—perhaps even more so, for Web sites and e-mail capabilities allow the easy and rapid promotion of virtually anything. Guidelines for recognizing and avoiding unreliable sites are suggested in the article on spotting a "quacky" Web site.

An editorial from *The New England Journal of Medicine* on alternative medicine offers a truly exquisite dissertation on the risks of untested and unregulated remedies, which often take the form of herbals and other dietary supplements. This is also the subject of an article by Stephen Barrett. Increasingly popular herbals are classified as food supplements under the Dietary Supplement Health and Education Act (DSHEA) of 1994, and currently account for about $1 billion in annual sales. Given that herbals have medicinal qualities, questions of safety and efficacy must be raised. Some argue that, because herbs are natural, safety is a non-issue, although this can be refuted easily by pointing out that the amanita mushroom and hurricanes are also quite natural but potentially deadly. To be sure, nearly one-third of modern drugs are derived from herbs and other plants, and undoubtedly more will be found to advance the modern medical arsenal against disease. But there is a clear distinction between pharmaceuticals, with carefully controlled active ingredients, and herbals, where the amounts of active ingredients depend more on how they are grown, harvested, and stored. Herbal literature is still grounded in folklore and tradition, not in scientific research. There are no guarantees of safety, and the consumer must decide if the risk is appropriate.

Two brief articles on ginkgo and ephedrine represent what is known about popular herbals. Widely used outside the United States, ginkgo extracts are touted to benefit circulatory and neurological problems. This might explain its advertised benefits for memory and Alzheimer's disease, but current studies are inconclusive. The botanical ephedrine, or ma huang, another supplement of Chinese origin, is clearly problematic. Possible adverse effects include heart attacks, strokes, seizures, psychosis, and death. Sold under such names as Cloud 9 and Herbal Ecstasy, ephedra is a stimulant that claims to improve strength and health, produce weight loss, and provide a high similar to that of cocaine.

Another promotional pitch pushes colloidal mineral supplements as the alternative cure-all for whatever is wrong with you. Once again, unfounded claims are made that our food lacks minerals and that these extremely small, negatively charged mineral particles are better absorbed. "Hard Facts on Colloidal Minerals" sets the record straight.

What we called "hyperactivity" in years past is now defined as Attention-Deficit/Hyperactivity Disorder (ADHD). It has been popular to promote the disproved theory that symptoms can be controlled through dietary changes, especially through the elimination of salicylates, artificial flavorings and colorings, or sugar. Numerous highly questionable products and therapies are also available for controlling children's behaviors.

A discussion of athletes and supplements is included in this unit because athletes typically are searching for a competitive edge and are extremely vulnerable to supplement promotionals. The assortment of promoted products ranges from amino acids for building muscle and creatine for a speedier recovery, to products claiming to energize the liver or burn fat. However, athletes should look to a good diet and within themselves, not into a bottle or box.

Finally, if you have wondered why most pharmacies appear to promote supplements and dubious alternative products, while nutritionists and this book take the opposite view, read the article on unethical behavior of pharmacists. When there is a conflict of interest, promoting sales and keeping a healthy bottom line often win.

# Twenty-Five Ways to Spot Quacks and Vitamin Pushers

**Stephen Barrett, M.D.**
**Victor Herbert, M.D., J.D.**

How can food quacks and other vitamin pushers be recognized? Here are 25 signs that should arouse suspicion.

### 1. When Talking about Nutrients, They Tell Only Part of the Story.

Quacks tell you all the wonderful things that vitamins and minerals do in your body and/or all the horrible things that can happen if you don't get enough. But they conveniently neglect to tell you that a balanced diet provides the nutrients people need and that the USDA food-group system makes balancing your diet simple.

### 2. They Claim That Most Americans Are Poorly Nourished.

This is an appeal to fear that is not only untrue, but ignores the fact that the main forms of bad nourishment in the United States are overweight in the population at large, particularly the poor, and undernourishment among the poverty-stricken. Poor people can ill afford to waste money on unnecessary vitamin pills. Their food money should be spent on nourishing food.

It is falsely alleged that Americans are so addicted to "junk" foods that an adequate diet is exceptional father than usual. While it is true that some snack foods are mainly "naked calories" (sugars and/or fats without other nutrients), it is not necessary for every morsel of food we eat to be loaded with nutrients. In fact, no normal person following the USDA food-group guidelines is in any danger of vitamin deficiency.

### 3. They Recommend "Nutrition Insurance" for Everyone.

Most vitamin pushers suggest that everyone is in danger of vitamin deficiency and should therefore take supplements as "insurance." Some suggest that it is difficult to get what you need from food, while others claim that it is impossible. Their pitch resembles that of the door-to-door huckster who states that your perfectly good furnace is in danger of blowing up unless you replace it with his product. Vitamin pushers will never tell you who *doesn't* need their products.

### 4. They Say That Most Diseases Are Due to Faulty Diet and Can Be Treated with "Nutritional" Methods.

This simply isn't so. Consult your doctor or any recognized textbook of medicine. They will tell you that although diet is a factor in some diseases (most notably coronary heart disease), most diseases have little or nothing to do with diet. Common symptoms like malaise (feeling poorly), fatigue, lack of pep, aches (including headaches) or pains, insomnia, and similar complaints are usually the body's reaction to emotional stress. The persistence of such symptoms is a signal to see a doctor to be evaluated for possible physical illness. It is not a reason to take vitamin pills.

### 5. They Allege That Modern Processing Methods and Storage Remove All Nutritive Value from Our Food.

It is true that food processing can change the nutrient content of foods. But the changes are not so drastic as the quack, who wants you to buy supplements, would like you to believe. While some processing methods destroy some nutrients, others add them. A balanced variety of foods will provide all the nourishment you need.

Quacks distort and oversimplify. When they say that milling removes B-vitamins, they don't bother to tell you that enrichment puts them back. When they

Reprinted with permission from *Quackwatch* (http://www.quackwatch.com). © 1998 by Stephen Barrett.

tell you that cooking destroys vitamins, they omit the fact that only a few vitamins are sensitive to heat. Nor do they tell you that these vitamins are easily obtained by consuming a portion of fresh uncooked fruit, vegetable, or fresh or frozen fruit juice each day. Any claims that minerals are destroyed by processing or cooking are pure lies. Heat does not destroy minerals.

## 6. They Claim That Diet Is a Major Factor in Behavior.

Food quacks relate diet not only to disease but to behavior. Some claim that adverse reactions to additives and/or common foods cause hyperactivity in children and even criminal behavior in adolescents and adults. These claims are based on a combination of delusions, anecdotal evidence, and poorly designed research.

## 7. They Claim That Fluoridation Is Dangerous.

Curiously, quacks are not always interested in real deficiencies. Fluoride is necessary to built decay-resistant teeth and strong bones. The best way to obtain adequate amounts of this important nutrient is to augment community water supplies so their fluoride concentration is about one part fluoride for every million parts of water. But quacks are usually opposed to water fluoridation, and some advocate water filters that remove fluoride. It seems that when they cannot profit from something, they may try to make money by opposing it.

## 8. They Claim That Soil Depletion and the Use of Pesticides and "Chemical" Fertilizers Result in Food That Is Less Safe and Less Nourishing.

These claims are used to promote the sale of so-called "organically grown" foods. If an essential nutrient is missing from the soil, a plant simply doesn't grow. Chemical fertilizers counteract the effects of soil depletion. Quacks also lie when they claim that plants grown with natural fertilizers (such as manure) are nutritionally superior to those grown with synthetic fertilizers. Before they can use them, plants convert natural fertilizers into the same chemicals that synthetic fertilizers supply. The vitamin content of a food is determined by its genetic makeup. Fertilizers can influence the levels of certain minerals in plants, but this is not a significant factor in the American diet. The pesticide residue of our food supply is extremely small and poses no health threat. Foods "certified" as "organic" are not safer or more nutritious than other foods. In fact, except for their high price, they are not significantly different.

## 9. They Claim You Are in Danger of Being "Poisoned" by Ordinary Food Additives and Preservatives.

This is another scare tactic designed to undermine your confidence in food scientists and government protection agencies as well as our food supply itself. Quacks want you to think they are out to protect you. They hope that if you trust them, you will buy their "natural" food products. The fact is that the tiny amounts of additives used in food pose no threat to human health. Some actually protect our health by preventing spoilage, rancidity, and mold growth.

## 10. They Charge That the Recommended Dietary Allowances (RDAs) Have Been Set Too Low.

The RDAs have been published by the National Research Council approximately every five years since 1943. They are defined as "the levels of intake of essential nutrients that, on the basis of scientific knowledge, are judged by the Food and Nutrition Board to be adequate to meet the known nutrient needs of practically all healthy persons." Neither the RDAs nor the Daily Values listed on food labels are "minimums" or "requirements." They are deliberately set higher than most people need. The reason quacks charge that the RDAs are to low is obvious: if you believe you need more than can be obtained from food, you are more likely to buy supplements.

## 11. They Claim That under Stress, and in Certain Diseases, Your Need for Nutrients Is Increased.

Many vitamin manufacturers have advertised that "stress robs the body of vitamins." One company has asserted that, "if you smoke, diet, or happen to be sick, you may be robbing your body of vitamins." Another has warned that "stress can deplete your body of water-soluble vitamins . . . and daily replacement is necessary." Other products are touted to fill the "special needs of athletes."

While it is true that the need for vitamins may rise slightly under physical stress and in certain diseases, this type of advertising is fraudulent. The average American—stressed or not—is not in danger of vitamin deficiency. The increased needs to which the ads refer are not higher than the amounts obtainable by proper eating. Someone who is really in danger of deficiency due to an illness would be very sick and would need medical care, probably in a hospital. But these promotions are aimed at average Americans who certainly don't need vitamin supplements to survive the common cold, a round of golf, or a job around the neighborhood! Athletes get more than enough vitamins when they eat the food needed to meet their caloric requirements.

Many vitamin pushers suggest that smokers need vitamin C supplements. Although it is true that smokers in North America have somewhat lower blood levels of this vitamin, these levels are still far above deficiency levels. In America, cigarette smoking is the leading cause of death preventable by self-discipline. Rather than seeking false comfort by taking vitamin C, smokers who are concerned about their health should stop smoking. Suggestions that "stress vitamins" are helpful against emotional stress are also fraudulent.

## 12. They Recommend "Supplements" and "Health Foods" for Everyone.

Food quacks belittle normal foods and ridicule the food-group systems of good nutrition. They may not tell you they earn their living from such pronouncements—via public appearances fees, product endorsements, sale of publications, or financial interests in vitamin companies, health-food stores, or organic farms.

The very term "health food" is a deceptive slogan. Judgments about individual foods should take into account how they contribute to an individual's overall diet. All food is health food in moderation, any food is junk food in excess. Did you ever stop to think that your corner grocery, fruit market, meat market, and supermarket are also health-food stores? They are—and they generally charge less than stores that use the slogan.

By the way, have you ever wondered why people who eat lots of "health foods" still feel they must load themselves up with vitamin supplements? Or why so many "health food" shoppers complain about ill health?

## 13. They Claim That "Natural" Vitamins Are Better than "Synthetic" Ones.

This claim is a flat lie. Each vitamin is a chain of atoms strung together as a molecule. Molecules made in the "factories" of nature are identical to those made in the factories of chemical companies. Does it makes sense to pay extra for vitamins extracted from foods when you can get all you need from the foods themselves?

## 14. They Suggest That a Questionnaire Can Be Used to Indicate Whether You Need Dietary Supplements.

No questionnaire can do this. A few entrepreneurs have devised lengthy computer-scored questionnaires with questions about symptoms that could be present if a vitamin deficiency exists. But such symptoms occur much more frequently in conditions unrelated to nutrition. Even when a deficiency actually exists, the tests don't provide enough information to discover the cause so that suitable treatment can be recommended. That requires a physical examination and appropriate laboratory tests. Many responsible nutritionists use a computer to help evaluate their clients' diet. But this is done to make dietary recommendations, such as reducing fat content or increasing fiber content. Supplements are seldom useful unless the person is unable (or unwilling) to consume an adequate diet.

Be wary, too, of questionnaires purported to determine whether supplements are needed to correct "nutrient deficiencies" or "dietary inadequacies." These questionnaires are scored so that everyone who takes the test is judged deficient. Responsible dietary analyses compare the individual's average daily food consumption with the recommended numbers of servings from each food group. The safest and best way to get nutrients is generally from food, not pills. So even if a diet is deficient, the most prudent action is usually diet modification rather than supplementation with pills.

## 15. They Say It Is Easy to Lose Weight.

Diet quacks would like you to believe that special pills or food combinations can cause "effortless" weight loss. But the only way to lose weight is to burn off more calories than you eat. This requires self-discipline: eating less, exercising more, or preferably doing both. There are about 3,500 calories in a pound of body weight. To lose one pound a week (a safe amount that is not just water), you must eat about five hundred fewer calories per day than you burn up. The most sensible diet for losing weight is one that is nutritionally balanced in carbohydrates, fats, and proteins. Most fad diets "work" by producing temporary weight loss—as a result of calorie restriction. But they are invariably too monotonous and are often too dangerous for long-term use. Unless a dieter develops and maintains better eating and exercise habits, weight loss on a diet will soon return.

The term "cellulite" is sometimes used to describe the dimpled fat found on the hips and thighs of many women. Although no medical evidence supports the claim, cellulite is represented as a special type of fat that is resistant to diet and exercise. Sure-fire cellulite remedies include creams (to "dissolve" it), brushes, rollers, "loofah" sponges, rubberized pants, and vitamin-mineral supplements with or without herbs. The cost of various treatment plans runs from a few dollars for a bottle of vitamins to many hundreds of dollars at a salon that offers heat treatments, massage, enzyme injections, and/or treatment with various gadgets. The simple truth about "cellulite" is that it is ordinary fat that can be lost only as part of an overall reducing program.

## 16. They Promise Quick, Dramatic, Miraculous Results.

Often the promises are subtle or couched in "weasel words" that create an illusion of a promise, so promoters can deny making them when the "feds" close in. False promises of cure are the quacks' most immoral practice. They don't seem to care how many people they break financially or in spirit—by elation over their expected good fortune followed by deep depression when the "treatment" fails. Nor do quacks keep count—while they fill their bank accounts—of how many people they lure away from effective medical care into disability or death.

Quacks will tell you that "megavitamins" (huge doses of vitamins) can prevent or cure many different ailments, particularly emotional ones. But they won't tell you that the "evidence" supporting such claims is unreliable because it is based on inadequate investigations, anecdotes, or testimonials. Nor do quacks inform you that megadoses may be harmful. Megavitamin therapy is nutritional roulette, and only the house makes the profit.

## 17. They Routinely Sell Vitamins and Other "Dietary Supplements" as Part of Their Practice.

Although vitamins are useful as therapeutic agents for certain health problems, the number of such conditions is small. Practitioners who sell supplements in their offices invariably recommend them inappropriately. In addition, such products tend to be substantially more expensive than similar ones in drugstores—or even health-food stores. You should also disregard any magazine or newsletter whose editor or publisher sells vitamins.

## 18. They Use Disclaimers Couched in Pseudomedical Jargon.

Instead of promising to cure your disease, some quacks will promise to "detoxify," "purify," or "revitalize" your body; "balance" its chemistry; bring it in harmony with nature; "stimulate" or "strengthen" your immune system; "support" or "rejuvenate" various organs in your body; or stimulate your body's power to heal itself. Of course, they never identify or make valid before-and-after measurements of any of these processes. These disclaimers serve two purposes. First, since it is impossible to measure the processes quacks allege, it may be difficult to prove them wrong. Moreover, if a quack is not a physician, the use of nonmedical terminology may help to avoid prosecution for practicing medicine without a license— although it shouldn't.

Some approaches to "detoxification" are based on notions that, as a result of intestinal stasis, intestinal contents putrefy, and toxins are formed and absorbed, which causes chronic poisoning of the body. This "autointoxication" theory was popular around the turn of the century but was abandoned by the scientific community during the 1930s. No such "toxins" have ever been found, and careful observations have shown that individuals in good health can vary greatly in bowel habits. Quacks may also suggest that fecal material collects on the lining of the intestine and causes trouble unless removed by laxatives, colonic irrigation, special diets, and/or various herbs or food supplements that "cleanse" the body. The falsity of this notion is obvious to doctors who perform intestinal surgery or peer within the large intestine with a diagnostic instrument. Fecal material does not adhere to the intestinal lining. Colonic irrigation is done by inserting a tube up to a foot or more into the rectum and pumping up to twenty gallons of warm water in and out. This type of enema is not only therapeutically worthless but can cause fatal electrolyte imbalance. Cases of death due to intestinal perforation and infection (from contaminated equipment) have also been reported.

## 19. They Use Anecdotes and Testimonials to Support Their Claims.

We all tend to believe what others tell us about personal experiences. But separating cause and effect from coincidence can be difficult. If people tell you that product X has cured their cancer, arthritis, or whatever, be skeptical. They may not actually have had the condition. If they did, their recovery most likely would have occurred without the help of product X. Most single episodes of disease end with just the passage of time, and most chronic ailments have symptoms-free periods. Establishing medical truths requires careful and repeated investigation—with well-designed experiments, not reports of coincidences misperceived as cause-and-effect. That's why testimonial evidence is forbidden in scientific articles, is usually inadmissible in court, and is not used to evaluate whether or not drugs should be legally marketable. (Imagine what would happen if the FDA decided that clinical trials were too expensive and therefore drug approval would be based on testimonial letters or interviews with a few patients.)

Never underestimate the extent to which people can be fooled by a worthless remedy. During the early 1940s, many thousands of people became convinced that "glyoxylide" could cure cancer. Yet analysis showed that it was simply distilled water! Many years before that, when arsenic was used as a "tonic," countless numbers of people swore by it even as it slowly poisoned them.

Symptoms that are psychosomatic (bodily reactions to tension) are often relieved by anything taken with a suggestion that it will work. Tiredness and other minor aches and pains may respond to any enthusiastically recommended nostrum. For these problems, even physicians may prescribe a placebo. A placebo is a substance that has no pharamacological effect on the condition for which it is used, but is given to satisfy a patient who supposes it to be a medicine. Vitamins (such as B12 shots) are commonly used in this way.

Placebos act by suggestion. Unfortunately, some doctors swallow the advertising hype or become confused by their own observations and "believe in vitamins" beyond those supplied by a good diet. Those who share such false beliefs do so because they confuse coincidence or placebo action with cause and effect. Homeopathic believers make the same error.

## 20. They Claim That Sugar Is a Deadly Poison.

Many vitamin pushers would have us believe that sugar is "the killer on the breakfast table" and is the underlying cause of everything from heart disease to hypoglycemia. The fact is, however, that when sugar is used in moderation as part of a normal, balanced diet, it is a perfectly safe source of calories and eating pleasure. In fact, if you ate no sugar, your liver would make it from protein and fat because your brain needs it. Sugar is a factor in the tooth decay process, but what counts is not merely the amount of sugar in the diet but how long any digestible carbohydrate remains in contact with the teeth. This, in turn, depends on such factors as the stickiness of the food, the type of bacteria on the teeth, and the extent of oral hygiene practiced by the individual.

## 21. They Display Credentials Not Recognized by Responsible Scientists or Educators.

The backbone of educational integrity in America is a system of accreditation by agencies recognized by the U.S. Secretary of Education or the Council on Postsec-

ondary Recognition and Accreditation. "Degrees" from nonaccredited schools are rarely worth the paper they are printed on. In the health field, there is no such thing as a reliable school that is not accredited.

Unfortunately, possession of an accredited degree does not guarantee reliability. Some schools that teach unscientific methods (chiropractic, naturopathy, acupuncture, and even quack nutritional methods) have achieved accreditation. Worse yet, a small percentage of individuals trained in reputable institutions (such as medical or dental schools or accredited universities) have strayed from scientific thought.

Since quacks operate outside of the scientific community, they also tend to form their own "professional" organizations. In some cases, the only membership requirement is payment of a fee. We and others we know have secured fancy "professional member" certificates for household pets by merely submitting the pet's name, address, and a check for $50. Don't assume that all groups with scientific-sounding names are respectable. Find out whether their views are scientifically based.

Some quacks are promoted with superlatives like "the world's foremost nutritionist" or "America's leading nutrition expert." There is no law against this tactic, just as there is none against calling oneself the "World's Foremost Lover." However, the scientific community recognizes no such title.

## 22. They Offer to Determine Your Body's Nutritional State with a Laboratory Test or a Questionnaire.

Various health-food industry members and unscientific practitioners utilize tests that they claim can determine your body's nutritional state and—of course—what products you should buy from them. One favorite method is hair analysis. For $25 to $50 plus a lock of your hair, you can get an elaborate computer printout of vitamins and minerals you supposedly need. Hair analysis has limited value (mainly in forensic medicine) in the diagnosis of heavy metal poisoning, but it is worthless as a screening device to detect nutritional problems. If a hair analysis laboratory recommends supplements, you can be sure that its computers are programmed to recommend them to everyone. Other tests used to hawk supplements include amino acid analysis of urine, muscle-testing (applied kinesiology), iridology, blood typing, "nutrient-deficiency" questionnaires, and "electrodiagnostic" gadgets.

## 23. They Claim They Are Being Persecuted by Orthodox Medicine and That Their Work Is Being Suppressed Because It's Controversial.

The "conspiracy charge" is an attempt to gain sympathy by portraying the quack as an "underdog." Quacks typically claim that the American Medical Association is against them because their cures would cut into the incomes that doctors make by keeping people sick. Don't fall for such nonsense! Reputable physicians are plenty busy. Moreover, many doctors engaged in prepaid health plans, group practice, full-time teaching, and government service receive the same salary whether or not their patients are sick—so keeping their patients healthy reduces their workload, not their income.

Quacks also claim there is a "controversy" about facts between themselves and "the bureaucrats," organized medicine, or "the establishment." They clamor for medical examination of their claims, but ignore any evidence that refutes them. The gambit "Do you believe in vitamins?" is another tactic used to increase confusion. Everyone knows that vitamins are needed by the human body. The real question is "Do you need additional vitamins beyond those in a well-balanced diet?" For most people, the answer is no. Nutrition is a science, not a religion. It is based upon matters of fact, not questions of belief.

Any physician who found a vitamin or other preparation that could cure sterility, heart disease, arthritis, cancer, or the like, could make an enormous fortune. Patients would flock to such a doctor (as they now do to those who falsely claim to cure such problems), and colleagues would shower the doctor with awards—including the Nobel Prize! And don't forget, doctors get sick, too. Do you believe they would conspire to suppress cures for diseases that also afflict them and their loved ones?

When polio was conquered, iron lungs became virtually obsolete, but nobody resisted this advancement because it would force hospitals to change. And neither will scientists mourn the eventual defeat of cancer.

## 24. They Warn You Not to Trust Your Doctor.

Quacks, who want you to trust them, suggest that most doctors are "butchers" and "poisoners." They exaggerate the shortcomings of our healthcare delivery system, but completely disregard their own—and those of other quacks. For the same reason, quacks also claim that doctors are nutrition illiterates. This, too, is untrue. The principles of nutrition are those of human biochemistry and physiology, courses required in every medical school. Some medical schools don't teach a separate required course labeled "Nutrition" because the subject is included in other courses at the points where it is more relevant. For example, nutrition in growth and development is taught in pediatrics, nutrition in wound healing is taught in surgery, and nutrition in pregnancy is covered in obstetrics. In addition, many medical schools do offer separate instruction in nutrition.

A physician's training, of course, does not end on the day of graduation from medical school or completion of specialty training. The medical profession advocates lifelong education, and some states require it for license renewal. Physicians can further their knowledge of nutrition by reading medical journals and textbooks, discussing cases with colleagues, and attending continuing education courses. Most doctors know what nutrients can and cannot do and can tell the difference between a real nutritional discovery and a piece of quack nonsense. Those who are unable to answer questions about dietetics (meal planning) can refer patients to someone who can—usually a registered dietitian.

Like all human beings, doctors sometimes make mistakes. However, quacks deliver mistreatment most of the time.

## 25. They Encourage Patients to Lend Political Support to Their Treatment Methods.

A century ago, before scientific methodology was generally accepted, valid new ideas were hard to evaluate and were sometimes rejected by a majority of the medical community, only to be upheld later. But today, treatments demonstrated as effective are welcomed by scientific practitioners and do not need a group to crusade for them. Quacks seek political endorsement because they can't prove that their methods work. Instead, they may seek to legalize their treatment and force insurance companies to pay for it. One of the surest signs that a treatment doesn't work is a political campaign to legalize its use.

# "How Quackery Sells"

## William T. Jarvis, Ph.D.
## Stephen Barrett, M.D.

Modern health quacks are supersalesman. They play on fear. They cater to hope. And once they have you, they'll keep you coming back for more . . . and more . . . and more. Seldom do their victims realize how often or how skillfully they are cheated. Does the mother who feels good as she hands her child a vitamin think to ask herself whether he really needs it? Do subscribers to "health food" publications realize that articles are slanted to stimulate business for their advertisers? Not usually.

Most people think that quackery is easy to spot. But it isn't. Its promoters wear the cloak of science. They use scientific terms and quote (or misquote) scientific references. On talk shows, they may be introduced as "scientists ahead of their time." The very word "quack" helps their camouflage by making us think of an outlandish character selling snake oil from the back of a covered wagon—and, of course, no intelligent people would buy snake oil nowadays, would they?

Well, maybe snake oil isn't selling so well, lately. But acupuncture? "Organic" foods? Mouthwash? Hair analysis? The latest diet book? Megavitamins? Stress formulas? Cholesterol-lowering teas? Homeopathic remedies? Nutritional "cures" for AIDS? Or shots to pep you up? Business is booming for health quacks. Their annual take is in the *billions!* Spot reducers, "immune boosters," water purifiers, "ergogenic aids," systems to "balance body chemistry," special diets for arthritis. Their product list is endless.

What sells is not the quality of their products, but their ability to influence their audience. To those in pain, they promise relief. To the incurable, they offer hope. To the nutrition-conscious, they say, "Make sure you have enough." To a public worried about pollution, they say, "Buy natural." To one and all, they promise better health and a longer life. Modern quacks can reach people emotionally. This article shows how they do it.

## Appeals to Vanity

An attractive young airline stewardess once told a physician that she was taking more than 20 vitamin pills a day. "I used to feel run-down all the time," she said, "but now I feel really great!"

"Yes," the doctor replied, "but there is no scientific evidence that extra vitamins can do that. Why not take the pills one month on, one month off, to see whether they really help you or whether it's just a coincidence. After all, $300 a year is a lot of money to be wasting."

"Look, doctor," she said. "I don't care what you say. I KNOW the pills are helping me."

How was this bright young lady converted into a true believer? First, an appeal to her curiosity persuaded her to try and see. Then an appeal to her vanity convinced her to disregard scientific evidence in favor of personal experience—to **think for herself.** Supplementation is encouraged by a distorted concept of **biochemical individuality**—that everyone is unique enough to disregard the Recommended Dietary Allowances (RDAs). Quacks won't tell you that scientists deliberately set the RDAs high enough to allow for individual differences. A more dangerous appeal of this type is the suggestion that although a remedy for a serious disease has not been shown to work for other people, **it still might work for you. (You are extraordinary!)**

A more subtle appeal to your vanity underlies the message of the TV ad quack: **Do it yourself—be your own doctor.** "Anyone out there have 'tired blood'?" he used to wonder. (Don't bother to find out what's wrong with you, however. Just try my tonic.) "Troubled with irregularity?" he asks. (Pay no attention to the doctors who say you don't need a daily movement. Just use my laxative.) "Want to kill germs on contact?" (Never mind that mouthwash doesn't prevent colds.) "Trouble sleeping?" (Don't bother to solve the underlying problem. Just try my sedative.)

## Turning Customers into Salespeople

Most people who think they have been helped by an unorthodox method enjoy sharing their success stories with their friends. People who give such **testimonials** are usually motivated by a sincere wish to **help their fellow humans.** Rarely do they realize how difficult it

Reprinted with permission from *Quackwatch* (http://www.quackwatch.com). © 1998 by Stephen Barrett.

is to evaluate a "health" product on the basis of personal experience. Like the airline stewardess, the average person who feels better after taking a product will not be able to rule out coincidence—or the placebo effect (feeling better because he thinks he has taken a positive step). Since we tend to believe what others tell us of personal experiences, testimonials can be powerful persuaders. Despite their unreliability, they are the cornerstone of the quack's success.

Multilevel companies that sell nutritional products systematically turn their customers into salespeople. "When you share our products," says the sales manual of one such company, "you're not just selling. You're passing on news about products you believe in to people you care about. Make a list of people you know; you'll be surprised how long it will be. This list is your first source of potential customers." A sales leader from another company suggests, "Answer all objections with testimonials. That's the secret to motivating people!"

Don't be surprised if one of your friends or neighbors tries to sell you vitamins. More than a million Americans have signed up as multilevel distributors. Like many drug addicts, they become suppliers to support their habit. A typical sales pitch goes like this: "How would you like to look better, feel better and have more energy? Try my vitamins for a few weeks." People normally have ups and downs, and a friend's interest or suggestion, or the thought of taking a positive step, may actually make a person feel better. Many who try the vitamins will mistakenly think they have been helped—and continue to buy them, usually at inflated prices.

## The Use of Fear

The sale of vitamins has become so profitable that some otherwise reputable manufacturers are promoting them with misleading claims. For example, for many years, Lederle Laboratories (makers of *Stresstabs*) and Hoffmann-La Roche advertised in major magazines that stress "robs" the body of vitamins and creates significant danger of vitamin deficiencies.

Another slick way for quackery to attract customers is the **invented disease**. Virtually everyone has symptoms of one sort or another—minor aches or pains, reactions to stress or hormone variations, effects of aging, etc. Labeling these ups and downs of life as symptoms of disease enables the quack to provide "treatment."

Food safety and environmental protection are important issues in our society. But rather than approach them logically, the food quacks exaggerate and oversimplify. To promote "organic" foods, they lump all additives into one class and attack them as "poisonous." They never mention that natural toxicants are

prevented or destroyed by modern food technology. Nor do they let on that many additives are naturally occurring substances.

Sugar has been subject to particularly vicious attack, being (falsely) blamed for most of the world's ailments. But quacks do more than warn about imaginary ailments. They sell "antidotes" for real ones. Care for some vitamin C to reduce the danger of smoking? Or some vitamin E to combat air pollutants? See your local supersalesperson.

Quackery's most serious form of fear-mongering has been its attack on water fluoridation. Although fluoridation's safety is established beyond scientific doubt, well-planned scare campaigns have persuaded thousands of communities not to adjust the fluoride content of their water to prevent cavities. Millions of innocent children have suffered as a result.

## Hope for Sale

Since ancient times, people have sought at least four different magic potions: the love potion, the fountain of youth, the cure-all, and the athletic superpill. Quackery has always been willing to cater to these desires. It used to offer unicorn horn, special elixirs, amulets, and magical brews. Today's products are vitamins, bee pollen, ginseng, Gerovital, pyramids, "glandular extracts," biorhythm charts, aromatherapy, and many more. Even reputable products are promoted as though they are potions. Toothpastes and colognes will improve our love life. Hair preparations and skin products will make us look "younger than our years." Olympic athletes tell us that breakfast cereals will make us champions. And youthful models reassure us that cigarette smokers are sexy and have fun.

False hope for the seriously ill is the cruelest form of quackery because it can lure victims away from effective treatment. Even when death is inevitable, however, false hope can do great damage. Experts who study the dying process tell us that while the initial reaction is shock and disbelief, most terminally ill patients will adjust very well as long as they do not feel abandoned. People who accept the reality of their fate not only die psychologically prepared, but also can put their affairs in order. On the other hand, those who buy false hope can get stuck in an attitude of denial. They waste not only financial resources but what little remaining time they have left.

## Clinical Tricks

The most important characteristic to which the success of quacks can be attributed is probably their ability to exude confidence. Even when they admit that a method is unproven, they can attempt to minimize this by mentioning how difficult and expensive it is to get something proven to the satisfaction of the FDA these days. If they exude **self-confidence** and enthusiasm, it is likely to be contagious and spread to patients and their loved ones.

Because people like the idea of making choices, quacks often refer to their methods as **"alternatives."** Correctly employed, it can refer to aspirin and Tylenol as alternatives for the treatment of minor aches and pains. Both are proven safe and effective for the same purpose. Lumpectomy can be an alternative to radical mastectomy for breast cancer. Both have verifiable records of safety and effectiveness from which judgments can be drawn. Can a method that is unsafe, ineffective or unproven be a genuine alternative to one that is proven? Obviously not.

Quacks don't always limit themselves to phony treatment. Sometimes they offer legitimate treatment as well—the quackery is promoted as **something extra.** One example is the "orthomolecular" treatment of mental disorders with high dosages of vitamins in addition to orthodox forms of treatment. Patients who receive the "extra" treatment often become convinced that they need to take vitamins for the rest of their life. Such an outcome is inconsistent with the goal of good medical care which should be to discourage unnecessary treatment.

The **one-sided coin** is a related ploy. When patients on combined (orthodox and quack) treatment improve, the quack remedy (e.g., laetrile) gets the credit. If things go badly, the patient is told that he arrived too late, and conventional treatment gets the blame. Some quacks who mix proven and unproven treatment call their approach **complementary** or **integrative therapy.**

Quacks also capitalize on the natural healing powers of the body by **taking credit** whenever possible for improvement in a patient's condition. One multi-level company—anxious to avoid legal difficulty in marketing its herbal concoction—makes no health claims whatsoever. "You take the product," a spokesperson suggests on the company's introductory videotape, "and tell me what it does for you." An opposite tack—**shifting blame**—is used by many cancer quacks. If their treatment doesn't work, it's because radiation and/or chemotherapy have "knocked out the immune system."

Another selling trick is the use of **weasel words.** Quacks often use this technique in suggesting that one or more items on a list is reason to suspect that you *may* have a vitamin deficiency, a yeast infection, or whatever else they are offering to fix.

The **disclaimer** is a related tactic. Instead of promising to cure your specific disease, some quacks will offer to "cleanse" or "detoxify" your body, balance its chemistry, release its "nerve energy," bring it in harmony with nature, or do other things to "help the body to heal itself." This type of disclaimer serves two purposes. Since it is impossible to measure the processes the quack describes, it is difficult to prove him wrong. In addition, if the quack is not a physician, the use of nonmedical terminology may help to avoid prosecution for practicing medicine without a license.

The **"money-back guarantee"** is a favorite trick of mail-order quacks. Most have no intention of returning any money—but even those who are willing know that few people will bother to return the product.

Another powerful persuader—**something for nothing**—is standard in ads promising effortless weight loss. It is also the hook of the telemarketer who promises a "valuable free prize" as a bonus for buying a water purifier, a six-month supply of vitamins, or some other health or nutrition product. Those who bite receive either nothing or items worth far less than their cost. Credit card customers may also find unauthorized charges to their account.

In a contest for patient satisfaction, art will beat science nearly every time. Quacks are masters at the art of delivering health care. The secret to this art is to make the patient believe that he is cared about as a person. To do this, quacks **lather love lavishly.** One way this is done is by having receptionists make notes on the patients' interests and concerns in order to recall them during future visits. This makes each patient feel special in a very personal sort of way. Some quacks even send birthday cards to every patient. Although seductive tactics may give patients a powerful psychological lift, they may also encourage over-reliance on an inappropriate therapy.

Psychologist Anthony R. Pratkanis, Ph.D., has identified nine strategies used to sell pseudoscientific beliefs and practices [Pratkanis AR. How to sell a pseudoscience, Skeptical Inquirer 19(4):19–25, 1995.]. They include setting phantom goals (such as better health, peace of mind, or improved sex life), making statements that tend to inspire trust ("supported by over 100 studies"), and fostering grandfalloons (proud and otherwise meaningless associations of people who share rituals, beliefs, jargon, goals, feelings, specialized information, and "enemies"). Multilevel sales groups, nutrition cultists, and crusaders for "alternative" treatments fit this description well.

## Handling the Opposition

Quacks are involved in a constant struggle with legitimate health care providers, mainstream scientists, government regulatory agencies and consumer protection groups. Despite the strength of this science-based opposition, quackery manages to flourish. To maintain their credibility, quacks use a variety of clever propaganda ploys. Here are some favorites:

**"They persecuted Galileo!"** The history of science is laced with instances where great pioneers and their discoveries were met with resistance. Harvey (nature of blood circulation), Lister (antiseptic technique) and Pasteur (germ theory) are notable examples. Today's quack boldly asserts that he is another example of someone ahead of his time. Close examination, however, will show how unlikely this is. First of all, the early pioneers who were persecuted lived during times that were much less scientific. In some cases, opposition to their ideas stemmed from religious forces. Secondly, it is a basic principle of the scientific method that the burden of proof belongs to the proponent of a claim. The ideas of Galileo, Harvey, Lister and Pasteur overcame their opposition because their soundness can be demonstrated.

A related ploy, which is a favorite with cancer quacks, is the charge of **"conspiracy."** How can we be sure that the AMA, the FDA, the American Cancer Society and others are not involved in some monstrous plot to withhold a cancer cure from the public? To begin with, history reveals no such practice in the past. The elimination of serious diseases is not a threat to the medical profession—doctors prosper by curing diseases, not by keeping people sick. It should also be apparent that modern medical technology has not altered the zeal of scientists to eliminate disease. When polio was conquered, iron lungs became virtually obsolete, but nobody resisted this advancement because it would force hospitals to change. Neither will medical scientists mourn the eventual defeat of cancer.

Moreover, how could a conspiracy to withhold a cancer cure hope to be successful? Many physicians die of cancer each year. Do you believe that the vast majority of doctors would conspire to withhold a cure for a disease which affects them, their colleagues and their loved ones? To be effective, a conspiracy would have to be worldwide. If laetrile, for example, really worked, many other nations' scientists would soon realize it.

Organized quackery poses its opposition to medical science as a philosophical conflict rather than a conflict about proven versus unproven or fraudulent methods. This creates the illusion of a "holy war" rather than a conflict that could be resolved by examining the facts.

Quacks like to charge that, **"Science doesn't have all the answers."** That's true, but it doesn't claim to have them. Rather, it is a rational and responsible process that can answer many questions—including whether procedures are safe and effective for their intended purpose. It is quackery that constantly claims to have answers for incurable diseases. The idea that people should turn to quack remedies when frustrated by science's inability to control a disease is irrational. Science may not have all the answers, but quackery has no answers at all! It will take your money and break your heart.

Many treatments advanced by the scientific community are later shown to be unsafe or worthless. Such failures become grist for organized quackery's public relations mill in its ongoing attack on science. Actually, "failures" reflect a key element of science: its willingness to test its methods and beliefs and abandon those shown to be invalid. True medical scientists have no philosophical commitment to particular treatment approaches, only a commitment to develop and use methods that are safe and effective for an intended purpose. When a quack remedy flunks a scientific test, its proponents merely reject the test.

Books espousing unscientific practices typically suggest that the reader consult a doctor before following their advice. This disclaimer is intended to protect the author and publisher from legal responsibility for any dangerous ideas contained in the book. Both author and publisher know full well, however, that most people won't ask their doctor. If they wanted their doctor's advice, they probably wouldn't be reading the book in the first place.

Sometimes the quack will say, "You may have come to me too late, but I will try my best to help you." That way, if the treatment fails, you have only yourself to blame. Patients who see the light and abandon quack treatment may also be blamed for stopping too soon.

## How to Avoid Being Tricked

The best way to avoid being tricked is to stay away from tricksters. Unfortunately, in health matters, this is no simple task. Quackery is not sold with a warning label. Moreover, the dividing line between what is quackery and what is not is by no means sharp. A product that is effective in one situation may be part of a quack scheme in another. (Quackery lies in the promise, not the product.) Practitioners who use effective methods may also use ineffective ones. For example, they may mix valuable advice to stop smoking with unsound advice to take vitamins. Even outright quacks may relieve some psychosomatic ailments with their reassuring manner.

This article illustrates how adept quacks are at selling themselves. Sad to say, in most contests between quacks and ordinary people, the quacks still are likely to win.

# Yet Another Study—Should You Pay Attention?

*How to know when to take health research news with a grain of salt*

*Hot Dogs Cause Cancer?
Researchers Say Yes*

*New warnings revive fears about
the danger of eating hot dogs,
particularly among children*

*Study Links Hot Dogs, Cancer
Ingestion by Children Boosts
Leukemia Risk, Report Says*

**S**O WENT headlines in the *Los Angeles Times,* the *New York Times,* and the *Washington Post* back in June of 1994. They came on the heels of three studies published simultaneously in a cancer research journal.

One of the studies found that children who eat more than 12 hot dogs a month have nine times the normal risk of developing childhood leukemia. The second suggested that children born to mothers who eat at least one frank a week during pregnancy have double the normal risk of developing brain tumors. The third traced brain tumors in children to *fathers* who ate hot dogs before conception. The risk of leukemia to children born of fathers who consumed hot dogs regularly was 11 times normal.

The problem: the three studies—and most certainly all the media commentary they attracted—were riddled with scientific holes.

To be sure, many of the reports in newspapers and other media outlets did point out weaknesses in the studies. But those weaknesses were strung between unnecessarily alarming headlines and warnings from researchers who, perhaps, had themselves experienced something of a knee-jerk reaction to the research. For instance, the concluding paragraph of the *New York Times* article leaves readers with this quoted advice about frankfurters from the former director of a cancer research center: "Reduce consumption of them as much as you can. They are a source of a possible cancer risk. I would not expose my children to it. It's like secondhand smoking."

Therein lies the difficulty at the heart of the matter. If scientists can't always look at research with a cool eye, how in the world are *you* supposed to? Following, **four questions to ask yourself as you read about study results or hear about them on the news.** They should help you put the latest reports into perspective as you try to make informed decisions about how to improve or maintain your lifestyle habits.

**1.** *What are the actual numbers as opposed to the relative numbers?* Let's say the hot dog research was airtight and children who eat franks more than a dozen times each month really are nine times (900 percent) more likely to get leukemia than children who eat them less often. The question is, how likely are children to develop leukemia to begin with?

They have a 0.3-in-1,000 chance. If you multiplied that number by nine to get the risk for children who have more than a dozen franks every month, the answer comes to roughly 2.5 in 1,000.

The point here is that even if something is many times more likely to happen under certain circumstances, that doesn't mean its potential influence is great enough to warrant changing the way you live your life.

Adding to the mathematical irrelevance of the findings is that there were only 17 children out of hundreds in the study who ate more than 12 franks each month—much too few to make any declarations about the dangers of hot dogs for the general population.

**2.** *What type of study was it?* There are three major types of human research—clinical trials, epidemiologic studies, and population-based intervention trials—and each has inherent strengths and limitations.

**Clinical trials** A clinical trial is an experiment conducted in a controlled setting, often a hospital, where researchers give a group of people treatment—such as a supplement, drug, or diet—and then measure their response. The iron absorption study discussed near the beginning of the News Bite at the top of page 2 in this issue is an example of a clinical trial.

Clinical trials are believed to yield very accurate results that can help establish cause-and-effect relationships between various substances or lifestyle activities and specific health outcomes. However, they tend to be conducted on restricted groups of people that include, for instance, just one age group, sex, or race. That allows the scientists to keep the study environment more "air-tight" so that variations within the population being studied don't confound the results. However, it means the results are not necessarily generalizable to all people. Clinical trials often need to be repeated in different groups with different genetic makeups and lifestyles before a recommendation for the general public can reliably be made.

**Epidemiologic studies** Epidemiologic studies look at much larger groups of people than clinical trials—up to tens of thousands of subjects. These are not experiments in which researchers control a certain aspect of the subjects' lives but, rather, make *observations* of free-living populations in which they search for relationships between lifestyle or genetic factors and the risk for chronic diseases. Harvard University's Nurses' Health Study, which looks at the lifestyles of some 90,000 women, is an example of epidemiologic research.

Because epidemiologic research is generally conducted on large groups of people, the results tend to be more generalizable to the population at large. However, epidemiology virtually never proves cause and effect; it can only

**Did you know...** Washing your hands for the 20 seconds recommended by the International Food Safety Council means you should be able to sing "Happy Birthday"

From *Tufts University Health & Nutrition Letter,* June 1998, p. 6. © 1998 by Tufts University Diet & Nutrition Letter. Reprinted by permission.

make *associations* on which other researchers might then decide to base a clinical trial to test whether "X" lifestyle actually leads to "Y" condition.

Granted, the more people in the study and the more tightly controlled it is for various lifestyle factors, the higher the chance that there really is something to any association found. But still, one can never automatically assume that an association proves a cause.

To show just how tenuous links brought to light in epidemiologic studies can be, scientists who published research on aspirin and heart disease in the prestigious journal *The Lancet* pointed out that according to one of their findings, people born under the signs of Gemini and Libra are likely to be harmed by taking aspirin rather than helped. If that piece of their research were serious science, the conclusion might be drawn by some that astrological influences directly affect health. The researchers highlighted the association specifically to point out the mistakes that could be made in viewing epidemiologic associations as fact.

### Population-Based Intervention Trials

Sort of a cross between an epidemiologic study and a clinical trial, a population-based intervention trial is a project in which large numbers of people live freely rather than in a controlled setting but are given either a treatment or a placebo and then observed to see whether a specific outcome occurs. A study of 29,000 male Finnish smokers that was released a few years ago, in which those who took beta-carotene turned out to be more likely to develop lung

cancer than those who didn't, is an example of an intervention trial.

The strength of such studies is that, like epidemiologic research, they can observe thousands of people. The drawback is that they cannot be as well-controlled as clinical trials. Thus, it may not always be the treatment that's having the effect (or the full effect) but something in the subjects' lifestyles that the scientists didn't account for.

**3.** *Does the study stand alone, or are its results corroborated by other pieces of research?* A single study hardly ever tells the whole story. While the goal of the media is to turn a piece of research into news—or at least to make news sound exciting—the goal of scientists is to add *incrementally* to a body of knowledge. In fact, before a scientist makes a recommendation, there must be supportive evidence from a variety of approaches so that the strengths of all of them combined compensate for the weaknesses in any single one. Clinical and epidemiologic studies are not the only kinds of investigations necessary. There is also research conducted with tissue cultures and with laboratory animals—which often doesn't make the front page or the 6 o'clock news.

Consider the hot dog research. The scientists who conducted it commented that perhaps chemicals in hot dogs called nitrites cause leukemia. One way they could test that theory would be to "contaminate" normal cells in the laboratory with various doses of nitrites and see whether the

cells mutated in such a way as to suggest that inside the body, the mutations would develop into leukemia.

They could also feed various doses of hot dogs—or of nitrites themselves—to laboratory animals and see if hot dog-nourished animals developed leukemia at a faster rate than those fed other meats. Cell culture studies and animal studies would also be necessary to help determine why hot dog-eating mothers raised their children's risk of developing brain cancer two-fold while hot dog-eating fathers raised the risk 11-fold. After all, for 9 months, a developing fetus is directly affected by everything its mother eats. Thus, without any clues to a plausible mechanism for how a father's frankfurter consumption could have so much more of an effect than a mother's, the numbers remain in the realm of fluke findings, and the hot dog hypothesis remains just that.

**4.** *Was the study published in a peer-reviewed journal?* Peer review is the process by which experts in a particular field review a study before it is accepted for publication in order to ensure that it was conducted appropriately. It is their express role to poke holes in the study's design or the researchers' interpretations. Only if they deem the study scientifically "clean" do the publication's editors print it. The journal in which the hot dog-leukemia research was published, *Cancer Causes and Control*, is not peer-reviewed. If it were, the research, riddled as it is with inconsistencies and faulty methodology, probably never would have made it into print.

## Mini-Glossary of Research Terms

**Placebo-controlled:** If a clinical trial or population-based intervention trial is placebo-controlled, that means there is a group similar to the treatment group that is given a mock pill, or placebo. The effect on the placebo group allows researchers to tell whether the actual treatment is having an effect or whether it's just the fact that their subjects are being treated; sometimes just being given a "sugar pill" provides a psychological boost that yields beneficial results.

**Double-blind:** A double-blind trial is one in which neither the study participants nor the researchers heading the study know who is getting the real treatment and who is getting the placebo until the experiment is over. As a result, the subjects can't knowingly alter their lifestyles during the trial to make the treatment more or less effective, and the researchers are prevented from reading into findings in order to come up with "expected" results.

**Prospective study:** In a prospective epidemiologic study, scientists look at a group of people at a specific point (or points) in time and then wait to see who gets what diseases before making associations between lifestyle and risk of illness. Harvard's Nurses' Health Study is prospective.

**Retrospective study:** In a retrospective study, researchers compare people with a disease or other condition to a similar group of people who aren't affected and then look backwards in time to see what differences in their lifestyles might have contributed to the different outcomes in their health status. Some retrospective studies are designed better than others. In the retrospective study that looked at pregnant women's consumption of hot dogs, mothers with teenage children were asked to recall what they ate as many as 14 years ago. (Can you remember what you ate last week?)

*twice* while soaping up. Try it—it takes longer than you think! You should wash from fingernails to forearms in hot, running water.

# How to Spot a "Quacky" Web Site

## Stephen Barrett, M.D.

The best way to avoid being quacked is to reject quackery's promoters. Each item listed below signifies that a web site is not a trustworthy information source.

## General Characteristics

• Any site used to market herbs or dietary supplements. Although some are useful, I do not believe it is possible to run a profitable business selling them without some form of deception. Deception includes (1) lack of full disclosure of the facts, (2) promotion or sale of products that lack a rational use, or (3) failure to provide advice indicating who should **not** use the products. During the past 25 years, I have never encountered a seller who did not do at least one of these three things.

• Any site used to market or promote homeopathic products. No such products have been proven effective.

• Any site that generally promotes "alternative" methods. There are more than a thousand "alternative" methods. The vast majority are worthless.

## False Statements about Nutrition

• Everyone should take vitamins.
• Vitamins are effective against stress.
• Taking vitamins makes people more energetic.

• Organic foods are safer and/or more nutritious than ordinary foods.
• Losing weight is easy.
• Special diets can cure cancer.
• Diet is the principal cause of hyperactivity.

## False Statements about "Alternative" Methods

• Acupuncture is effective against a long list of diseases.
• Chelation therapy is an effective substitute for bypass surgery.
• Chiropractic treatment is effective against a large number of diseases.
• Herbs are generally superior to prescription drugs.
• Homeopathic products are effective remedies.
• Spines should be checked and adjusted regularly by a chiropractor.

## False Statements about Other Issues

• Fluoridation is dangerous.
• Immunizations are dangerous.
• Mercury-amalgam ("silver") fillings should be removed because they make people sick.
• All teeth with root canals should be removed because they make people sick.

Reprinted with permission from *Quackwatch (http://www.quackwatch.com). © 1998 by Stephen Barrett.*

# ALTERNATIVE MEDICINE — THE RISKS OF UNTESTED AND UNREGULATED REMEDIES

WHAT is there about alternative medicine that sets it apart from ordinary medicine? The term refers to a remarkably heterogeneous group of theories and practices — as disparate as homeopathy, therapeutic touch, imagery, and herbal medicine. What unites them? Eisenberg et al. defined alternative medicine (now often called complementary medicine) as "medical interventions not taught widely at U.S. medical schools or generally available at U.S. hospitals."[1] That is not a very satisfactory definition, especially since many alternative remedies have recently found their way into the medical mainstream. Medical schools teach alternative medicine, hospitals and health maintenance organizations offer it,[2] and laws in some states require health plans to cover it.[3] It also constitutes a huge and rapidly growing industry, in which major pharmaceutical companies are now participating.[4]

What most sets alternative medicine apart, in our view, is that it has not been scientifically tested and its advocates largely deny the need for such testing. By testing, we mean the marshaling of rigorous evidence of safety and efficacy, as required by the Food and Drug Administration (FDA) for the approval of drugs and by the best peer-reviewed medical journals for the publication of research reports. Of course, many treatments used in conventional medicine have not been rigorously tested, either, but the scientific community generally acknowledges that this is a failing that needs to be remedied. Many advocates of alternative medicine, in contrast, believe the scientific method is simply not applicable to their remedies. They rely instead on anecdotes and theories.

In 1992, Congress established within the National Institutes of Health an Office of Alternative Medicine to evaluate alternative remedies. So far, the results have been disappointing. For example, of the 30 research grants the office awarded in 1993, 28 have resulted in "final reports" (abstracts) that are listed in the office's public on-line data base.[5] But a Medline search almost six years after the grants were awarded revealed that only 9 of the 28 resulted in published papers. Five were in 2 journals not included among the 3500 journal titles in the Countway Library of Medicine's collection.[6-10] Of the other four studies, none was a controlled clinical trial that would allow any conclusions to be drawn about the efficacy of an alternative treatment.[11-14]

It might be argued that conventional medicine relies on anecdotes, too, some of which are published as case reports in peer-reviewed journals. But these case reports differ from the anecdotes of alternative medicine. They describe a well-documented new finding in a defined setting. If, for example, the *Journal* were to receive a paper describing a patient's recovery from cancer of the pancreas after he had ingested a rhubarb diet, we would require documentation of the disease and its extent, we would ask about other, similar patients who did not recover after eating rhubarb, and we might suggest trying the diet on other patients. If the answers to these and other questions were satisfactory, we might publish a case report — not to announce a remedy, but only to suggest a hypothesis that should be tested in a proper clinical trial. In contrast, anecdotes about alternative remedies (usually published in books and magazines for the public) have no such documentation and are considered sufficient in themselves as support for therapeutic claims.

Alternative medicine also distinguishes itself by an ideology that largely ignores biologic mechanisms, often disparages modern science, and relies on what are purported to be ancient practices and natural remedies (which are seen as somehow being simultaneously more potent and less toxic than conventional medicine). Accordingly, herbs or mixtures of herbs are considered superior to the active compounds isolated in the laboratory. And healing methods such as homeopathy and therapeutic touch are fervently promoted despite not only the lack of good clinical evidence of effectiveness, but the presence of a rationale that violates fundamental scientific laws — surely a circumstance that requires more, rather than less, evidence.

Of all forms of alternative treatment, the most common is herbal medicine.[15] Until the 20th century, most remedies were botanicals, a few of which were found through trial and error to be helpful. For example, purple foxglove was found to be helpful for dropsy, the opium poppy for pain, cough, and diarrhea, and cinchona bark for fever. But therapeutic successes with botanicals came at great human cost. The indications for using a given botanical were ill defined, dosage was arbitrary because the concentrations of the active ingredient were unknown, and all manner of contaminants were often present. More important, many of the remedies simply did not

From *The New England Journal of Medicine*, September 17, 1998, pp. 839-841. © 1998 by the Massachusetts Medical Society. All rights reserved. Reprinted by permission.

work, and some were harmful or even deadly. The only way to separate the beneficial from the useless or hazardous was through anecdotes relayed mainly by word of mouth.

All that began to change in the 20th century as a result of rapid advances in medical science. The emergence of sophisticated chemical and pharmacologic methods meant that we could identify and purify the active ingredients in botanicals and study them. Digitalis was extracted from the purple foxglove, morphine from the opium poppy, and quinine from cinchona bark. Furthermore, once the chemistry was understood, it was possible to synthesize related molecules with more desirable properties. For example, penicillin was fortuitously discovered when penicillium mold contaminated some bacterial cultures. Isolating and characterizing it permitted the synthesis of a wide variety of related antibiotics with different spectrums of activity.

In addition, powerful epidemiologic tools were developed for testing potential remedies. In particular, the evolution of the randomized, controlled clinical trial enabled researchers to study with precision the safety, efficacy, and dose effects of proposed treatments and the indications for them. No longer do we have to rely on trial and error and anecdotes. We have learned to ask for and expect statistically reliable evidence before accepting conclusions about remedies. Without such evidence, the FDA will not permit a drug to be marketed.

The results of these advances have been spectacular. As examples, we now know that treatment with aspirin, heparin, thrombolytic agents, and beta-adrenergic blockers greatly reduces mortality from myocardial infarction; a combination of nucleoside analogues and a protease inhibitor can stave off the onset of AIDS in people with human immunodefiency virus infection; antibiotics heal peptic ulcers; and a cocktail of cytotoxic drugs can cure most cases of childhood leukemia. Also in this century, we have developed and tested vaccines against a great many infectious scourges, including measles, poliomyelitis, pertussis, diphtheria, hepatitis B, some forms of meningitis, and pneumococcal pneumonia, and we have a vast arsenal of effective antibiotics for many others. In less than a century, life expectancy in the United States has increased by three decades, in part because of better sanitation and living standards, but in large part because of advances in medicine realized through rigorous testing. Other countries lagged behind, but as scientific medicine became universal, all countries affluent enough to afford it saw the same benefits.

Now, with the increased interest in alternative medicine, we see a reversion to irrational approaches to medical practice, even while scientific medicine is making some of its most dramatic advances. Exploring the reasons for this paradox is outside the scope of this editorial, but it is probably in part a matter of disillusionment with the often hurried and impersonal care delivered by conventional physicians, as well as the harsh treatments that may be necessary for life-threatening diseases.

Fortunately, most untested herbal remedies are probably harmless. In addition, they seem to be used primarily by people who are healthy and believe the remedies will help them stay that way, or by people who have common, relatively minor problems, such as backache or fatigue.[1] Most such people would probably seek out conventional doctors if they had indications of serious disease, such as crushing chest pain, a mass in the breast, or blood in the urine. Still, uncertainty about whether symptoms are serious could result in a harmful delay in getting treatment that has been proved effective. And some people may embrace alternative medicine exclusively, putting themselves in great danger. In this issue of the *Journal,* Coppes et al. describe two such instances.[16]

Also in this issue, we see that there are risks of alternative medicine in addition to that of failing to receive effective treatment. Slifman and her colleagues report a case of digitalis toxicity in a young woman who had ingested a contaminated herbal concoction.[17] Ko reports finding widespread inconsistencies and adulterations in his analysis of Asian patent medicines.[18] LoVecchio et al. report on a patient who suffered central nervous system depression after ingesting a substance sold in health-food stores as a growth hormone stimulator,[19] and Beigel and colleagues describe the puzzling clinical course of a patient in whom lead poisoning developed after he took an Indian herbal remedy for his diabetes.[20] These are without doubt simply examples of what will be a rapidly growing problem.

What about the FDA? Shouldn't it be monitoring the safety and efficacy of these remedies? Not any longer, according to the U.S. Congress. In response to the lobbying efforts of the multibillion-dollar "dietary supplement" industry, Congress in 1994 exempted their products from FDA regulation.[21,22] (Homeopathic remedies have been exempted since 1938.[23]) Since then, these products have flooded the market, subject only to the scruples of their manufacturers. They may contain the substances listed on the label in the amounts claimed, but they need not, and there is no one to prevent their sale if they don't. In analyses of ginseng products, for example, the amount of the active ingredient in each pill varied by as much as a factor of 10 among brands that were labeled as containing the same amount.[24] Some brands contained none at all.[25]

Herbal remedies may also be sold without any knowledge of their mechanism of action. In this issue of the *Journal,* DiPaola and his colleagues report that the herbal mixture called PC-SPES (PC for prostate cancer, and *spes* the Latin for "hope") has substantial estrogenic activity.[26] Yet this substance is promoted as bolstering the immune system in patients with prostate cancer that is refractory to treatment with estrogen.[27] Many men taking PC-SPES have thus received varying amounts of hormonal treatment without knowing it, some in addition to the estrogen treatments given to them by their conventional physicians.

The only legal requirement in the sale of such products is that they not be promoted as preventing or treating disease.[28] To comply with that stipulation, their labeling has risen to an art form of doublespeak (witness the name PC-SPES). Not only are they sold under the euphemistic rubric "dietary supplements," but also the medical uses for which they are sold are merely insinuated. Nevertheless, it is clear what is meant. Shark cartilage (priced in a local drugstore at more than $3 for a day's dose) is promoted on its label "to maintain a proper bone and joint function," saw palmetto to "promote prostate health," and horse-chestnut seed extract to "promote . . . leg vein health." Anyone can walk into a health-food store and unwittingly buy PC-SPES with unknown amounts of estrogenic activity, plantain laced with digitalis, or Indian herbs contaminated with heavy metals. Caveat emptor. The FDA can intervene only after the fact, when it is shown that a product is harmful.[28]

It is time for the scientific community to stop giving alternative medicine a free ride. There cannot be two kinds of medicine — conventional and alternative. There is only medicine that has been adequately tested and medicine that has not, medicine that works and medicine that may or may not work. Once a treatment has been tested rigorously, it no longer matters whether it was considered alternative at the outset. If it is found to be reasonably safe and effective, it will be accepted. But assertions, speculation, and testimonials do not substitute for evidence. Alternative treatments should be subjected to scientific testing no less rigorous than that required for conventional treatments.

Marcia Angell, M.D.
Jerome P. Kassirer, M.D.

## REFERENCES

**1.** Eisenberg DM, Kessler RC, Foster C, Norlock FE, Calkins DR, Delbanco TL. Unconventional medicine in the United States — prevalence, costs, and patterns of use. N Engl J Med 1993;328:246-52.
**2.** Spiegel D, Stroud P, Fyfe A. Complementary medicine. West J Med 1998;168:241-7.
**3.** Cooper RA, Stoflet SJ. Trends in the education and practice of alternative medicine clinicians. Health Aff (Millwood) 1996;15(3):226-38.
**4.** Canedy D. Real medicine or medicine show? Growth of herbal remedy sales raises issues about value. New York Times. July 23, 1998:D1.
**5.** National Institutes of Health, Office of Alternative Medicine. Grant award and research data. Bethesda, Md.: Office of Alternative Medicine. (See: http://altmed.od.nih.gov/oam/research/grants.)
**6.** Chou CK, McDougall JA, Ahn C, Vora N. Electrochemical treatment of mouse and rat fibrosarcomas with direct current. Bioelectromagnetics 1997;18(1):14-24.
**7.** Olson M, Sneed N, LaVia M, Virella G, Bonadonna R, Michel Y. Stress-induced immunosuppression and therapeutic touch. Alternative Ther Health Med 1997;3(2):68-74.
**8.** Shaffer HJ, LaSalvia TA, Stein JP. Comparing Hatha yoga with dynamic group psychotherapy for enhancing methadone maintenance treatment: a randomized clinical trial. Alternative Ther Health Med 1997;3(4):57-66.
**9.** Walker SR, Tonigan JS, Miller WR, Corner S, Kahlich L. Intercessory prayer in the treatment of alcohol abuse and dependence: a pilot investigation. Alternative Ther Health Med 1997;3(6):79-86.
**10.** Richardson MA, Post-White J, Grimm EA, Moye LA, Singletary SE, Justice B. Coping, life attitudes, and immune responses to imagery and group support after breast cancer treatment. Alternative Ther Health Med 1997;3(5):62-70.
**11.** Reid SA, Duke LM, Allen JB. Resting frontal electroencephalographic asymmetry in depression: inconsistencies suggest the need to identify mediating factors. Psychophysiology 1998;35(4):389-404.
**12.** Crawford HJ, Knebel T, Kaplan L, et al. Hypnotic analgesia. 1. Somatosensory event-related potential changes to noxious stimuli and 2. Transfer learning to reduce chronic low back pain. Int J Clin Exp Hypn 1998;46:92-132.
**13.** Shannahoff-Khalsa DS, Beckett LR. Clinical case report: efficacy of yogic techniques in the treatment of obsessive compulsive disorders. Int J Neurosci 1996;85:1-17.
**14.** Prasad KN, Hernandez C, Edwards-Prasad J, Nelson J, Borus T, Robinson WA. Modification of the effect of tamoxifen, *cis*-platin, DTIC, and interferon-$\alpha$2b on human melanoma cells in culture by a mixture of vitamins. Nutr Cancer 1994;22:233-45.
**15.** Brody JE. Alternative medicine makes inroads, but watch out for curves. New York Times. April 28, 1998:F7.
**16.** Coppes MJ, Anderson RA, Egeler RM, Wolff JEA. Alternative therapies for the treatment of childhood cancer. N Engl J Med 1998;339:846-7.
**17.** Slifman NR, Obermeyer WR, Aloi BK, et al. Contamination of botanical dietary supplements by *Digitalis lanata*. N Engl J Med 1998;339:806-11.
**18.** Ko RJ. Adulterants in Asian patent medicines. N Engl J Med 1998;339:847.
**19.** LoVecchio F, Curry SC, Bagnasco T. Butyrolactone-induced central nervous system depression after ingestion of RenewTrient, a "dietary supplement." N Engl J Med 1998;339:847-8.
**20.** Beigel Y, Ostfeld I, Schoenfeld N. A leading question. N Engl J Med 1998;339:827-30.
**21.** Wittes B. FDA exemption sought for self-help medicines. The Recorder. October 7, 1994:2.
**22.** Dietary Supplement Health and Education Act of 1994. (Public Law 103-417.)
**23.** Wagner MW. Is homeopathy 'new science' or 'new age'? Sci Rev Alternative Med 1997;1(1):7-12.
**24.** Herbal roulette. Consumer Reports. November 1995:698.
**25.** Cui J, Garle M, Eneroth P, Björkhem I. What do commercial ginseng preparations contain? Lancet 1994;344:134.
**26.** DiPaola RS, Zhang H, Lambert GH, et al. Clinical and biologic activity of an estrogenic herbal combination (PC-SPES) in prostate cancer. N Engl J Med 1998;339:785-91.
**27.** Anticancer botanicals that work supportively with chemotherapy: PCSpes. Alternative Medicine Digest. November 1997:84-5.
**28.** Love LA. The MedWatch Program. Clin Toxicol 1998;36:263-7.

## The 'Dietary Supplement' Mess
### Commission Report Issued

### by **Stephen Barrett**, MD

In the early 1990s, Congress began considering two bills to greatly strengthen the ability of federal agencies to combat health frauds. One would have increased the FDA's enforcement powers as well as the penalties for violating the Food, Drug, and Cosmetic Act. The other would have amended the Federal Trade Commission Act to make it illegal to advertise nutritional or therapeutic claims that would not be permissible on supplement labels. During the same period, the FDA was considering tighter regulations for these labels.

> *The end result was a law that greatly weakened the FDA's ability to protect consumers.*

Alarmed by these developments, the health-food industry and its allies urged Congress to "preserve the consumer's freedom to choose dietary supplements." To whip up their troops, industry leaders warned retailers that they would be put out of business. Consumers were told that unless they took action, the FDA would take away their right to buy vitamins. These claims, although bogus, generated an avalanche of communications to Congress.

The end result was a law that greatly weakened the FDA's ability to protect consumers. Called the Dietary Supplement Health and Education Act (DSHEA) of 1994, it defined "dietary supplements" as a separate regulatory category and liberalized what information could be distributed by their sellers.

It also created an NIH Office of Dietary Supplements and directed the President to appoint a Commission on Dietary Supplement Labels to recommend ways to implement the act. The Commission's recommendations were released on June 24, 1997. (See "Recommendations from the Dietary Supplement Commission.")

### Expanded Definition

The Food, Drug, and Cosmetic Act defines "drug" as any article (except devices) "intended for use in the diagnosis, cure, mitigation, treatment, or prevention of disease" and "articles (other than food) intended to affect the structure or function of the body." These words permit the FDA to stop the marketing of products with unsubstantiated "drug" claims on their labels.

To evade the law's intent, the supplement industry is organized to ensure that the public learns of "medicinal" uses that are not stated on product labels. This is done mainly by promoting the ingredients of the products in books, magazines, newsletters, booklets, lectures, radio and television broadcasts, and oral claims made by retailers.

DSHEA worsened this situation by increasing the amount of misinformation that can be directly transmitted to prospective customers. It also expanded the types of products that could be marketed as "supplements." The most logical definition of "dietary supplement" would be something that supplies one or more essential nutrients missing from the diet. DSHEA went far beyond this to include vitamins; minerals; herbs or other botanicals; amino acids; other dietary substances to supplement the diet by increasing dietary intake; and any concentrate, metabolite, constituent, extract, or combination of any such ingredients. Although

many such products (particularly herbs) are marketed for their alleged preventive or therapeutic effects, DSHEA has made it difficult or impossible for the FDA to regulate them as drugs. Since its passage, even hormones, such as DHEA and melatonin, are being hawked as supplements. DSHEA also prohibits the FDA from banning dubious supplement ingredients as "unapproved food additives." The FDA considered this strategy more efficient than taking action against individual manufacturers who made illegal drug claims. Since DSHEA's passage, the only way to banish an ingredient is to prove it is unsafe. Ingredients that are useless but harmless are protected.

### 'Nutritional Support' Statements

DSHEA allows dietary supplements to bear "statements of support" that: (1) claim a benefit related to classical nutrient deficiency disease, (2) describe how ingredients affect the structure or function of the human body, (3) characterize the documented mechanism by which the ingredients act to maintain structure or function, or (4) describe general well-being from consumption of the ingredients. The statement "calcium builds strong bones and teeth" is said to be a classic example of an allowable structure/function statement for a food. What constitutes an allowable statement for a supplement has not been specified either by law or by regulation.

To be legal, a "nutritional support" statement must not be a "drug" claim. In other words, it should not suggest that the product or ingredient is intended for prevention or treatment of disease.

The Dietary Supplement Commission expressed concern that "some statements of nutritional support are in fact akin to drug claims." Some members be-

Reprinted with permission from *Nutrition Forum*, July/August 1997, pp. 25–29. © 1997 by Prometheus Books, 59 John Glenn Drive, Amherst, NY 14228.

# *Major Recommendations from the Dietary Supplement Commission*

## Safety

- Safety of supplement products must be assured.
- The FDA, the supplement industry, scientific groups, and consumer groups should work together to expand and improve postmarketing surveillance, including adverse reporting systems.
- Product information should include appropriate warnings.
- The FDA should take swift enforcement action to address safety issues, such as those posed by ephedra-containing products. The agency should be given additional resources to do this.

## Health Claims

- The approval process for health claims should be the same for dietary supplements and conventional foods.
- The standard of "significant scientific agreement" is appropriate but should not require unanimous or near unanimous support.
- To determine whether significant scientific agreement exists for particular claims, the FDA should obtain broad input and use appropriate outside expert panels.

## Statements of Nutritional Support

- Statements of nutritional support should provide useful information about the product's intended use.
- Statements of nutritional support should be supported by scientifically valid evidence substantiating that the statements are truthful and not misleading
- Structure/function statements should not suggest disease prevention or treatment.
- Statements that mention a body system, organ, or function affected by a supplement using such terms as "stimulate," "maintain," "support," "regulate," or "promote" can be appropriate when the statements do not suggest disease prevention or treat-

ment or use for a serious health condition beyond the ability of the consumer to evaluate.

- Statements should not be made for products to "restore" normal or "correct" abnormal function where the abnormality implies the presence of disease. (For example, a claim to "restore" normal blood pressure when the abnormality implies hypertension.)
- Statements of nutritional support are not to be drug claims. They should not refer to specific diseases, disorders, or classes of diseases and should not use such drug-related terms as "diagnose," "treat," "prevent," "cure," or "mitigate."

## Substantiation of Nutritional Support Statements

- The Dietary Supplement Health and Education Act (DSHEA) requires manufacturers marketing supplements labeled for "nutritional support" to notify the Secretary of Health and Human Services within 30 days after marketing of a product bearing such a statement. To satisfy this requirement, the notice should include: (1) the identity of the ingredient(s) for which the statement is made, (2) the product's intended use, including recommended dosage, (3) appropriate contraindications or warnings, (4) a brief summary of the evidence and conclusions about safety and effectiveness of the stated dosage, and (5) a consumer version of the evidence on which any claim is made.
- DSHEA requires manufacturers marketing supplements labeled for "nutritional support" to have substantiation. To satisfy that requirement, the manufacturer's substantiation files should contain: (1) a copy of the notification letter, (2) key evidence, including an interpretive summary by a qualified individual, (3) the identity and quantity of the pertinent dietary ingredients, (4) evidence substantiating the

ingredient's safety, (5) assurance that good manufacturing practices were followed, and (6) the qualifications of the individual(s) who reviewed the evidence for safety and effectiveness. A consumer version of the evidence should be made available to the public for each product bearing a statement of nutritional support. This version should not state or imply use for preventing or treating disease.

## Publications Connected to Sales

- Articles provided to consumers must be balanced and truthful. The FDA should promptly issue warnings or undertake enforcement action if it becomes aware of violations.
- The FDA should monitor practices in this area and issue guidelines as needed.

## Botanical Products

- The FDA should establish an OTC review panel to review botanical products intended for preventive or therapeutic use.
- For products unable to meet FDA review requirements, creation of an alternative approval system should be considered.

## Assessment of Consumer Education

- Research should be done to determine whether consumers want and can use information required by existing FDA regulations, DSHEA requirements, and Dietary Supplement Commission recommendations. This would include statements of nutritional support as well as point-of-sale literature.

## Expert Evaluation

- The dietary supplement industry should consider establishing an expert advisory committee to provide scientific review of label statements and claims and guidance on safety and appropriate labeling. Such a committee might be supported by one or more trade associations or might be established as an independent entity funded by grants and/or fees for services.

lieve that claims related to organs (such as "supports the eyes" or "supports the cardiovascular system") are really drug claims and that DSHEA has created a loophole for such claims. Some members are particularly concerned about statements that mention an acute effect on the structure or function of a major system (such as "reduces heart rate").

Actually, few statements about the biochemical or physiologic properties of nutrients have practical value for consumers. By definition, every essential nutrient is important to proper body function. Simple statements about nutrient function are more likely to be misleading than helpful. A statement such as "vitamin A is essential to good eye function" could suggest: (1) people need to take special steps to be sure they get enough, (2) extra vitamin A may enhance eyesight, and (3) common eye problems may be caused by vitamin A deficiency or remedied by taking supplements. To be completely truthful, a "nutritional support" statement about vitamin A would have to counter all three misconceptions and indicate that people eating sensibly don't need to worry about whether their vitamin A intake is adequate. In other words, truthful statements about nutrient supplements would have to indicate who doesn't need them. No vitamin manufacturer has ever done this or ever will.

Since herbs are not nutrients, the concept of "nutritional support" statements for herbs is absurd. The Dietary Supplement Commission noted: "Many botanicals now are being marketed with statements of nutritional support that suggest only indirectly the type of therapeutic use that is traditional for the product. . . . Most Commissioners believe direct therapeutic statements . . . may be more informative." The Commission's report urges the FDA to develop a review process that could enable herbs that have substantiated therapeutic use to be marketed as over-the-counter drugs.

A recent ad in *Veggie Life* magazine illustrates the absurdities that DSHEA has spawned. The headline states: "IT PROTECTS YOUR HEART THE WAY FORT KNOX PROTECTS GOLD." The body of the ad states: "MaxiLIFE Cardio Protector nutritionally supports healthy cardiovascular function on a whole new level of potency.* That's because it's no ordinary formula, but a nutritional all-star team of cardioprotective agents." The asterisk refers to the disclaimer that DSHEA requires with "support" statements: "This statement has not been evaluated by the Food and Drug Administration. The product is not intended to diagnose, treat, cure or prevent any disease." The Fort Knox analogy, which suggests complete cardioprotection, is printed in half-inch type. The disclaimer is in 4-point type, which is barely visible.

Under some circumstances, some ingredients in Cardio Protector might help protect a person's heart. Its B vitamins, for example, could lower elevated blood homocysteine levels, which are a risk factor for coronary artery disease. However, there is no reason for people whose homocysteine level is normal to use this product. The dozen or so other ingredients have little or no proven value for cardioprotection. People really interested in protecting their heart should follow an individually designed program based on risk-factor analysis. For these reasons, I believe that Cardio Protector has no rational use. Its manufacturer, Twin Laboratories of Ronkonkema, New York, also markets Prostate Protector and Brain Protector.

Under DSHEA, manufacturers who make statements of "nutritional support" must have substantiation that such statements are truthful and not misleading. The law also requires that the Secretary of Health and Human Services be notified no later than 30 days after the first marketing of a supplement for which the statement is being made. The law does not define substantiation.

## Publications Connected to Sales

Historically, the FDA has considered literature used directly in connection with the sale of a product to be "labeling" for the product. DSHEA exempts publications from "labeling" if they: (1) are not false or misleading, (2) do not promote a particular manufacturer or brand, (3) present a "balanced" view of pertinent scientific information, and (4) are physically separated from the items discussed. However, since most "dietary supplements" are either useless, irrationally formulated, and/or overpriced, the supplement industry has little reason to provide literature that is not misleading.

The Dietary Supplement Commission concluded that the criteria listed above would be difficult to apply, particularly the requirement for balance. "Balance" is difficult or impossible to define, and standards, if they are developed, would be difficult to enforce. Moreover, no federal agency has the resources to regulate what individual retailers do in their stores.

## Further Weakening Proposed

The Nutrition Labeling and Education Act of 1990 prohibits misleading health claims on foods. It requires such claims to be supported by "significant scientific agreement" and be cleared by the FDA before use in the marketplace. Section 618 of the FDA Modernization and Accountability Act (S. 830) would eliminate preclearance and enable claims to be based on statements by any federal agency, even if the agency's position is counter to the prevailing scientific view or fails to take overall diet into account. (Currently, for example, even though some agencies have recommended eating a low-fat diet, the FDA does not permit health claims to be made for low-fat foods that are very high in sodium.) The Food and Nutrition Labeling Group, a 21-member coalition of prominent professional and consumer organizations, has vigorously objected to Section 618.

## The Bottom Line

The FDA has never had enough resources to cope with the enormous amount of deception in the supplement and health-food marketplace. DSHEA has made the problem worse. If I were FDA Commissioner, I would drop any pretense of being able to protect the public. Instead, I would announce that unless Congress provides an adequate law, the FDA cannot protect the public from the deceptive marketing of what DSHEA calls "dietary supplements."

**See Addendum.**

*Stephen Barrett, MD, a retired psychiatrist, is a board member of the National Council Against Health Fraud and webmaster of Quackwatch (***http://www.quackwatch.com***), a guide to quackery, health frauds, and intelligent decision making.*

# ADDENDUM

## Table 1

## Innovations in DSHEA Compared to Prior Law (NLEA and FDCA)

| Issue | Provisions Under Prior Law | DSHEA |
|---|---|---|
| Definition of dietary supplement. | Only essential nutrients such as vitamins, minerals, and proteins considered. | Adds amino acids, herbs, botanicals, or similar substances or mixtures intended to supplement the diet, and concentrates, metabolites, constituents, extracts or combinations thereof, designed to increase total daily intake in pill, capsule, tablet, powder, or liquid form. |
| Regulatory framework for assuring safety of products. | More; FDA had more authority to regulate products such as herbs or certain dietary supplements that might be harmful. They could be classified as "food additives" of "new drugs" under the FDCA which required premarket approval. New ingredients in dietary supplements were regulated under the 1958 Food Additive Amendments to the FDCA. | Less; dietary supplements are no longer subject to premarket safety evaluations required of new food or for new uses of old ingredients. Also, regulatory avenues are more circumscribed by the new law for these products. Other safety provisions of the FDCA must be met. |
| Guidelines for literature now displayed where label and supplements are sold. | Publications such as articles, book chapters, or abstracts of peer reviewed scientific papers were considered labeling and regulated as such when provided in connection with the sale of dietary supplements. | Such information not considered part of the label and is not regulated as such as long as the publications are not false and misleading, do not promote a particular brand or manufacturer and are displayed so as to present a balanced view of the relevant scientific information, physically separate from the dietary supplement. |
| Use of claims and supporting nutritional statements. | Only appropriate health claims authorized by the FDA allowed for products qualified to bear the health claim. | Nutritional statements allowed without prior approval by FDA. Statements about classical nutrient deficiency disease allowed if the prevalence of the disease in the U.S. is disclosed. Supplement's effects on the structure or function of the body or well-being achieved by consumption of the dietary ingredient are allowed if manufacturer can substantiate that the statements are true and not misleading, and the product label bears the disclaimer that the statement has not been evaluated by FDA, and that the product is not intended to diagnose, treat, cure or prevent any disease. (Note: Structure function claims are not considered health claims.) |

Source: *Nutrition & the M.D.*, May 1997, p. 3.

## Table 2

## Comparisons of Labeling and Health Claims for Foods Under NLEA and for Dietary Supplements Under DSHEA

| Issue | NLEA | DSHEA |
|---|---|---|
| Definitions | "High potency" not permitted under proposed regulations on foods. Antioxidant content claims permissible on both foods and supplements. | Regulations to define such terms as "high potency" (100% or more the RDI for vitamins and minerals or 100% of the DRV for protein or fiber for at least two-thirds of the nutrients present in the product). Definitions of "antioxidant" (vitamins C, E, beta carotene) provided. |
| Claims permitted | Certain preapproved disease prevention claims permitted on food packages, when nutrient-disease relationship supported by significant scientific agreement. | Includes all NLEA health claims, a benefit related to "classical nutrient deficiency disease" and discloses its prevalence in U.S.: <br>• Describes role of nutrient/dietary ingredient intended to affect structure or function in humans (that is a statement of how nutrition is supported). <br>• Characterizes the documented mechanism by which nutrient acts to maintain structure or function. <br>• Describes general well-being from consuming supplement. |
| Ingredient labeling | Required on most food products. | Ingredients not marketed in U.S. before passage of DSHEA permitted unless they contain substances that have not been present in the food supply as a material used for food in a form, or they are in a form that has been chemically altered. If there is evidence that the supplement will reasonably be expected to be safe when used as directed, and the manufacturer provides the FDA with information on which the manufacturer has concluded that the dietary supplement is expected to be safe, it will be permitted. |
| Reference daily intakes (RDIs) | RDI's are new food label reference values for nutrients, replacing the USRDA's. They did not exist until 1997. | More nutrients have RDIs and % DV can now be stated when present. RDI's may appear on nutrition facts panel as % of Daily Value (DV) for protein and 26 vitamins and minerals. Recently added K, selenium, manganese, chromium, molybdenum, and chloride. No RDI for fluoride. |
| Nutrient labeling for non-nutrient ingredients | Not allowed | Dietary ingredients that are not nutrients can be displayed prominently on the label following nutrient ingredients. |
| Nutrition labeling | Information on dietary ingredients for which reference daily intakes (RDI) are available or daily reference values (DRV). RDI that are not available appear only in the ingredient label, not within the nutrition facts panel. | Supplements must bear supplement facts with dietary ingredients for which FDA has established DVs listed first. DSHEA also permits the label to include information on substances that are not nutrients listed next. For example, herbal substances may now be listed on the label panel, and the source of the substance may also be listed. |

Source: *Nutrition & the M.D.,* May, 1997, p. 5.

# Minding Your Memory with Ginkgo?

That the quest for a memory enhancer has focused on the ancient ginkgo biloba tree has lyrical symbolism. For if any tree could be a repository of memory, it would be the ginkgo—a primitive but lasting specimen with an evolutionary history dating back 230 million years. With age, almost everyone experiences some difficulty recalling names and words. But are ginkgo biloba extracts, which are marketed as memory boosters, an elixir for this "normal" memory loss—not to mention the 4 million Americans suffering from the disabling dementia of Alzheimer's disease?

The supplements are certainly being snatched up as though they are. Americans spent more than $100 million last year on this supposed brain booster, which is widely used in Europe as a treatment for cognitive problems, such as memory loss. While no well-designed studies have evaluated ginkgo for people who are simply forgetful, a recent study looking at it as a treatment for dementia showed encouraging, if preliminary, results. Unfortunately, there is no evidence that the mild benefits found in the study translate into memory aids for those without dementia. And people with Alzheimer's disease or other forms of dementia should discuss ginkgo extracts—and other drugs approved by the Food and Drug Administration—with their doctor before deciding on treatment.

## AN ANCIENT HISTORY

In its native Asia, extracts of the ginkgo biloba, or maidenhair, tree are used for ailments ranging from asthma to hypertension. In Germany and France, standardized ginkgo extracts are among the most commonly prescribed drugs for circulatory and neurological problems. Ginkgo extracts contain a variety of active ingredients that appear to act in concert to induce antioxidant and anti-inflammatory effects. Both of these

properties could account for its supposed benefits to the brain. Some studies show that it may relax blood vessels, reduce clotting, and reduce the abnormalities that afflict the brain in those with Alzheimer's disease.

The study mentioned earlier, published in the *Journal of the American Medical Association (JAMA)*, is the first American trial to rigorously examine ginkgo. The study evaluated 309 patients with mild to severe dementia from Alzheimer's disease and other causes. Patients received either EGb 761, an extract of the plant commonly used in Europe, or a placebo. Subjects were evaluated every three months for a year. Of the 202 patients who completed the trial, cognitive performance and social functioning were more likely to stabilize or improve in the ginkgo-takers than in those taking the placebo. The improvements tended to be modest, but they were significant enough to be noticed by those caring for the patients. The extract had few side effects.

## THE BOTTOM LINE

These results suggest that ginkgo is aiding some people. The questions are who? and why? Subjects in the study

had dementia—but that could result from a variety of causes besides Alzheimer's disease, including treatable ones, such as depression or side effects from medications. Also, because ginkgo side effects were not really a concern, the high drop-out rate in the study suggests that many people quit because they experienced no benefit. For these reasons, most medical experts are not ready to fully embrace ginkgo. "Ginkgo may be a mild memory enhancer. But it's also possible that, in this study, alleviating depression, or simply energizing patients, led to secondary memory gains," says *Health After 50* board member Dr. Peter Rabins, a geriatric psychiatrist at Johns Hopkins.

For now, people with Alzheimer's disease will gain more from the prescription drugs tacrine (Cognex) and donepezil (Aricept), which have been more extensively studied and are approved by the FDA. "This study did not show that ginkgo is an alternative to these medications," says Dr. Rabins. The most encouraging news for Alzheimer's patients right now is that the arsenal of proven medications is soon to increase: Several new medications submitted to the FDA are likely to be approved in the near future.

*Action* STEPS → **Taking Ginkgo**

▼ There is no evidence that ginkgo biloba enhances memory in those with normal memory loss.
▼ If you are truly concerned about memory loss, consult your physician to rule out a treatable cause, such as depression, or other conditions that merit comprehensive medical planning and care, such as Alzheimer's disease.
▼ Because ginkgo reduces blood clotting, it should be used cautiously if you already take blood-thinning medications, such as aspirin or warfarin.
▼ If you do decide to try ginkgo, dosages are uncertain. Most trials have used 120 to 160 mg of ginkgo extract a day, divided into three doses. Subjects in the *JAMA* study took 120 mg. A four- to six-week course of treatment is required to determine effectiveness. But how long to continue the supplement is unknown.
▼ Because ginkgo is not regulated by the FDA, active ingredients may vary among brands.

Reprinted with permission from *The Johns Hopkins Medical Letter: Health After 50,* February 1998, p. 3. © 1998 by MedLetter Associates. To order a one-year subscription, call 800-829-9170.

# HEALTH & FITNESS

# Ephedrine's deadly edge

BY MICHELE PULLIA TURK

Roughly one in three U.S. adults swallows some kind of dietary supplement every day or so. It might be no more than an extra dose of vitamin C. It might be a substance that is harmless but whose claimed salutary effects are based more on faith than on facts. Or, in some cases, it just might kill them.

For several years, products containing ephedrine, a powerful stimulant extracted from a Chinese herb variously called ma huang or ephedra, have been especially hot. Health food stores, supermarkets, and pharmacies are stocked with ephedra-based products whose labels suggest victory over a bulging waistline, greater energy, even enhanced potency. Ephedrine stimulates the heart and central nervous system; thus the use of such products by teenagers as a legal high.

Unlike drugs, ephedra-based products don't have to be shown to be safe or effective, because herbs, vitamins, and minerals were classified as dietary supplements by the Dietary Supplement Health and Education Act of 1994. The Food and Drug Administration cannot regulate dietary supplements unless it can marshal evidence that a product is unsafe ["Nature's Remedies," May 19].

The FDA has been trying to build just such a case against ephedrine. Since 1993, the agency has compiled more than 800 reports of "adverse reactions" to ephedra-based products, including strokes, high blood pressure, heart palpitations, seizures, and heart attacks (box, "Read before you swallow"). Dietary supplements that contain ephedrine have been linked, according to the FDA, to three dozen deaths, including that of Peter Schlendorf, a college student who apparently overdosed during spring break in Florida last year on Ultimate Xphoria.

One reason the FDA believes such preparations pose a danger is that the amount of ephedrine in different products' recommended dosages varies widely and can be hard to gauge. Bottles standing side by side may supply doses of 1 to 110 milligrams of ephedrine. The ephedrine content usually is stated not directly but as a percentage of the ma huang. Sometimes even the quantity of ma huang is unspecified, leaving the amount of ephedrine in a dose an open question.

A casual inspection suggests that most ephedra-based products include six to 20 other ingredients as well. An inquiry by the FDA confirmed that. Most, for example, also include botanical sources of caffeine, such as kola nut and guarana; adding this stimulant may increase the effect of the ephedrine.

Last week, mounting concerns about ephedrine prompted the Presidential Commission on Dietary Supplement Labels, a panel established as part of the 1994 law, to recommend that consumers be provided with detailed label information and warnings about the risk of exceeding the label dosage. While most ephedrine-based products carry a note or warning, the language is not always direct. The "note" on one product, for example, states that it "should not be taken by those wishing to eliminate the stimulants caffeine and ephedrine from their diets."

**Initial salvo.** The commission's recommendation is far more modest than the FDA's proposal earlier in June to enhance the safety of herbal supplements containing ephedrine—the first time the FDA has exercised its regulatory powers under the 1994 law. Under the proposal, dietary supplements that blend ephedrine with sources of caffeine and those that provide 8 milligrams or more of ephedrine per dose would be prohibited. Product labels would caution consumers not to ingest more than 24 milligrams of ephedrine per day or to use the product for more than seven days. The FDA also would require warning pregnant women and individuals with medical problems like hypertension, heart conditions, neurologic disorders, and diabetes to avoid ephedrine. The final recommendations should be released in the fall.

Following the death of Peter Schlendorf, Florida, Nebraska, and New York were among the states that banned the sale of at least some ephedrine products. In its report, the presidential commission urged the FDA to response more swiftly to reports that a product might

## Following Peter Schlendorf's death, Florida, Nebraska, and New York banned the sale of at least some ephedrine products.

be harmful. "The FDA and industry should work out a system of monitoring and responding to adverse reactions," says Annette Dickinson, a commission member and director of scientific and regulatory affairs for the Council for Responsible Nutrition, a dietary supplement trade group.

**Why take them?** Whether ephedra-based dietary supplements even do what they are perceived as doing is questionable. The FDA's latest advisory committee found little evidence that ephedra-based supplements are effective at triggering weight loss, for example.

"The reason people lose weight when they take ephedrine is that they can't get the utensils to their mouths because their hands are shaking so much," says Varro Tyler, an authority on medicinal plants who served on a previous FDA committee that investigated ephedrine. Dickinson refers to "a body of evidence and consumer experience that suggests benefits for weight loss and sports nutrition." But she adds that

"the question is whether any benefit outweighs the risks in the general population."

Using ephedrine as an approved aid to weight control is more common in Europe, where journal reports have

### Read before you swallow

*The Food and Drug Administration has gathered more than 800 reports of "adverse reactions" associated with over-the-counter products that contain ephedrine. The largest two categories are cardiovascular and neurological. The most significant problems:*

**CARDIOVASCULAR REPORTS**

- Heart attack
- Abnormal heartbeat
- Stroke
- Death
- Weakened heart muscle

**NEUROLOGICAL REPORTS**

- Psychiatric episodes (psychosis, suicidal impulses, depression)
- Seizure
- Dizziness
- Loss of consciousness

shown that ephedrine combined with caffeine and aspirin can help obese people lose weight. Few U.S. studies have been done; ephedra cannot be patented, which reduces the incentive for individual manufacturers to conduct research.

The Ephedra Research Foundation, a coalition of manufacturers and distributors, is funding a $600,000 study of products that combine ephedra with kola nut for the purpose of weight loss. Conducted jointly by Harvard and Vanderbilt medical schools, the study will investigate formulations similar to current over-the-counter versions for effectiveness against obesity. It is expected to be finished by the end of the year—but its results are unlikely to bring the scrutiny to a close.

# Hard Facts on Colloidal Minerals
## Cure-all or crushed rocks?
### by Beth Fontenot, MS, RD

Colloidal mineral supplements are the current craze in "alternative" nutrition, promising to cure what ails you—and to confuse consumers. They are simply extra-small mineral particles suspended in a solution, and they are being promoted as the cure for acne, anemia, brittle nails, birth defects, cancer, constipation, depression, diabetes, goiter, graying hair, hair loss, hyperactivity, impotence, infertility, memory loss, PMS, and wrinkles.

Colloidal minerals are sold largely by multi-level marketing companies under such names as Clark's Mineral Formula, Mineral Toddy, Mineral Solutions, and Micro-Mins. They sell for up to $50 for a month's supply. The fact that these products are sold by multilevel marketing companies should make one skeptical, and the numerous claims made by the marketers are dubious at best.

## The Sales Pitch

The story behind colloidal minerals goes like this: In 1925, a Paiute Indian led an ailing Utah rancher, Thomas Clark, to a legendary spring known for its healing powers. Soon after drinking from the spring, Clark was healed of his ailment. As Clark followed the spring back into the mountains, he discovered a deposit of minerals that was later determined to be the re-

*They are being promoted as the cure for acne, anemia, birth defects, cancer, constipation, depression, diabetes, goiter, hyperactivity, impotence, infertility, memory loss, PMS, and wrinkles.*

mains of a prehistoric rain forest. He created a "miracle tonic" by extracting the minerals from the spring and passed it among his friends who reportedly experi-

enced remarkable results. Many manufacturers tout their product as coming from this "original source," but similar deposits are said to be found in a few other areas of the world.

Collodial minerals, which have been described by some as "mud" or "crushed rocks," are sold as elixirs, capsules, and oral sprays. The mineral content varies by product, but the ingredient lists all read like the Periodic Table of Elements: aluminum, arsenic, cadmium, lead, lithium, platinum, silver, titanium, as well as an assortment of others less familiar minerals.

The promoters maintain that our soil is so depleted that the food we eat is lacking in the minerals our bodies need, and furthermore, we absorb only about 5% of the minerals we do get from food. A multitude of diseases and medical conditions, as well as deaths, are due to mineral deficiencies, they say.

The promotional materials declare that colloidal minerals have a natural negative charge that enhances their absorption as well as the transport and availability of other nutrients. Toxins and heavy metals are supposedly attracted to this negative charge and are flushed from the body. In addition, the marketers assert that the small size of colloidal minerals, as opposed to the elemental minerals found in over-the-counter supplements, makes

From *Nutrition Forum,* September/October 1997, pp. 33-34. © 1997 by Prometheus Books, 59 John Glenn Drive, Amherst, NY 14228. Reprinted by permission of the publisher.

them more easily absorbed by the cells of the body. The ads also carefully point out that toxicity is not a concern, and one company's ad states that their product contains only "truly organic" minerals.

## Reality Check

The claims for these mineral products are nothing more than imaginative sales gimmicks. Absorption of a nutrient is not affected by its charge, and even if colloidal minerals are better absorbed (and experts dispute that fact), that would not make them desirable. Some minerals are toxic at high levels, and many of those present in the products are not recognized as essential to humans. The fact is that for many minerals, absorption by the body is largely regulated by the need for the mineral. And as for the claim about "truly organic" minerals, the fact is that minerals are *inorganic*. (Organic materials contain carbon atoms, and inorganic materials do not.)

No scientific evidence can be found to support any of the claims made by the marketers of these products, including the claim regarding mineral deficiencies in foods.

Currently, there are 16 minerals recognized as essential to humans. The Committee on Dietary Allowances of the National Academy of Sciences has established a Recommended Dietary Allowance (RDA) for the major minerals calcium, phosphorus, and magnesium, and for the best-known trace minerals iron, zinc, iodine, and selenium. Estimated Minimum Requirements have been established for sodium, potassium, and chloride. Other minerals such as copper, manganese, fluoride, chromium, and molybdenum are known to be essential, and an Estimated Safe and Adequate Daily Dietary Intake (ESADDI) is published for these. Arsenic, nickel, silicon, and boron are recognized as essential to animals, but are not firmly established as essential for humans. Very little is known about the need for cadmium, cobalt, lead, lithium, tin, and vanadium. At this time, the evidence that these are essential is weak.

Minerals play a critical role in the maintenance of health as well as in the management of some disease states. The fact that minerals are required only in small amounts and that they can be toxic in excess raises substantial concern about the indiscriminate use of supplements. There are mechanisms in the body that regulate the absorption and excretion of excessive amounts of the essential minerals; however, there does not appear to be such a mechanism for regulating the absorption and excretion of nonessential minerals. There also exists the potential for adverse mineral interactions and imbalances to occur in the body when mineral supplements are used haphazardly.

The bottom line is that a healthy diet that provides a wide variety of foods from both plant and animal sources is the safest, least expensive, and most practical way to ensure an adequate intake of the minerals required by the human body. The claims for colloidal minerals are just too hard to swallow.

---

*Beth Fontenot is a nutrition consultant and freelance nutrition writer in Lake Charles, LA. She serves on the adjunct faculty at both McNeese State University in Lake Charles and Lamar University in Orange, TX.*

# Can Nutrition Cure ADHD?
## *The facts about diets and dietary supplements*
### by **Beth Fontenot**, MS, RD

**F**ew medical conditions lend themselves to more unproven claims, distortions of the truth, and controversial therapies than does Attention-Deficit/Hyperactivity Disorder (ADHD). Numerous dietary interventions and nutritional supplements have been claimed to ease or cure ADHD. Unfortunately, the promise of a quick solution or a cure that doesn't involve the use of drugs is often irresistible for vulnerable, well-meaning parents, even if that "solution" has no scientific basis or is outright quackery.

The American Psychiatric Association's *Diagnostic and Statistics Manual* (*DSM-IV*) lists three categories of ADHD: (1) predominantly inattentive type, (2) predominantly hyperactive-impulsive type, and (3) combined type. Specific criteria must be met for the diagnosis of each type. In most cases, the cause of the condition is unknown, but it is believed that ADHD may be the result of organic, genetic, and psychosocial factors.

Standard therapy for ADHD involves the use of stimulant medications such as Ritalin or Dexedrine, behavioral management, and/or special education. Various "natural" treatments have also been proposed, including defined diets, elimination diets, dietary supplements, megavitamin therapy, and herbal therapy.

## Salicylates and Sugar

Benjamin Feingold, MD, was the first person to implicate diet as the primary cause of hyperactivity and advocate the use of a defined diet. The Feingold Diet, popularized in the 1970s, was based on the idea that hyperactivity in children was caused by salicylates (found naturally in some fruits and vegetables) and artificial colorings and flavorings in the food supply. The diet required that all of these substances be removed from a child's diet. Dr. Feingold estimated that 50% of his hyperactive patients responded favorably to this diet.

But there was a problem with Dr. Feingold's research. It was based on un-controlled trials of children he had treated. Controlled double-blind challenge studies have not supported Dr. Feingold's claims. In addition, his diet is very difficult to follow since many foods that a child typically eats contain some type of additive, though the diet itself is not harmful. Nevertheless, many families follow the diet, and Feingold Associations are still active in some parts of the country.

Another food that has been implicated as a cause of ADHD in most children is sugar. However, there is no good evidence to support this claim. A meta-analysis in the *Journal of the American Medical Association* (*JAMA*: 1617–1621, November 22–29, 1995) examined 16 articles reporting on 23 separate studies on the relationship between sugar and the behavior and cognition of children. The authors found that sugar did not affect the behavior or cognitive performance of children.

Many parents firmly believe that an excess of sugary foods causes hyperactivity or inattentive behavior in their children. In fact, avoiding sugar is one of the more popular pieces of advice that parents with ADHD children receive. Questions remain as to why the results of controlled studies differ from the impression of parents. It may be that popular folklore or publicity proposing a link between sugar and behavior may encourage parents to expect adverse behavior and selectively focus on it. In addition, high-sugar foods are commonly consumed at parties and gatherings where children tend to get excited, and parents may connect the intake of sugar with "hyperactive" behavior.

## Dubious Products

A search on the Internet for nutritional treatments for ADHD uncovers numerous supplements claimed to relieve the symptoms of ADHD, improve a child's attentiveness, or control a child's behavior. These products cover the supplement spectrum: antioxidants, amino acids, herbs, vitamins, minerals, and an array of other dietary supplements, some with questionable ingredients.

One such product that is highly promoted for the treatment of ADHD is "Pycnogenol," a commercial mixture of bioflavonoids that appears to exhibit antioxidative activity in animal studies. Bioflavonoids are naturally available from vegetables, and are found in the white matter inside the peel of citrus fruits. The impact of large amounts of bioflavonoids on the human body is unknown, as is their usefulness.

Advertisements for "Pycnogenol" state that it is a patented extract from the bark of the French Maritime Pine Tree, and it is described as "the most potent, natural antioxidant compound ever discovered." According to its promoters, "Pycnogenol" is important to brain function because it protects the brain cells from compounds that circulate in the blood. There is no evidence that Pycnogenol is effective to use, and reports of its beneficial effects on ADHD are strictly anecdotal.

Still another product which claims to be beneficial for children with ADHD is "beCALM'd." This product is sold by Technology Services Team, a multilevel marketing company. It is supposed to increase the production of neurotransmitters which will supposedly allow the brain to function better. The ad on the Internet states that beCALM'd is a patented "precise combination of amino acids, vitamins, and minerals."

The ingredients of beCALM'd include l-glutamine, d-phenylalanine, calcium, magnesium, chromium, folic acid, and vitamins A and B$_6$. The promoters for this product claim that in order to get enough of the right combination of these nutrients for the brain to function properly, one would need to consume "several pounds of fish, whole milk, cheese, and 2 or 3 pounds of turkey per day." In fact, the nutrient ingredients in beCALM'd are all available in adequate amounts in a balanced diet with normal portion sizes, and there is no known

From *Nutrition Forum*, May/June 1998, pp. 19, 22. © 1998 by Prometheus Books, 59 John Glenn Drive, Amherst, NY 14228. Reprinted by permission of the publisher.

magic combination of nutrients that will make the brain work better.

Vaxa International, a "homeopathic nutraceutical company," has its version of a defined diet for ADHD on the Internet. The diet requires eliminating many foods including dairy products, all yellow foods (like corn and squash), and fruit juices. The company claims that a high-protein shake for breakfast made with coffee and a protein powder is needed "to feed the brain." The ADHD program also encourages the use of colloidal minerals (see *Nutrition Forum*, September/October, 1997) and one or more of its three supplemental products, depending on which symptoms of ADHD need to be treated.

One of these supplements is "Attend"—claimed to be a "brain fertilizer." It is composed of amino acids, essential fatty acids, lipid complexes, homeopathic medicines, hormone precursors, and precursors to neurotransmitters. Vaxa's "Extress" is a supplement purported to be helpful with temper problems because it contains branched-chain amino acids. There is no scientific evidence that any of these products are effective.

There are also various herbal therapies that are supposed to treat ADHD. Gingko biloba, capsicum, veratrum album, eleuthrero (Siberian ginseng), and evening primrose oil are just some of the botanicals that are advertised as beneficial for treating the symptoms of ADHD. But there is no evidence that any herb is beneficial in the treatment of ADHD. Without adequate testing, quality controls, and standardization of the active principles in herbs, parents just can't be sure of what they are purchasing and what they are giving their children.

Megavitamin therapy has also been proposed for the management of ADHD. Megavitamin therapy is defined as using one or more vitamins in doses at least 10 times the recommended dietary allowance. Some studies have reported benefit from megavitamin therapy for the management of ADHD, but these were poorly designed and lacked appropriate controls.

A study published in *Advances in Neurology* (58:303–310, 1992) was designed to determine whether megavitamin therapy could have a positive effect on children with ADHD. Forty-one children participated in the randomized, controlled trial, which monitored physical, behavioral, and biochemical parameters. The study concluded that megavitamin therapy was ineffective in the management of ADHD and posed a danger because of the potential for hepatotoxicity.

## Advice from the Experts

The American Academy of Pediatrics has concluded that special diets and supplements do not relieve the symptoms of ADHD and warns that food modification alone should not be used as treatment for ADHD.

A statement from a National Institutes of Health Consensus Conference said that defined diets should not be universally used in the treatment of childhood hyperactivity, and a defined diet should not be initiated until a child and his family have been fully and appropriately evaluated and all traditional therapeutic options considered.

Some of the best advice for parents and professionals on the issue of nutrition and ADHD appeared in an article published in the *Journal of Child Neurology* (10 Suppl 1:S96–100, January 1995). The author says that professionals should be informed about controversial treatments proposed for children with learning disabilities so that they can educate parents on the facts about these treatments. The author also advises parents of children with learning disabilities not to accept controversial treatments without question and not to put their children through unproven treatments that are unlikely to help.

---

**A Cautionary Note**

Because the Feingold Diet does no physical harm, it might appear to be helpful in some instances. However, the potential benefits should be weighed against the potential harm of (1) teaching children that their behavior and school performance are related to what they eat rather than what they feel, (2) undermining their self-esteem by implanting notions that they are unhealthy and fragile, (3) creating situations in which their eating behavior or fear of chemicals are regarded as peculiar by other children, and (4) depriving them of the opportunity to receive appropriate professional help. —*Stephen Barrett, MD*

---

*Beth Fontenot is a nutrition consultant and freelance nutrition writer in Lake Charles, LA. She serves on the adjunct faculty at McNeese State University in Lake Charles, TX.*

# Don't Buy Phony 'Ergogenic Aids'

## The real story vs. a mountain of hype

### by Stephen Barrett, MD

More than a hundred companies are marketing phony "ergogenic aids," combinations of various vitamins, minerals, amino acids, and other "dietary supplements" claimed to build muscles and/or enhance athletic performance. In 1991, researchers from the U.S. Centers for Disease Control and Prevention surveyed 12 popular health and bodybuilding magazines (one issue each) and found ads for 89 brands and 311 products with a total of 235 unique ingredients. *Health Foods Business* estimates that in 1996, total sales of such products through health-food stores exceeded $204 million. They are also sold through pharmacies and superstores.

### The Start of 'Ergogenic' Myths

The notion that massive amounts of protein are necessary during training have evolved from the ancient beliefs that great strength could be obtained by eating the raw meat of lions, tigers, or other animals that displayed great fighting strength. Today, although few athletes consume raw meat, the idea that "you are what you eat" is still widely promoted by food faddists.

During the 1900s, when muscles were discovered to contain protein, athletes and coaches mistakenly concluded that protein was the principal component. (Actually, it is water.) These protein beliefs were further reinforced during the 1930s by Bob Hoffman (1899–1985) and later by Joe Weider (1923–), both of whom published magazines that catered to bodybuilders and weightlifters. They asserted that athletes have special protein needs, that protein

supplements have special muscle-building and health-giving powers, and that the most efficient way to get enough protein is by using supplements. The scientific facts are otherwise. Muscle-building is not caused by eating extra protein. It is stimulated by increased muscular work. Once basic protein needs have been met, the small additional amount needed during intense training is easily obtainable from a balanced diet. Few Americans fail to consume adequate amounts of protein.

> *Hoffman and Weider asserted that protein supplements have special muscle-building and health-giving powers.*

Hoffman marketed supplement products and bodybuilding equipment through his York Barbell Company of York, Pennsylvania. A prolific writer, he published two magazines and more than 30 books on fitness and nutrition. For many years, York Barbell's nutritional products were promoted with false and misleading claims. In 1960, the company was charged with misbranding its Energol Germ Oil Concentrate because literature accompanying the oil claimed falsely that it could prevent or treat more than 120 diseases and conditions, including epilepsy, gallstones, and arthritis. In 1961, 15 other York Barbell products were seized as misbranded. In 1968, a larger number of products came under at-

tack by the government for similar reasons. In 1972, the FDA seized three types of York Barbell protein supplements, charging that they were misbranded with false and misleading bodybuilding claims. In 1974, the company was again charged with misbranding Energol and protein supplements. The oil had been claimed to be a special source of vigor and energy. False bodybuilding claims had been made for the protein supplements.

Despite his many brushes with the law, Hoffman achieved considerable professional prominence. During his athletic career, first as an oarsman and then as a weightlifter, he received over 600 trophies, certificates, and awards. He was the Olympic weightlifting coach from 1936 to 1968 and was a founding member of the President's Council on Physical Fitness and Sports.

Weider began bodybuilding as a teenager and was 16 when he launched a newsletter called *Your Physique*. A few years later, he started a company that sold bodybuilding equipment and instructional booklets through the mail. In 1946, Joe's brother Ben joined the business, and they set up the International Federation of Bodybuilders, which promotes the sport worldwide and sponsors competitions. According to press reports, their business empire now grosses over $500 million annually.

Weider Health & Fitness is the dominant player in the sports-supplement marketplace. It publishes seven magazines, sells bodybuilding equipment, broadcasts "Muscle Magazine" on ESPN, and sponsors many athletic and aerobic events throughout the year. The magazines are *Muscle & Fitness, Shape, Flex, Living Fit, Men's Fitness, Prime Health & Fitness,* and *Senior*

Reprinted with permission from *Nutrition Forum*, May/June 1997, pp. 17, 19-21, 24. © 1997 by Prometheus Books, 59 John Glenn Drive, Amherst, NY 14228.

*Golfer.* The supplements include Anabolic Mega-Pak, Dynamic Life Essence, Dynamic Super Stress-End, Dynamic Power Source, Dynamic Driving Force, Dynamic Fat Burners, Dynamic Liver Concentrate Energizer, Dynamic Sustained Endurance, Dynamic Recupe, Dynamic Body Shaper, and Dynamic Muscle Builder. None of these products appears capable of doing what its name suggests, and none contains any nutrients not readily obtainable from a balanced diet.

> *None of these products appears capable of doing what its name suggests.*

In 1984, the FTC charged that ads for Anabolic Mega-Pak (containing amino acids, minerals, vitamins, and herbs) and Dynamic Life Essence (an amino acid product) had been misleading. The FTC complaint was settled in 1985 when Weider and the company agreed not to falsely claim that these products can help build muscles or are effective substitutes for anabolic steroids. They also agreed to pay a minimum of $400,000 in refunds or (if refunds did not reach this figure) to fund research on the relationship of nutrition to muscle development. Although the forbidden claims no longer appear in Weider ads, similar messages appear in articles in the magazines and are implied by endorsements and pictures of muscular athletes as well as by names of the products themselves. False and misleading claims have also appeared in a series of 18 booklets published in 1990 by Weider Health & Fitness and marketed through GNC stores.

## The Market Grows

During the 1970s, in addition to protein supplements and assorted vitamins, the main products touted to athletes were wheat germ oil and bee pollen (falsely claimed to boost energy and endurance). In the early 1980s, Weider Health & Fitness introduced an "Olympians" line said to have been developed by working closely with "Olympians and nutritional researchers." Most were sustained-release vitamin concoctions that included an exotic ingredient or two. As public interest in fitness grew, several drug companies began falsely claiming that multivitamin or "stress" supplements were just what active people needed.

*Life Extension,* by Durk Pearson and Sandy Shaw, was published in 1982 and was followed by appearances by the authors on hundreds of radio and television talk shows. The book claimed that supplements of certain amino acids would cause the body to release growth hormone, which would produce muscle growth and fat loss with little or no effort. These claims were based on faulty extrapolations of experiments in which animals were given large does of these amino acids by injection. Swallowing amino acids does not cause humans to release growth hormone.

> *False and misleading claims have also appeared in a series of 18 booklets published in 1990 by Weider Health & Fitness and marketed through GNC stores.*

But the massive publicity garned by Pearson and Shaw inspired the health-food industry to market hundreds of new products for athletes and would-be dieters. Many of these products are falsely claimed to be "natural steroids" or "steroid substitutes." In the ensuing years, scores of other useless ingredients have been added to "ergogenic aids."

Some manufacturers make no claims in their ads but imply them in product names. Many use pictures of athletes to convey their messages. Some make explicit claims in their ads or product literature, while others use simple puffery. Several have published charts suggesting which products are good for specific purposes. Some even market products for specific sports.

## Just the Facts

Athletes who eat a balanced diet don't need extra protein or vitamins. In *The Complete Sports Medicine Book for Women,* sports medicine specialist Gabe Mirkin, MD, and gynecologist Mona Shangold, MD, explain why: "You don't need much extra protein even to enlarge your muscles. For example, 1 pound of muscle contains only about 100 grams of protein, since it is composed of more than 72% water. So if you are gaining 1 pound of muscle every week in an excellent strength training program, you are adding only about 100 grams of protein each week, or about 15 grams of protein each day. Two cups of corn and beans will meet this need—far less than you would expect. In addition, requirements for only four vitamins increase with exercise: thiamin, niacin, riboflavin, and pantothenic acid. These vitamins are used up minimally in the breakdown of carbohydrates and, to a small degree, protein for energy. But you will find them abundantly in food. Furthermore, deficiencies of these vitamins have never been reported in athletes."

What about other products? The most thorough investigation has been conducted by David Lightsey, MD, an exercise physiologist and nutritionist who coordinates the National Council Against Health Fraud's Task Force on Ergogenic Aids. During the past several years, he has telephoned more than 100 companies that market "ergogenic aids." In a recent interview, Lightsey told me: "In each case, I told a company representative that I had been asked to collect data on the company's product(s) and issue a formal report. After they described the alleged benefits, I would ask how data supporting these claims were collected. As my questions became more specific, their responses became more vague. Some said they could not be more specific because they did not wish to reveal trade secrets.

---

## Hot but risky?

Creatine has been described as the "hottest" ergogenic supplement of the decade. It is popular because it can increase endurance and speed recovery from strenuous activities, which can enhance strength training for certain sports. However, a significant percentage of users experience cramps, muscle spasms, and pulled muscles. Scientific studies have shown that depletion of creatine stores may be associated with the onset of muscle fatigue and that supplementation can increase muscle creatine levels after a few days. The increase was greatest among vegetarians who were found to have the lowest stores. It is not known whether people with adequate dietary intake to begin with run the greatest risk of trouble with supplements. The NCAA Committee on Competitive Safeguards and Medical Aspects of Sports has urged that research be done to determine whether long-term use is safe and whether certain individuals might be predisposed to negative side effects.

"I ended each interview with a request for written documentation. Fewer than half sent anything. Most of the studies they sent were poorly designed and proved nothing. The few that were well designed did not support product claims but were taken out of context.

"Some companies claimed that one team or another was using their products. In each such case, I contacted the team management and learned that although one or more players used the company's products, the management had neither endorsed the products nor encouraged their use."

Lightsey believes there are two reasons why many athletes believe that various products have helped them: (1) use of the product often coincides with natural improvement due to training, and (2) increased self-confidence or a placebo effect inspires greater performance. Any such "psychological benefit," however, should be weighed against the dangers of misinformation, wasted money, misplaced faith, and adverse physical effects—both known and unknown—that can result from megadoses of nutrients. Moreover, how many people who are involved in fitness programs or recreational sports need a placebo for inspiration?

## Lack of Action

Little government effort has been made to protect consumers from wasting money on "sports nutrient" products. The FTC took the action noted above against Weider Health & Fitness, the market leader. In 1986, the agency acted against A. H. Robins and its subsidiary, the Viobin Corporation, which had been making false claims for wheat germ oil products for more than 15 years. The case was settled with a consent agreement prohibiting representations that the oil could help consumers improve endurance, stamina, vigor, or other aspects of athletic fitness, or that its active ingredient "octacosanol" is related in any way to body reaction time, oxygen uptake, oxygen debt, or athletic performance.

In 1992, the New York City Department of Consumer Affairs (DCA) published a report called "Magic Muscle Pills! Health and Fitness Quackery in Nutrition Supplements." DCA investigators found that manufacturers they contacted for information about their products were unable to provide a single published report from a scientific journal to back the claims that their products could benefit athletes.

Along with its report, DCA issued "Notices of Violation" to six companies whose products it had investigated. It also warned consumers to beware of terms like "fat burner," "fat fighter," "fat metabolizer," "energy enhancer," "performance booster," "strength booster," "ergogenic aid," "anabolic optimizer," and "genetic optimizer." Calling the bodybuilding supplement industry "an economic hoax with unhealthy consequences," DCA officials urged the FDA and FTC to stop the "blatantly druglike claims" and false advertising used to promote these products.

In 1994, the FTC reached a consent agreement under which General Nutrition, Inc., paid $2.4 million to settle charges that it had falsely advertised 41 products, most of which had been packaged by other manufacturers. The products included Weider's Super Fat Burners, eleven other "muscle builders," and five other phony "ergogenic aids." No action was taken against the other manufacturers. The FTC's staff is well aware that the "sports nutrition" marketplace needs cleaning up, but it lacks the resources to pursue the majority of offenders. A Trade Regulation Rule that would govern the entire industry could make enforcement more efficient, but the agency has expressed no interest in this approach.

The FDA has the legal right to ban claims that the products stimulate hormone activity or alter the body's metabolism. (Claims of this type enable the agency to classify them as drugs and ban unapproved uses.) In 1994, David Lightsey and I petitioned the FDA to ban all ingredients in these products that had not been proven safe and effective for their intended use and to issue a public warning that the FDA does not recognize them as effective. The agency replied that our petition "did not contain scientific evidence that the claims described in the petition were such that products are . . . unapproved new drugs" and that it "did not provide scientific evidence that would allow the FDA to evaluate the validity of the claims."

*Dr. Barrett is board chairman of Quackwatch, Inc., and a board member of the National Council Against Health Fraud. His best-known book is The Vitamin Pushers: How the "Health Food" Industry Is Selling America a Bill of Goods (Prometheus, 1994).*

# The Unethical Behavior of Pharmacists

## *How to market dubious supplements and unproven remedies*

### by Stephen Barrett, MD

Most pharmacists who work in retail pharmacies have a serious potential conflict of interest. On the one hand, they are professionals, expected to be knowledgeable about drugs and to dispense them in a responsible and ethical manner. On the other hand, their income depends on the sale of products. Before the FDA's OTC (Over-the-Counter) Drug Review drove most of the ineffective ingredients out of OTC drug products, few pharmacists protested or attempted to protect their customers from wasting money on products that were ineffective, unnecessary, or irrationally formulated.

During the mid-1980s, two dietitians examined the labels of vitamin products at five pharmacies, three groceries, and three health-food stores in New Haven, CT. Products were considered appropriate if they contained between 50% and 200% of the U.S. RDAs and no more than 100% of others for which Estimated Safe and Adequate Daily Dietary Intakes exist. Only 16 out of 105 (15%) of the multivitamin/mineral products met these criteria (*Journal of the American Dietetic Association* 7:341–343, 1987).

Today the situation appears worse. Although OTC drugs are generally effective, nearly all pharmacies still carry irrational supplements, and many stock dubious herbal and homeopathic products as well. Chain drugstores are more likely to do so than individually owned stores.

> *Nearly all pharmacies still carry irrational supplements, and many stock dubious herbal and homeopathic products as well.*

## Marketing Ploys

Pharmacy schools appear to teach the facts needed to advise people that "nutrition insurance" is rarely needed, that "stress" supplements are a scam, and that doses above the RDAs are seldom appropriate. Yet pharmacists throughout America seem content to sell supplements to people who don't need them. Their professional journals rarely contain articles criticizing the fraud involved, and their trade publications talk mainly about vitamin promotion. In fact, most pharmacy trade publications carry articles urging pharmacists to compete with health-food retailers by using similar propaganda techniques!

Many pharmacies display posters or flyers telling what vitamins do in the body. Some also list the problems that occur with nutrient deficiencies. These items are obviously intended to promote sales by inducing customers to think that (a) if a little is good, more is better, and/or (b) if they have any of the symptoms listed, a vitamin might be the answer to their problem.

Many vitamin promoters suggest that being busy, skipping meals, or "eating on the run" places people at risk for dietary deficiency. According to this notion, busy people don't take the time to consume nourishing food. These claims are misleading because preparing or eating a balanced diet takes no more time than preparing or eating an unbalanced diet.

Major vitamin manufacturers and trade associations play a significant role in spreading misinformation. During the early 1980s, for example, Hoffman-La Roche advertised that "busy" people should take supplements. An article in a pharmacy trade publication later revealed that these ads were intended to influence pharmacists (who advise many customers) as well as the general public. During the same period, until stopped by the New York State Attorney General, Lederle Laboratories marketed Stresstabs with misleading claims that "stress robs the body of nutrients."

In 1989, the Council for Responsible Nutrition (CRN), a nutritional supplement industry association that mainly represents

From *Nutrition Forum*, January/February 1998, pp. 1-2, 4. © 1998 by Prometheus Books, 59 John Glenn Drive, Amherst, NY 14228. Reprinted by permission of the publisher.

large manufacturers, began advertising that virtually everyone has a "vitamin gap." During the mid-1980s, market research had found that most Americans felt they were getting adequate nutrition from their diet. CRN's "Vitamin Gap" campaign was designed to convince people that supplements were still needed. First it falsely suggested that vitamins could help against stress. Then it falsely suggested that most Americans were not getting enough in their diet.

Lederle used the "vitamin gap" theme in a Centrum ad in the June 1997 *Journal of the American Dietetic Association.* Centrum is a sensibly formulated multivitamin/multimineral product that costs about 10¢ per day. However, the ad suggested that the majority of Americans are not getting the nutrients they need in their diet and should use Centrum to bridge the alleged "gaps." According to the ad: "Statistics show that 9 out of 10 Americans don't get all the nutrients they need from what they eat, and, in fact, are missing out on important vitamins and minerals."

This statement was based on an analysis of data collected between 1976 and 1980 from the Second National Health and Nu-

❧

*If asked directly for advice, most pharmacists will answer to the best of their ability. However, many are poorly informed.*

trition Examination Survey. The survey found that only 9% of the participants remembered consuming the recommended five portions of fruits and vegetables on the day covered by the survey (*American Journal of Public Health* 80:1443–1449, 1990). This does not mean that people who reported less were deficient in vitamins or minerals. Dietary surveys that measure nutrient intake for a single day or even a few days are not suitable for determining the overall quality of an individual's diet. Ade-

quate nutrient intake can be achieved with fewer than the "recommended" number of portions of fruits and vegetables. Furthermore, Americans are eating more fruits and vegetables than they did 20 years ago. CRN used the same faulty reasoning to justify its original campaign.

CRN has produced two brochures that the National Association of Chain Drug Stores distributed to retail pharmacies. One contains a chart of "the health benefits of vitamins and minerals" and subtly suggests that many people don't get enough. Both refer to research developments and speculations that higher-than-RDA levels of various nutrients might help prevent disease. Both state that "appropriate use of nutritional supplements should be part of a healthy lifestyle," but neither provides the information an individual would need to judge whether supplementation makes sense. Both are posted to CRN's Web site (**http://www.crnusa.org/Consumer.htm**).

## Investigative Reports

If asked directly for advice, most pharmacists will answer to the best of their ability. However, many are poorly informed.

---

# Making Up for Lost Revenues

Pharmacy trade publications, such as *Natural Pharmacist,* suggest that "natural products" offer opportunities to make up for prescription drug revenues lost as a result of managed care and other cost-containment programs. One pharmacy supplier aligned with this trend is The JAG Group of San Clemente, California. According to its Web site (**http://www.jagenterprises.com/servmain.htm**), "natural products offer profit margins greater than those for prescription drugs." JAG's comprehensive program features:

- Product lines that typically produce a 100% markup or more.
- A three-day seminar covering "the importance of wellness" and how to "use natural products to prevent and/or improve chronic disease states."
- WellStore Software designed as a sales and marketing tool to: (1) capture customer information, including e-mail address, (2) categorize products to market directly to customer needs, (3) provide thank-you notes to encourage loyalty, (4) provide product information to print for customers, and (5) track patient-health histories to create fee-for-service revenue.
- Pharmacist Plus™ Software with causes, signs, and symptoms of 223 common ailments and specific dietary, homeopathic, and herbal recommendations. (I believe that providing such information to customers would be outside the scope of pharmacy practice and would constitute the illegal practice of medicine and would violate state laws against theft by deception. Furthermore, homeopathic products have no proven effectiveness.)

- Drug Depletion Software telling "what supplements patients need to replace vital nutrients that are depleted by many of the prescription drugs they are taking." (I do not believe there are many situations in which this is important.)
- Nutritional Analysis Software (an electronic nutritionist) to allow the pharmacist to charge a fee for providing consultations to patients—including assessment of "nutritional needs that best fit your patient's gender, age, lifestyle, analysis of food intake and identification of nutritional deficiencies" and "recommendations for optimum nutrient levels to maintain good health." (I do not believe any software can do this.)
- A TV commercial, radio spots, newspaper and yellow page ads, doctor letters, and a column that can be published under the pharmacist's own name.
- A personalized Internet Web page, which adds the pharmacist to a list of "complementary and natural healthcare practitioners worldwide" so that "when someone searches for a natural healthcare practitioner, they will find you." (I do not believe that pharmacists are qualified or legally permitted to be "natural healthcare practitioners.")
- An in-store display unit designed to let customers see a variety of products, books, and services in one place.
- Answers to questions needed "when a customer is standing in front of you" or when "you want to know about a new fad or product your customer just asked you about."
- "The best experts in the fields of pharmacy, natural products, and complementary medicine available" by picking up the phone or accessing the Internet.—**SB**

In 1985, reporters from *Consumer Reports* magazine visited 30 drugstores in Pennsylvania, Missouri, and California. The reporters complained of feeling tired or nervous, and asked whether a vitamin product might help. Seventeen were sold a vitamin product, and one was sold an amino acid preparation. Only 9 of the 30 pharmacists suggested that a doctor be consulted (*Consumer Reports* 51:170–175, 1986).

In 1987, two pharmacy school professors sent a questionnaire to 1000 pharmacists in the Detroit metropolitan area and received 197 responses. Among the 116 who identified their five most-common reasons for recommending vitamins or minerals, 66 (56%) listed fatigue and 57 (49%) listed stress (*Journal of Clinical Pharmacy and Therapeutics* 15:141–146, 1990). Neither reason is valid. In response to a question about homeopathy, 27.4% said it was "useful," 18.3% judged it "useless," and 54.3% "didn't know" (*Journal of Clinical Pharmacy and Therapeutics* 15:131–139, 1990).

## What Happened to Ethics?

Merlin Nelson, MD, Pharm.D., coauthor of the above-mentioned survey, has asked pharmacists why they promote and sell food supplements to healthy individuals who don't need them. He concluded: "The most common reason is greed. Advertising creates a demand that the pharmacist can supply and make a profit. 'If I don't sell them, they'll just go to my competition down the street,' is a common response. Pharmacists are apparently more interested in a sale than in the patient's welfare. . . .

"Rather than just recommending a multivitamin to patients concerned about obtaining enough vitamins in their diet, pharmacists should offer sound nutritional advice or provide referrals to experts in nutrition such as registered dietitians" (*American Pharmacy* NS28(10) 34–36, 1988).

Pharmacists are also the only recognized health professionals who sell tobacco products, which cause more death and years of lost life than any other consumer product. Although some pharmacists have stopped, the majority do not consider tobacco sales unethical. Nelson is one of only a handful of pharmacists who have criticized the misleading promotions of supplement manufacturers. As far as I can tell, no professional pharmacy organization has ever done so.

The American Pharmaceutical Association's code of ethics does not state that pharmacists have a duty to prevent dubious products from lining their shelves. Five states have laws declaring it illegal for pharmacists to sell ineffective products, but these laws have never been applied to the sale of OTC products.

I believe that pharmacists have as much of an ethical duty to discourage use of inappropriate products as physicians do to advise against unnecessary surgery or medical care. Very few pharmacists do so. Pharmacy journal editors ignore this problem. Hospital-based pharmacists generally exhibit a higher standard of practice, but very few of them are speaking out about the problems described in this article.

---

*Stephen Barrett, MD, is a retired psychiatrist who resides in Allentown, Pennsylvania. His 44 books include* The Vitamin Pushers: How the "Health Food" Industry Is Selling America a Bill of Goods.

## Unit Selections

## Key Points to Consider

❖ Should more be done about hunger in the United States? Whose responsibility is it, that of the government or of the private sector? How could you help?

❖ What should be the roles of the United States and other developed countries in solving world hunger? To what extent should countries be expected to solve their own problems?

❖ What criteria would you use to decide when to help another country and how much?

❖ How well has the Food and Agriculture Organization (FAO) addressed concerns about hunger and malnutrition in its World Food Summit? What else would you have included or expressed differently? Why?

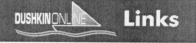 **Links** **www.dushkin.com/online/**

32. **Population Reference Bureau**
    *http://www.prb.org*
33. **World Health Organization**
    *http://www.who.ch/Welcome.html*
34. **World Hunger Year**
    *http://www.iglou.com/why/ria.htm*
35. **WWW Virtual Library: Demography & Population Studies**
    *http://coombs.anu.edu.au/ResFacilities/DemographyPage.html*

These sites are annotated on pages 4 and 5.

*If you give me a fish, I will eat for a day.
And you will have my thanks, and I'll be on my
way. If you teach me to fish, you'll bring me
dignity, For I can feed myself, through all eternity.*
*—Don Ferrens, 1990*

The World Food Summit met in Rome in November of
1996 and was attended by officials from nearly 200
nations. They declared that all people have the right to
be free from hunger through access to safe, nutritious,
and culturally acceptable food. In making this declaration, officials pledged to work together to provide a
political environment within which they could implement
economic and social policies capable of delivering this
promise. Permeating the discussions was an emphasis
on changing world trade policies as the key to
improving food access. They did not sign a binding
agreement.

There was, moreover, disagreement with the
conclusions of the World Food Summit. Meeting nearby
were those who represented a variety of secular and
religious organizations that work directly with people.
They claimed that food security is not a supply
problem, to be solved by controlling the population
growth of undeveloped countries and expanding the
capital-intensive agriculture of the industrialized world,
as the Summit had declared. Rather, they contended,
food security is a demand problem, to be solved by
distributing food more fairly, reducing overconsumption
by affluent nations, and improving sustainable
smallholder agriculture.

Nor is there agreement over the extent of global
hunger. Agencies such as the Food and Agriculture
Organization (FAO) of the United Nations report that
14 percent of the world's population, or 800 million
people, do not have enough food to meet basic needs.
UNICEF (United Nations International Children's Emergency Fund) says that among the malnourished are half
of all children younger than 5 years in South Asia and
one-third of those in sub-Saharan Africa. Yet others
argue that the data upon which these conclusions have
been reached are both flawed and inadequate, that we
simply don't know what the nutritional needs of people
are, and that we don't have adequate information
about their health status to make judgments.

There is little disagreement, however, over the costs
of hunger and malnutrition. A 1998 fact sheet from
the UNICEF states that "Malnutrition contributes to over
6 million child deaths each year, 55% of the nearly
12 million deaths among children under 5 in developing countries." Malnourished children live out their
lives with disabilities and weakened immune systems.
As adults they are more subject to heart disease,
diabetes, and hypertension. Their motivation and
curiosity are dulled, reducing the exploratory activities
that result in normal mental and cognitive development.
In turn, this robs their countries of innovative and
rational leadership and undermines the world struggle
for peace and equality.

The first article in this unit, "Winning the Food
Race," will address aspects of food security. When
population growth exceeds current food production
and/or food distribution, some people inevitably will
get food of insufficient quantity or quality. Somehow
agricultural practices that can be sustained locally over
time must be implemented in order to achieve a constant food supply. This article lists the pledges made by
the FAO in Rome to reduce hunger and malnutrition

and, in very broad terms, a plan of action to accomplish these objectives.

Hunger and malnutrition result from too few calories
or low intakes of nutrients. The lack of a single nutrient
can result in an obvious deficiency such as goiter or
rickets. Mild to moderate deficiencies that are hardly
observable but that significantly impair health are just as
likely. The causes are complex. Malnutrition and hunger
are a result of disease, unsafe water, and poor
sanitation. They follow war and environmental disasters.
They are a consequence of discrimination against
women, who often lack access to education and good
information and have difficulty finding gainful employment. They result from too little purchasing power and
poor distribution of the food that is available. And they
are found in all corners of the world.

But hunger is more than a physical phenomenon.
Two articles about famine in the Sudan and the effects
of hunger on children describe the physical and
emotional impact of hunger where it happens. Hunger
respects no geographical boundaries, and although it is
most common in Africa, it is known on every continent
and in every country. Famines have been frequent
throughout history, and they bring an acute focus to
hunger. Between 1845–1850, the Irish potato famine
resulted in thousands of deaths and huge numbers of
immigrants to the United States. Millions of Ethiopians
and citizens of other parts of Africa have died during
recent years. China has faced periodic famines throughout the nineteenth and twentieth centuries. India now
claims to be self-sufficient in food production, but it has
not solved the problem of chronic hunger.

In spite of decidedly greater wealth, hunger is also
visible in developed countries. Among the poor in the
United Kingdom, increased risks of premature births,
obesity, and hypertension can be documented. Stunting
among young children in the Russian Federation
increased from 9 to 15 percent in a recent two-year
period. Even in the United States, an estimated 13
million children under age 12 get insufficient food.
Experts say that U.S. hunger differs from hunger in
developing countries in that its cause is poverty uncomp-
licated by natural disasters, war, or an undeveloped
economy. More Americans go to bed hungry now than
in the mid-1980s, and millions in our country are said
to have food insecurity.

Food programs that are intended to supplement the
family's food budget sometimes become the primary
source of food. WIC (an aid program for women,
infants, and children) in particular has been documented to be extremely cost-effective, saving 3 dollars
in potential medical costs for every dollar spent,
according to the General Accounting Office. But even
Federal Food Assistance Programs such as WIC and
food stamps do not reach all of the needy. Since
1980, private sector emergency feeding programs such
as soup kitchens, food pantries, and homeless shelters
have multiplied all over the country. Many of them
report turning people away or closing temporarily due
to increased demand and dwindling resources.

It would be unfair to leave the impression that no
global progress is evident. Bolivia is the first country to
declare that iodized salt has virtually eliminated iodine
deficiency as a public health problem. Fortification
programs elsewhere are saving hundreds of thousands of
children from deficiencies. Community volunteer programs
in a number of countries are monitoring growth rates,
promoting breast feeding, and reducing malnutrition.

# *Winning the Food Race*

**In many developing countries rapid population growth makes it difficult for food production to keep up with demand. Helping couples prevent unintended pregnancies by providing family planning would slow the growth in demand for food. This would buy time to increase food supplies and improve food production technologies while conserving natural resources.**

While the global economy produces enough food to feed the world's 6 billion people—if food could be better distributed—many people lack access to enough food for a healthy life. In particular, the UN Food and Agriculture Organization (FAO) has identified 82 poor countries that are at particular risk. These countries face rapid population growth, do not produce enough food domestically, confront serious constraints to producing more food, and cannot import enough to make up the deficit.

## Hunger Widespread

In poor countries, especially where population is growing rapidly, hunger and malnutrition are often critical problems. An estimated two billion people suffer from malnutrition and dietary deficiencies. More than 840 million people—disproportionately women and girl children— suffer chronic malnourishment. Each year about 18 million people, mostly children, die from starvation, malnutrition, and related causes.

The World Food Summit in 1996 focused international attention on the concept of *food security*—access by all people to "safe and nutritious food to maintain a healthy and active life," according to FAO. Worrisome trends in agricultural production and current international trade policies raise questions about whether food production and distribution can improve fast enough to overtake population growth and reach the goal of food security.

## Discouraging New Trends

From the 1960s until a few years ago, world food supply kept pace with population growth. New agricultural technologies, better seed varieties, and irrigation—the Green Revolution—expanded the food supply. At the same time, in many developing countries contraceptive use has risen substantially, and fertility has fallen rapidly, amounting to a reproductive revolution. Between 1985 and 1995, however, in 64 of 105 countries studied by FAO, food pro-

duction lagged behind population growth. Africa now produces nearly 30% less food per person than in 1967. Moreover, trying to meet the rising demand for food is leading people to overuse the world's finite resource base. Most developing countries already are cultivating virtually all arable land. In some areas fertile soils are being exploited faster than they can regenerate. Fresh water supplies are becoming degraded or exhausted. Yields from capture fisheries have fallen. Such trends make it increasingly difficult to meet the world's food needs.

## Steps to Food Security

Winning the food race requires a coordinated approach to increase agricultural production, improve food distribution, manage resources, and provide family planning. Also providing education and health care is essential to improve people's well-being and thus promote productivity and sustainable resource use. Along with better food distribution, achieving food security requires addressing the needs of small farmers and raising agricultural productivity while preserving soil and water resources.

The ultimate outcome of the race to achieve food security is likely to depend on answers to the following questions:

- Will a new Green Revolution dramatically increase crop yields and keep up with growth in demand?

- Will resource degradation, waste, and pollution be reduced, and by how much?

- How soon will the reproductive revolution lead to replacement-level fertility worldwide?

Recent fertility declines have raised the hope that world population can stabilize some time in the next century. The sooner the world reaches replacement-level fertility of about two children per couple, the sooner world attention could shift away from the need to increase food production continually and toward improving the quality of life for all.

From *Population Reports*, Series M, No. 13, December 1997, pp. 3-7. © 1997 by Johns Hopkins University School of Public Health, Population Information Program, Baltimore. Reprinted by permission.

# *Population Growth And Food Needs*

In many developing countries rapid population growth makes it difficult for agricultural production to keep pace with the rising demand for food. Most developing countries already are cultivating virtually all arable land and are bringing ever more marginal land under cultivation.

"Unfortunately, population growth continues to outstrip food availability in many countries," reported Jacques Diouf, director-general of the United Nations Food and Agriculture Organization (FAO), at the 1996 World Food Summit in Rome (99). For example, between 1985 and 1995, food production lagged behind population growth in 64 of 105 developing countries studied by FAO (114). Among regions, Africa fared the worst. Food production per person fell in 31 of 46 African countries (114, 119).

Concerns about lagging agricultural production and rapid population growth, as well as inadequate food distribution systems, have focused international attention on the concept of *food security* (43, 97, 99). FAO defines food security as a "state of affairs where all people at all times have access to safe and nutritious food to maintain a healthy and active life" (99). By this definition about two billion people—one person in every three—lack food security. Either they cannot grow enough food themselves, or they cannot afford to purchase enough in the domestic marketplace. As a result, they suffer from micronutrient and protein energy deficiencies in their diets (98, 132, 133).

Although the global economy probably produces enough food to feed the nearly 6 billion people in the world and even more, if it were distributed equitably, this food is not readily available to many millions of people. Natural resources, population, and agricultural production technologies are distributed unevenly around the world. Some countries produce more food than they need for domestic use, while others do not produce enough to assure access to adequate diets for all of their people (69). Thus better distribution of food is an essential component of any world strategy to improve food security (109) (see p. 204).

While the way most people live and work has little impact on food distribution policies, people in their everyday lives do make a great difference in the demand for and supply of food, both as consumers and producers. While changes in food distribution policies are decided in national capitals and at international negotiations, communities and individuals can do much themselves to influence the demand for and supply of food. Therefore programs and policies that enable people to improve agricultural productivity, manage natural resources, and plan their families are essential to improving food security.

■

## Population: The Demand Side

Population growth, along with changes in people's living standards and dietary preferences, largely determine changes in the demand for food (3, 69, 99). Throughout history societies have raced to keep the food supply equal to or ahead of population growth. The race has not always been won, as the history of widespread malnutrition and famines attests (69).

Currently, world population is growing by over 80 million people a year—that is, by one billion people every 12 to 13 years (121). Such change is unprecedented. It was not until about 1800 that the world's total population reached 1 billion. It took approximately another century to reach 2 billion. In the past 50 years more people have been added to the world's population than during the previous 4 million years.

The world's population is expected to reach 6 billion in 1999 (36). According to UN projections, by 2025 the world would contain over 8 billion people, of whom some 6.8 billion would live in developing countries (120, 121).

Since the 1960s the rate of population growth has slowed. In what demographers have termed a reproductive revolution, fertility in developing countries has declined as contraceptive use has risen. Family planning programs have helped millions of couples avoid unintended pregnancies and thus have contributed importantly to reducing fertility rates (30, 74, 80). Because of family planning programs in the past, the world now contains 400 million fewer people than it would otherwise (7).

World population is growing by 1.5% per year today compared with 2% per year in the 1960s. In some developing countries, however, primarily in sub-Saharan Africa, population is still growing at 2% to 3.5% per year, rates at which populations would double in 20 to 35 years (72, 120, 121). Even growth rates of 2% or less create a powerful momentum for future population increase, particularly as they are applied to ever larger numbers of people.

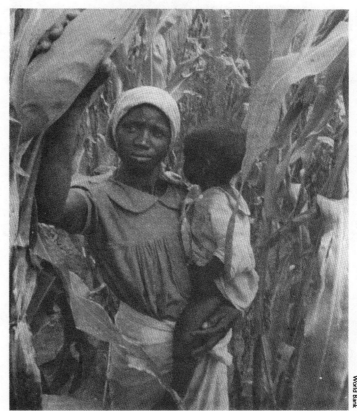

*In Malawi a farmer examines her corn ready for harvest. Throughout history societies have raced to keep the food supply equal to or ahead of population growth. The race has not always been won.*

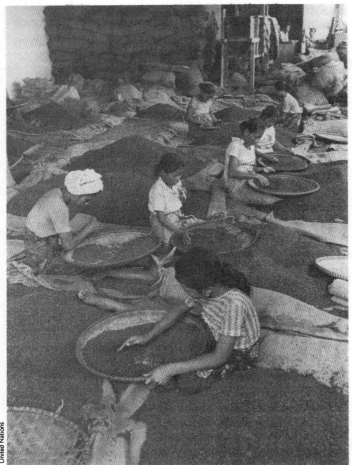

*Many developing countries export one or two basic raw materials such as rubber or cacao, making them vulnerable to price changes. These women are cleaning peppercorns in a factory in Indonesia.*

**Changing diets.** As living standards have risen in many parts of the world, more people have chosen to eat meat and dairy products regularly rather than to continue living almost entirely on grains such as rice, corn (maize), and wheat. As people consume meat and dairy products instead of consuming grain directly, more grain must be produced to maintain the same caloric value. When used to feed livestock, grain provides humans less than half as much food energy as when consumed by people directly (11, 31).

Reflecting changing diets as well as population increases, the world's consumption of meat has nearly quadrupled in the second half of this century—from an estimated 44 million metric tons in 1950 to about 200 million metric tons in 1995. Today nearly 40% of the world's grain production goes to feed livestock (11, 12). This trend makes it more difficult to feed the world's poor, who often cannot afford to eat meat at all.

■

## Food Production: The Supply Side

For most of the past 50 years food production has outpaced rising demand. World population has doubled since World War II, but food production has tripled (22, 47, 83). In the developing world the daily calories available per person increased from an average of 1,925 calories in 1961 to 2,540 in 1992 (128). World food production has expanded since the early 1960s due mainly to the Green Revolution—adoption of crop rotation, the production and use of petroleum-based fertilizers and chemical pesticides, expanded irrigation, and the introduction of genetically superior, disease-resistant cultivars (cultivated crops) (83, 94, 98, 99, 130).

The trend may now be changing for the worse, however. Since about 1990 global grain production has risen only slightly and, despite slower rates of population growth, grain supplies per capita have fallen. In the worst case, Africa now produces nearly 30% *less* food per person than it did in 1967 (54, 117). The reasons for the change in the trend include not only rapid population growth on the demand side, but also higher population densities in traditional agricultural areas, fragmentation of small farmsteads, poor land management, and inappropriate agricultural and economic policies, all of which suppress supply (47, 117).

With one-third of world population lacking food security now, FAO estimates that world food production would have to double to provide food security for the 8 billion people projected for 2025 (98, 99). By 2050, when world population is projected to be over 9 billion, the situation would be even more challenging. At current levels of consumption, without allowing for additional imports of food, Africa would have to increase food production by 300% to provide minimally adequate diets for the 2 billion people projected in 2050; Latin America would have to increase food production by 80% to feed a projected 810 million people; and Asia's food production would have to grow by 70% to feed the 5.4 billion people projected. Even North America would have to increase food production by 30% to feed a projected 384 million people in 2050 (36, 85).

Rapid population growth not only pushes up demand for food but may also be starting to diminish supply as well (8, 33, 35, 99). As people try to obtain higher yields from heavily used natural resources, soil loss worsens, fresh water becomes scarcer, and pollution increases. As a result the developing world's capacity to expand food production may well be shrinking, not expanding (8, 22, 53, 65, 97, 100).

■

## Food Distribution

Food security could be improved for millions of people if food from countries with a surplus were better distributed to countries where there are food deficits—that is, countries that do not produce enough food to meet domestic needs (59, 98, 99, 117). The international trade system, however, works against the ability of poor countries to meet their food needs with imports.

Most rich countries produce enough food for themselves and for export as well. Affluent manufacturing countries that are not self-sufficient in food production can afford to import as much food as they need, and more. Also, developed countries protect their agricultural sectors with various economic incentives and trade barriers—including price supports for key commodities, such as wheat and corn, and tariffs to shield domestic growers from cheaper imports.

In contrast, the poorest countries, particularly those with food deficits, usually export only one or two raw commodities, such as rubber or cacao. When prices of export commodities decline on the world market, or when prices of vital imported supplies rise, they are hit hard (54). During the

1980s raw commodities exported by developing countries lost 40% of their value in relation to the manufactured goods that these countries imported (98). Between 1982 and 1992 the real value of cacao fell by 60%, cotton by 40%, and natural rubber by 45% (54). In 1991—just one year—Africa lost an estimated US$5.6 billion because of declines in commodity prices (50). Recently, however, some raw commodity prices have risen, providing relief to developing-country trade balances (83).

Declining commodity prices usually are good for consumers in wealthy countries, but in poor countries small-scale farmers suffer (108). In the 1970s and 1980s, for example, while real farm incomes increased substantially in most developed countries, real income from agriculture dropped for the average farmer in the developing world (98). To maintain their purchasing power, these poor farmers often try to bring more marginal land into production, even though this land yields less per hectare. Farmers may be pushed off their land altogether to make room for export-driven agriculture, as governments try to make up the shortfall in international trade revenues (50, 82).

National governments and international organizations can help to improve food distribution systems and can adopt new policies that make food more available and affordable. Over the long run, FAO argues, increased regional trade and cooperation are important to raising living standards in poor countries (99) and to providing more affordable food. In addition, better world markets for developing-country agricultural produce could help provide more jobs in these nations, raise incomes, reduce hunger, and minimize pressures from subsistence farming on the resource base (83).

At the same time, however, FAO contends that international trade alone "cannot solve the problems of poverty and access [to food] which are the keys to food security" (99). Given current population growth trends and land degradation patterns, FAO has warned that "future nutritional requirements challenge...both food production and environmental capabilities" (100).

■

## Conflicting Predictions

For the past two decades food prices generally have fallen. Between 1981 and 1990, for example, the price of staple foods fell by close to 40% on world markets (83). Because this figure is an average, however, it masks price increases that have occurred in a number of developing countries in recent years.

In 1995 world grain prices soared by roughly half as world grain reserves fell to just 231 million metric tons, only enough to meet needs for 48 days and well below the minimum food cushion of 60 days advised by FAO (51). The shortfall in grain production and the rise in prices appear to have been temporary, largely the result of three years of poor harvests, stockpiling, a shift to production of other crops as price subsidies were cut in Europe and North America, and substantial declines in food production in the former Soviet Union (20, 137).

Expert opinion is divided on the long-term outlook for food prices, reflecting differences of opinion about production capacities and environmental limits. FAO, the World Bank, and the International Food Policy Research Institute expect food prices to decline, following the basic trend of the past two decades (47, 83, 137). According to the Worldwatch Institute, however, food prices could rise over the next two decades in response to falling production per capita and rapid growth in food demand in developing countries (10).

The Japanese Ministry of Agriculture has forecast a doubling of world grain prices by 2010 and more than doubling of prices for wheat and rice (using 1992 as the base year). Unlike other forecasts, this one takes into account such factors as decreasing availability of arable land and fresh water and the mounting environmental costs of using more and more fertilizers and pesticides (10, 52). Soil erosion and degradation already have reduced agricultural productivity on about one-third of the world's cropland (98).

■

## Carrying Capacity

Logically, population growth must stop at some point, or the earth would become overcrowded and its resources eventually would be depleted. The term "carrying capacity" refers to the number of people that the earth can support on a sustained basis—that is, support indefinitely at a constant standard of living without destroying the natural resource base. There is no way to predict how large the population could become, however, before it overwhelmed the planet. Nor is there any way to predict the quality of life in the future under the almost infinite variety of scenarios for population growth, consumption patterns, food production, technological change, natural resource use, air and water pollution, land degradation, and many other factors (15, 33, 42).

The question of carrying capacity has been debated for 200 years, since 1798, when the English economist Thomas Malthus published his *Essay on the Principle of Population as It Affects the Future Improvement of Society*. Malthus reasoned that, since productive land and potable water are finite resources, population growth inevitably would outstrip the food and water supply at some point. Mass starvation and anarchy would follow (57).

The Middle Ages in Europe provided many tragic examples for Malthus. Europe's population had risen from about 36 million in the year 1000 to 80 million in 1300, while new technology, or innovations of any kind, were unknown. By 1300 good farmland was virtually exhausted. As more people tried to live from the same amount of cropland, food prices rose beyond the reach of the poor (that is, beyond the reach of nearly everyone except the clergy and nobility). Devastating famines ravaged the land in 1316 and 1317. Then in 1346 the Black Plague struck. By the end of the century it had killed one-third of the entire population of Europe (69).

Malthus failed to anticipate the subsequent leaps in agricultural technology and economies of scale that have enabled world population to rise to nearly six billion. Today, however, scientists warn that the planet may be increasingly at risk in the future. As biologists Peter Vitousek and colleagues argue, at current levels of population and technology, human activities cause "rapid, novel, and substantial changes" to the earth's ecosystems. These include degrading soil and water supplies; altering nature's cycles, largely by releasing enormous amounts of carbon dioxide into the atmosphere; and destroying or altering biological resources, even driving some plant and animal species into extinction. Reducing the pace of human impact on the earth's natural systems might

# Figure 1. Chronic Undernutrition

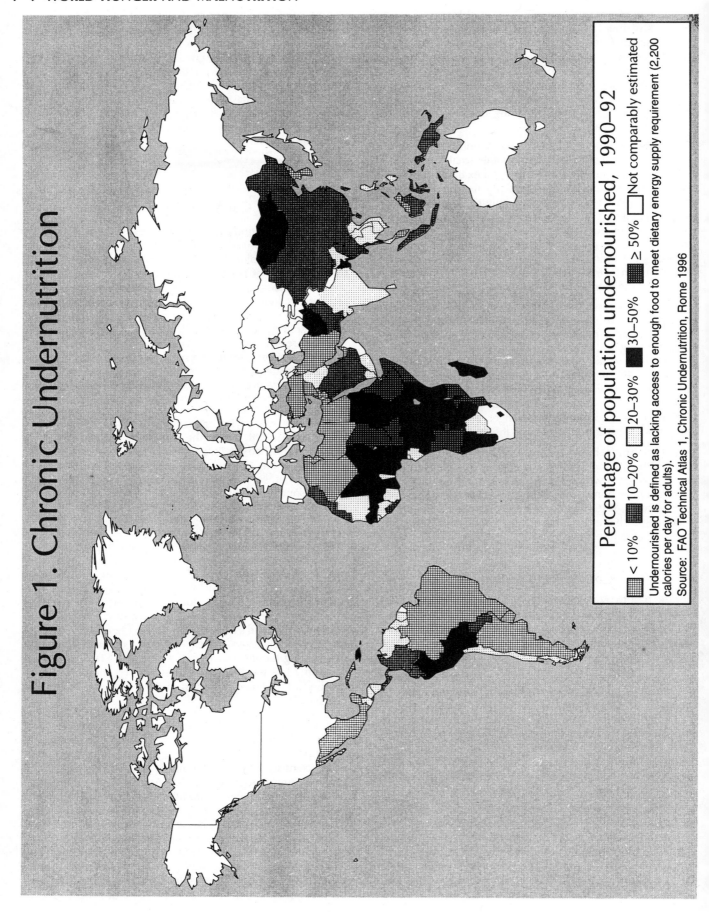

Percentage of population undernourished, 1990–92

☐ < 10%   ▨ 10–20%   ☐ 20–30%   ■ 30–50%   ▦ ≥ 50%   ☐ Not comparably estimated

Undernourished is defined as lacking access to enough food to meet dietary energy supply requirement (2,200 calories per day for adults).

Source:   FAO Technical Atlas 1, Chronic Undernutrition, Rome 1996

give natural systems more time to adjust. The two basic ways of slowing the growth in human effects on the Earth, they advise, are to slow population growth and to use resources more efficiently (124).

While no one can accurately predict the distant future, the final outcome of the race between population growth and food supply is likely to hinge on the answers to several questions:

- Will a new Green Revolution dramatically increase crop yields and keep up with growth in demand (65, 66, 84)?
- How soon will the reproductive revolution lead to replacement-level fertility worldwide (2, 33, 35, 80, 113)?
- Will resource degradation, waste, and environmental pollution be reduced, and by how much (19, 25, 73)?
- Can poor countries help small-scale and subsistence farmers (including women) become more productive and better off without overexploiting nonrenewable natural resources (99, 131)?
- Will international trade policies be reformed to improve the flow of food across national borders?

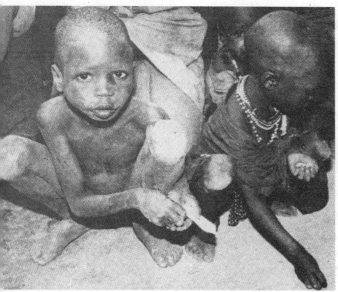

...many parts of sub-Saharan Africa, people often go without enough ...od. Worldwide, each year about 18 million people, most of them ...ildren, die from starvation, malnutrition, and related causes.

# Steps Toward Food Security

The World Food Summit in 1996 focused new attention on achieving food security (see "Excerpts from the World Food Summit"). What can countries and communities do to help reach food security?

Achieving food security over the long term depends partly on slowing population growth (6, 97, 110). Providing family planning to all couples who want it would go far to reducing fertility rates and slowing population growth in many developing countries (79, 125). An estimated 100 million married women, and probably millions of other women, are interested in avoiding pregnancy but are not currently using contraception (79).

At the same time, a second Green Revolution could increase yields and buy more time for world population eventually to stabilize. In this revolution practicing sustainable agriculture—that is, protecting natural resources from becoming increasingly degraded and polluted—will be essential. Also, developing countries can explore new ways to help meet their food needs. These include improving yields on marginal land, farming forests, expanding aquaculture, rediscovering forgotten foods, and encouraging urban agriculture.

■

## A Sustained Reproductive Revolution?

What are the prospects for slowing population growth through a sustained reproductive revolution in developing countries? The world's population has become so large that even small *rates* of growth still mean rapid increases in *absolute numbers* of people—a more relevant measure of food demand than growth rates (74). For example, the population of India, estimated at 970 million in mid-1997, is growing at an annual pace of 1.9%. At this rate India's population has a net gain of 18 million people each year (118). If the 1.9% rate were to continue, India's population would double in 36 years, reaching 1.9 billion in 2033. Also, following three decades of an intense government effort to limit the number of children per family, China has a population growth rate of 1.1% per year. Even at this rate, there are another 12 to 13 million mouths to feed in China each year (12).

At current fertility rates in most developing countries, women give birth to an average of more than three children over their lifetimes. In some countries women average five or six children, or even seven children in a few countries. These numbers, of course, far exceed "replacement-level" fertility of about two children per woman—the fertility rate at which population growth would level off and population size would eventually stabilize. Even if the next generation has fewer children than the previous one, the population will grow as long as couples average more than two children each.

Because of high fertility in the past, most developing country populations are young. In the developing world as a whole, half of the population is under age 23 (122). In sub-Saharan Africa children under age 15 comprise almost 40% of the population (2). As young people reach childbearing age themselves, most will have several children of their own. Even after fertility falls to replacement level, it takes at least another generation or two for population size to stabilize. Also, it takes at least 15 years for the smaller size of age groups to have an appreciable effect on food demand and resource needs (33).

Time is of the essence. Each 20-year delay in reaching replacement-level fertility of about two children per woman would add at least 1 billion people to the world's eventual stable population size (33). If replacement-level fertility were reached worldwide by the end of this decade—which is virtually impossible—world population would eventually level off at less than 9 billion. If, at the other extreme, replacement level were not reached until the year 2080—which might be the case if family planning programs did not expand to meet the needs of larger populations and the rising interest in contraception—the world's ultimate population size would be at least 14 billion (33, 36). The actual date—and thus the ultimate world population size—is likely to be somewhere in between.

# Excerpts from the World Food Summit

Source: United Nations Food and Agriculture Organization 1996 (109)

## Declaration

We, the Heads of State and Government, or our representatives, gathered at the World Food Summit at the invitation of the Food and Agriculture Organization of the United Nations, reaffirm the right of everyone to have access to safe and nutritious food....

We consider it intolerable that more than 800 million people throughout the world, and particularly in developing countries, do not have enough food to meet their basic nutritional needs. This situation is unacceptable. Food supplies have increased substantially, but constraints on access to food and continuing inadequacy of household and national incomes to purchase food, instability of supply and demand, as well as natural and man-made disasters, prevent basic food needs from being fulfilled.

The problems of hunger and food insecurity have global dimensions and are likely to persist and even increase dramatically in some regions unless urgent, determined, and concerted action is taken, given the anticipated increase in the world's population and the stress on natural resources....

Increased food production, including staple food, must be undertaken. This should happen within the framework of sustainable management of natural resources, elimination of unsustainable patterns of consumption and production, particularly in industrialized countries, and early stabilization of the world population.

We acknowledge the fundamental contribution to food security by women, particularly in rural areas of developing countries, and the need to ensure equality between men and women. Revitalization of rural areas must also be a priority to enhance social stability and help redress the excessive rate of rural-urban migration confronting many countries....

We agree that trade is a key element in achieving food security. We agree to pursue food trade and overall trade policies that will encourage our producers and consumers to utilize available resources in an economically sound and sustainable manner....

Particular attention should be given to those who cannot produce or procure enough food for an adequate diet, including those affected by war, civil strife, natural disasters, or climate-related ecological changes. We are conscious of the need for urgent action to combat pests, drought, and natural resource degradation including desertification, overfishing, and erosion of biological diversity....

We pledge our actions and support to implement the World Food Summit Plan of Action.

—Rome, November 13, 1996

## Plan of Action

1 The Rome Declaration on World Food Security and the World Food Summit Plan of Action lay the foundations for diverse paths to a common objective—food security at the individual, household, national, regional and global levels. ...Coordinated efforts and shared responsibilities are essential....

2 Poverty eradication is essential to improve access to food. The vast majority of those who are undernourished either cannot produce or cannot afford to buy enough food. They have inadequate access to means of production such as land, water, inputs, improved seeds and plants, appropriate technologies, and farm credit....

3 A peaceful and stable environment in every country is a fundamental condition for the attainment of sustainable food security.... Farmers, fishers, and foresters, and other food producers and providers, have critical roles in achieving food security, and their full involvement and enablement are crucial for success.

4 Poverty, hunger and malnutrition are some of the principal causes of accelerated migration from rural to urban areas in developing countries. The largest population shift of all times is now under way. Unless these problems are addressed in an appropriate and timely fashion, the political, economic and social stability of many countries and regions may well be seriously affected, perhaps even compromising world peace....

5 Availability of enough food for all can be attained. The 5.8 billion people in the world today have, on an average, 15% more food per person than the global population of 4 billion people had 20 years ago. Yet, further large increases in world food production, through the sustainable management of natural resources, are required to feed a growing population and achieve improved diets....

6 Harmful seasonal and inter-annual instability of food supplies can be reduced. Progress should include minimizing the vulnerability to and impact of climate fluctuations and pests and diseases....

7 Unless national governments and the international community address the multifaceted causes underlying food insecurity, the number of hungry and malnourished people will remain very high in developing countries, particularly in Africa south of the Sahara; and sustainable food security will not be achieved. This situation is unacceptable. This Plan of Action envisages an ongoing effort to eradicate hunger in all countries, with an immediate view to reducing the number of undernourished people to half their present level no later than 2015, and a mid-term review to ascertain whether it is possible to achieve this target by 2010....

## Commitments: Population and Food

**Commitment One:**
**The Basis for Action**
"A growing world population and the urgency of eradicating hunger and malnutrition call for determined policies and effective actions."

**Commitment One:**
**Objectives and Actions: objective 1.2 (c)**
"Fully integrate population concerns into development strategies, plans, and decision-making, including factors affecting mirgration, and devise appropriate population policies, programmes and family planning services, consistent with the Report and the Programme of Action of the International Conference on Population and Development, Cairo 1994."

**Commitment Two:**
**Objectives and Actions: objective 2.4 (a)**
"Promote access for all people, especially the poor and members of vulnerable and disadvantaged groups to primary health care, including reproductive health services consistent with the Report and the Programme of Action of the International Conference on Population and Development, Cairo 1994."

If fertility were to decline to replacement level by the year 2050, the world population would be about 9.4 billion, according to the UN "medium" projection, the case considered most likely to occur. In this case world population would level off at 11.6 billion around the year 2100 (3, 36). To reach replacement-level fertility by 2050 would require that contraceptive prevalence—the percentage of married women of reproductive age using contraception—rise from the 1990 level of about 50% in developing countries to 73% by 2025, matching current levels in developed countries. The reproductive revolution is most likely to be sustained if commitment to family planning programs in developing countries expands to meet people's increasing interest in having smaller families and the large amount of unmet need for family planning, (78, 79).

## ■
## A Second Green Revolution?

To help bring food security to the 8 billion people projected in 2025, the world needs another Green Revolution (18, 87, 111), as many delegates to the World Food Summit urged (24, 65). The Green Revolution that began in the 1960s has helped keep food supply ahead of rising demand over the past 30 years. By doubling and tripling yields, it bought time for developing countries to start dealing with rapid population growth.

But the Green Revolution represented only a "temporary success," as Norman Borlaug, the Danish-American plant geneticist who was one of its architects, noted upon receiving the 1970 Nobel Peace Prize for his contribution (25). Borlaug pointed out that it is not enough to boost yields on existing cropland; slowing population growth also is crucial.

The first Green Revolution raised the productivity of the three main staple food crops—rice, wheat, and corn (83, 99). Between 1950 and 1990 grain yields increased by nearly two and a half times, from 1.06 metric tons per hectare to 2.52 tons (98). A second revolution also must raise the productivity of other important food crops such as sorghum, millet, and cassava—foods produced and consumed mainly by the world's poor (45, 55, 98, 99).

So far, the outlook for a second Green Revolution is uncertain. Because most increases in food supplies must come from currently cultivated land, raising productivity will require new technologies and better farming practices. Poor people, however, cannot afford the large amounts of fertilizers, pesticides, and other agricultural inputs that increased yields in the first Green Revolution (46). Moreover, the population of developing countries is much larger than it was in the 1960s, the amount of arable land per person is less, and natural resources are more degraded. Nevertheless, three recent developments are promising:

- **Super rice.** The International Rice Research Institute (IRRI) in the Philippines has developed a new strain of super rice capable of boosting yields by 25%, amounting to an extra 100 million metric tons a year—enough to feed an additional 450 million people. This rice does not promise to produce well on marginal land, however, and therefore its use may be limited to well-irrigated bottom land (61, 64, 66).

- **Improved corn.** The International Center for the Improvement of Maize and Wheat in Mexico has engineered several improved varieties of corn that could increase yields by up to 40%. These varieties could be grown on marginal land under difficult growing conditions and thus could be raised by poor farmers. If widely used, the new varieties could feed an additional 50 million people a year (34).

- **A new potato.** The International Potato Centre in Peru claims that, for an investment of US$25 million, it could produce a new potato that would be resistant to a virulent form of potato blight that has reached every continent except Australia (64).

These developments, encouraging as they are, could well be offset, however, if current patterns of soil degradation and damaging agricultural practices continue.

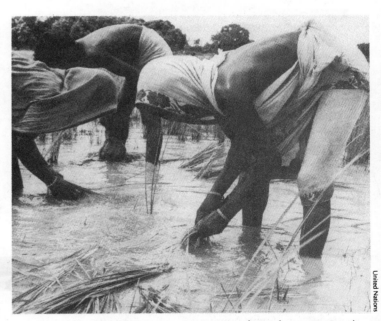

*Workers plant rice cuttings at an experimental rice farm near Bombay, India, in 1962. The Green Revolution that began in the 1960s has helped keep food production ahead of population growth. But it amounts to only a temporary success. Now, a second Green Revolution is needed.*

## ■
## Protecting Natural Resources

In many areas the two natural resources most essential to agricultural production—arable land and fresh water—are becoming degraded and polluted (see pp. 11 and 13). Unless steps are taken soon to reverse this course, the risks of irreversible damage to the resource base will increase.

**Land resources.** Adopting such soil conservation measures as matching crops closely to soil types, using farming methods appropriate to the terrain, enhancing the soil with organic matter, terracing steep hillsides, ringing farm plots with soil-anchoring trees, and managing watersheds better can reduce loss of productive agricultural land due to soil erosion and degradation (98). Farmers also can protect the land by adopting low-till or no-till farming and rotating crops, thus giving soils a chance to recover nutrients.

In many degraded areas land rehabilitation has proved to be so time-consuming, labor-intensive, and expensive that it is virtually impossible. India, for example, has grappled with land degradation in arid and semi-arid regions for decades but with little result (98). Other places, however, have had more success. In 1979, for example, after an extensive land rehabilitation project, China increased food production by some 70% in Mizhi County on the Loess Plateau. The project, carried out in cooperation with the United Nations Development Program, helped farmers turn steep slopes over to permanent vegetation, terrace other slopes, and control gully erosion by erecting small dams of rocks and sandbags. Many farmers also replaced annual crops with perennials, such as alfalfa, which hold the soil in place (98).

**Water resources.** The world needs a "blue revolution" as much as it needs another Green Revolution. Based on the UN medium population projection, over 4 billion people would be affected by water shortages in the year 2050. By then, for example, in Nigeria only about 900 cubic meters would be available per person, compared with 3,200 cubic meters per person in 1990 (26).

A water-short world is an unstable world. More than 200 river systems cross international borders; nearly 100 countries share just 13 major rivers and lakes (26, 73). Water use practices in upstream countries can affect water supplies in downstream countries. Disputes can arise, especially where countries with rapid population growth and limited arable land and water supplies vie for access to water. For example, Ethiopia plans to divert more of the Blue Nile's waters for irrigated agriculture, while Egypt, downstream, depends on the Nile's waters for its very existence (41).

Instead of a "first come, first served" approach to water management, countries and regions need to manage distribution and use of water resources to ensure that everyone gets a fair share. Guaranteeing access to water supplies also would help food-deficit countries improve their agricultural production. Some countries have successfully negotiated agreements over use of water resources—for example, India and Bangladesh, which share the Ganges, the largest and most important river on the Indian subcontinent (14).

With the prospect of less water per person, countries must conserve available water resources and manage them better than in the past. Many strategies and technologies exist to help save water and distribute it equitably. These include building reservoirs and small catchment dams to collect water during the rainy season for use during the dry season, allowing aquifers to recharge, reducing leaks in urban water pipes, protecting watersheds by planting trees to reduce erosion, and recycling municipal waste water for agricultural use (98, 99).

Since irrigation water is wasted almost everywhere, there is great scope in the short run for water conservation in agriculture (97, 98, 99). In particular, the following steps can encourage efficient use of water and can promote conservation:

- Improving the design of irrigation systems and using technologies better suited to climate and terrain can greatly reduce waste and improve crop yields. For example, Israeli farmers use drip irrigation: each plant receives water through its own little drip tube. With this technique they have increased the efficiency of irrigation by as much as 95%. Over the past 20 years Israel's food production has doubled without using any more water (26).

- Pricing water at its real value, instead of subsidizing it, can have an immediate effect on water use, encouraging farmers to save water and use it more efficiently (73).

- For some agricultural purposes waste water from households and municipalities ("brown water") can substitute for fresh water. For example, in Calcutta sewage lagoons are used to raise carp and irrigate vegetable gardens (26). In most cases sewage water needs to be pretreated in order to eliminate pathogens.

- Water harvesting and low-cost irrigation schemes can help poor farmers meet their water needs. Water harvesting involves digging holes to collect runoff for irrigating crops, pastures, and trees during dry months. Where this technique has been used, as in Kenya, Burkina Faso, and Niger, crop yields are twice those produced by dryland farming methods (99).

- Reforesting upland watersheds can reduce water runoff and raise soil moisture levels, helping to recharge groundwater aquifers and capturing more water for human use (26, 99).

In the long run, countries must design and implement strategies to manage entire watersheds. In some cases, where two or more countries share watersheds, management efforts need to transcend national borders (97).

■

## Exploring Other Food Options

Still other options to help meet food needs at the national or local level include improving yields on marginal land, farming forests, expanding aquaculture, rediscovering forgotten foods, and encouraging urban agriculture. Innovative approaches that increase agricultural productivity while protecting the natural resource base also can help.

**Improving yields on marginal land.** FAO estimates that there may be some two billion hectares of marginal land that could be converted to agriculture, but three-quarters of it is too dry, too steep, too wet, too cold, or too shallow to support sustainable food production (98, 99). There is some scope for introducing more efficient farming techniques to help subsistence farmers working marginal lands, however.

For example, the International Institute of Tropical Agriculture has pioneered "alley farming," which could substitute for slash-and-burn, shifting cultivation on fragile and highly erodible tropical soils. Alley farming is now being introduced in over 20 countries in Africa and Asia (48). The concept is simple: leguminous crops, such as mucuna, which fix nitrogen and improve soil organic matter, are planted between rows of food crops, such as peas and beans. The legumes help hold the soil in place and improve nutrient content while preventing weeds from taking root. If crops are used in the right combination, alley farming can greatly improve yields on poor soils in hilly regions and thus reduce the need to clear forests for farmland.

**Farming forests.** Forests are generally worth more standing and managed sustainably than when cut down for short-term profit. For example, in Peru harvesting forest products from one hectare could be worth over US$400 annually, year after year. Logging the same area and selling the timber would yield a one-time return of $1,000 (98). FAO studies in Peru, the Brazilian Amazon, the Philippines, and Indonesia suggest that harvesting forest products on a sustainable basis is twice as productive in the long-run as clearing forests for agricultural and grazing land (99). Cleared land often takes 50 to 100 years to recover. Furthermore, once forest is cleared, the biological diversity of secondary growth never matches that of pristine wilderness (35).

Many plant products found in forests are harvested for food. These include mushrooms, coconuts, saps, and gums. The sago palm is a food staple for more than 300,000 Melanesians. Grasses, foliage, and bamboo are used as animal fodder and for building materials. Forests contain thousands of different species of plants that could be used for medicines and pharmaceuticals. For example, a derivative of the rosy periwinkle, found in Madagascar, has improved the survival of children suffering from leukemia. Taxol, found in the western yew, which grows in the forests of the American northwest, is being used in anti-cancer drugs (54).

Forest plants and trees are also exploited for horticulture and extractive products such as natural rubber, oils, and resins. Some 1.5 million people in the Brazilian Amazon derive a major portion of their income from harvesting natural rubber and other forest products (98). Vines and fibers are used in furniture making. Rattan supports a thriving furniture industry in Southeast Asia, bringing in US$2 billion a year (98, 99).

**Expanding aquaculture.** About 17% of the world's animal protein for human consumption comes from fish. In some Asian countries that figure is over 50%. Between 1984 and 1994 the amount of fish and other products farmed in the sea and from freshwater ponds more than doubled, rising from 10 million metric tons to 23 million metric tons (98, 99).

In the developing world, where the world's aquaculture and mariculture industries are concentrated, most fish farming operations are for export and not for local consumption. Exports of such species as shrimp, prawns, and grouper bring in substantial foreign exchange earnings for a number of poor countries. Where farming fish for local consumption has been tried, the results have been encouraging.

For example, faced with the loss of their livelihoods because of overfishing and increased competition from commercial trawlers, poor fishing communities in Capiz Province, on the island of Panay, the Philippines, turned to fish farming and

crab fattening. The mariculture operations were established by the women of these fishing villages with loans and technical assistance from the Philippine offices of FAO and the United Nations Population Fund. As part of the project, the women were offered family planning, and in a few years over half were using contraception. With smaller families, the women's health is better, they are able to earn more money, and their children are able to stay in school longer (40).

**Rediscovering forgotten foods.** Another way to help make up for food shortages, especially in the world's poorest countries, is to rediscover forgotten traditional food plants. Amaranth and quinoa, two grains that historically were cultivated by the Incas of Peru and the Aztecs of Mexico, provide examples. Both grains are versatile and nutritious foods, containing more high-quality protein than most other commercial grains, including corn, rice, and wheat (127). Moreover, both grow well under difficult conditions. Amaranth thrives in hot climates. The quinoa plant, because it is frost-resistant, can be grown at high altitudes (39).

**Encouraging urban agriculture.** As cities continue to expand in developing countries, people are growing more and more food in urban areas (37). Worldwide, some 200 million city dwellers are growing food, providing about 1 billion people with at least part of their food supply (63, 93).

The scale of urban agriculture varies a great deal, including household gardens covering no more than 20 square meters, small commercial operations occupying 200 to 1,000 square meters, and greenhouses that cover 20 to 30 hectares. Some urban farmers raise fish, shellfish, and aquatic plants in small tanks, ponds, sewage lagoons, and estuaries. Others use vacant city lots to grow vegetables and fruits. Still others keep guinea pigs, rabbits, and chickens in cages hung on walls or grow vegetables using hydroponic techniques (63, 93).

Urban farmers produce impressive amounts of food. In Accra, Ghana, for example, urban gardens supply the city with 90% of its vegetables. In Dar-es-Salaam, Tanzania, one adult in every five grows fruits or vegetables. Over 60% of the area around Bangkok has been devoted to vegetable gardens, cultivated mostly by women and children (63, 93).

**Adopting new approaches.** Some countries with traditional farming systems are improving yields with new approaches that use low-level agricultural inputs—fertilizing with animal wastes instead of chemicals, recycling nutrients, conserving water, and selecting a variety of crops well-suited to soil conditions and climate (98, 99, 110, 111, 112). In Indonesia, for example, the Javan rice crop was nearly wiped out in 1984 by a plague of pesticide-resistant brown plant hoppers. In response, the government introduced a new approach, Integrated Pest Management (IPM) (127).

IPM involves taking several related steps—preserving natural pest predators, using pest-resistant seed varieties, and drastically reducing the amount of chemical pesticides used. Using this approach, the infestation of brown plant hoppers was controlled with only minimal crop losses (98). Within a few years, Javanese farmers who used the IPM methods had higher yields than those who continued to spray their crops with pesticides (98).

# Bibliography

An asterisk (*) denotes an item that was particularly useful in the preparation of this issue of ***Population Reports.***


1. ALAN GUTTMACHER INSTITUTE (AGI). Hope and realities—Closing the gap between women's aspirations and their reproductive experiences. New York, AGI, 1995. p. 7-41.
2. ASHFORD, L.S. New perspectives on population: Lessons from Cairo. Population Bulletin 50(1): 2-40. March 1995.
3. BENDER, W. and SMITH, M. Population, food and nutrition. Population Bulletin 51(4): 2-43. February 1997.
4. BENDER, W. and SMITH, M. Feeding the future. Population Today 25(3): 4-5. March 1997.
5. BONGAARTS, J. Population growth and global warming. Prepared for the 1992 annual meeting of the Population Association of America, Denver, April 30-May 2, 1992. 23 p.
* 6. BONGAARTS, J. Population pressure and the food supply system in the developing world. New York, Population Council, March 1996. p. 3-30.
7. BONGAARTS, J., MAULDIN, W.P., and PHILLIPS, J.F. The demographic impact of family planning programs. Studies in Family Planning 21(6): 299-310. November-December 1990.
8. BOJO, J.P. Economics and land degradation. Ambio 20(2): 75-79. April 1991.
9. BROWN, L. The agricultural link: How environmental deterioration could disrupt economic progress. Washington, D.C., Worldwatch Institute, August 1997. (Worldwatch paper 136) 68 p.
10. BROWN, L. Japanese government breaks with World Bank food forecast. World Watch, May-June, 1996. p. 6-7.
* 11. BROWN, L. Tough choices—Facing the challenge of food scarcity. New York, Norton, 1996. p. 20-135.
12. BROWN, L. Who will feed China? Wake-up call for a small planet. New York, Norton, 1995. 141 p.
13. BROWN, L. and KANE, H. Full house. New York, Norton, 1994. p. 21-223.
14. BURNS, J. Sharing Ganges waters, India and Bangladesh test the depth of cooperation. New York Times, May 25, 1997. p. 6.
15. COHEN, J. How many people can the earth support? New York, Norton, 1995. p. 25-260.
16. CONSULTATIVE GROUP ON INTERNATIONAL AGRICULTURAL RESEARCH (CGIAR). The forgotten farmer: Plant genetic resources, women and the CGIAR. Rome, CGIAR, 1996. 16 p.
17. COSTANZA, R., D'ARGE, R., DE GROOT, R., et al. The value of the world's ecosystem services and natural capital. Nature 387(6630): 253-260. May 15, 1997.
18. DANISH 92-GROUP. Food security—Sustainable options. Copenhagen, Danish 92-Group, 1996. p. 1-11.
* 19. DOOS, B. Environmental degradation, global food production and risk for large-scale migrations. Ambio 23(2): 124-130. March 1994.
20. ECONOMIST. Will the world starve? Feast and famine. Economist, November 16, 1996. p. 21-23.
21. EDWARDS, R. Tomorrow's bitter harvest. New Scientist, August 17, 1996. p. 14-15.
* 22. EHRLICH, A. Building a sustainable food system. In: Smith, P., ed. The world at the crossroads—Towards a sustainable, equitable and liveable world. London, Earthscan, 1994, p. 21-35.
23. EHRLICH, P. and EHRLICH, A. The population explosion. New York, Simon and Schuster, 1990. 251 p.
24. ELLIOTT, J. The greening of the green revolution. Food Summit Watch, November 13, 1996. p. 1 & 7.
* 25. ENGELMAN, R. and LEROY, P. Conserving land: Population and sustainable food production. Washington, D.C., Population Action International, 1995. p. 8-42.
* 26. ENGELMAN, R. and LEROY, P. Sustaining water: Population and the future of renewable water supplies. Washington, D.C., Population Action International, 1993. p. 7-47.
27. ENVIRONMENT LIAISON CENTRE INTERNATIONAL (ELCI). The struggle against desertification—Combating degradation in Africa's drylands. Nairobi, ELCI, 1995. p. 7-32.
* 28. FALKENMARK, M. and WIDSTRAND, C. Population and water resources: A delicate balance. Population Bulletin. Washington, D.C., Population Reference Bureau, 1992.
29. FEDER, B. Sowing preservation—Towns are slowing invasion of farms by bulldozers. New York Times, March 20, 1997. p. D1, 19.
30. FREEDMAN, R. and BLANC, A.K. Fertility transition: An update. International Family Planning Perspectives 18(2): 44-50, 72. June 1992.
* 31. GARDNER, G. Shrinking fields: Cropland loss in a world of eight billion. Washington, D.C., Worldwatch Institute, July 1996. p. 12-31.
32. GARDNER, R. and BLACKBURN, R. Migrants, refugees, and internally displaced persons: A new focus for reproductive health programs. Population Reports, Series J, No. 45. Baltimore, Johns Hopkins School of Public Health, Population Information Program. 1996.
* 33. GREEN, C.P. The environment and population growth: Decade for action. Population Reports, Series M, No. 10. Baltimore, Johns Hopkins School of Public Health, Population Information Program, May 1992. 32 p.
34. GRIER, P. Hardier corn can feed more hungry people. Christian Science Monitor, July 13, 1994. p. 8.
* 35. HARRISON, P. The third revolution: Environment, population and a sustainable world. London, I.B. Tauris, 1992. p. 43, 282.
36. HAUB, C. New UN projections depict a variety of demographic futures. Population Today 25(4): 1-3. April 1997.
37. HELMORE, K. and RATTA, A. The surprising yields of urban agriculture. Choices, April 1995. p. 22-27.
38. HINRICHSEN, D. Coastal waters of the world: Trends, threats and strategies. (To be published by Island Press, 1997).
39. HINRICHSEN, D. Forgotten foods. People & the Planet 4(4): 25. 1995.
40. HINRICHSEN, D. Where women take control. People & the Planet 3(1): 22-23. 1994.
41. HINRICHSEN, D. The world's water woes. International Wildlife 26(4): 22-27. July-August 1996.
42. HINRICHSEN, D. Computing the risks. International Wildlife 26(2): 22-35. March-April 1996.
43. HOLLOWAY, N. Agriculture—No pain, no gain. Far Eastern Economic Review, November 16, 1995. p. 88-94.
44. INTERNATIONAL CENTER FOR AGRICULTRUAL RESEARCH IN THE DRY AREAS (ICARDA). Biodiversity: A key to food security. Aleppo, Syria, ICARDA, 1996. p. 5-18.
45. INTERNATIONAL CENTER FOR TROPICAL AGRICULTURE (CIAT). CIAT in perspective 1995-96. Cali, Colombia, CIAT, 1996. 43 p.
46. INTERNATIONAL FUND FOR AGRICULTURAL DEVELOPMENT (IFAD). Workshop on approaches to rural poverty alleviation in SADC countries. Cape Town, South Africa, IFAD, February 19-22, 1996. p. 5-11.
* 47. INTERNATIONAL FOOD POLICY RESEARCH INSTITUTE (IFPRI). A 2020 Vision for food, agriculture, and the environment. Washington, D.C., IFPRI, 1995. p. 1-45.
48. INTERNATIONAL INSTITUTE OF TROPICAL AGRICULTURE (IITA). Dealing with the issues of our times. Ibadan, Nigeria, IITA, June 1994. 14 p.
49. KARL, M. The crucial role of women in food security. Quezon City, Philippines, Isis International-Manila, 1996. 22 p.
50. KIBIRIGE, J. Population growth, poverty and health. Social Science and Medicine 45(2): 247-259. 1997.
51. KLEINER, K. Panic as grain stocks fall to all time low. New Scientist, February 3, 1996. p. 10.
52. KYODO NEWS. Grain prices could double by 2010. Kyodo News, December 25, 1995.
53. LEAN, G. The era of scarcity is upon us. Our Planet, 8(4): 10-12. 1996.
* 54. LEAN, G. and HINRICHSEN, D. Atlas of the environment. New York, Harper Perennial, 1994. 184 p.
55. LEARY, W. E. Research yields underused sources of food in Africa: Grains. New York Times, April 23, 1996. p. C4.
* 56. LINCOLN, D. Reproductive health, population growth, economic development and environmental change. In: Environmental Change and Human Health. London, Wiley, 1993. p. 197-214.
57. MALTHUS, T. R. An essay on the principle of population. New York, W.W. Norton & Co., 1976.
58. MENSEN IN NOOD (MN). CARITAS NEDERLAND. Food security, only a woman's job? Gender and food security. Amsterdam, MN, September 1996. p. 5-20.
59. MIES, M. A breakdown in relations—Women, food security and trade. Quezon City, Philippines, Isis International-Manila, 1996. 18 p.
60. MOFFETT, G. Global population growth: 21st century challenges. New York, Foreign Policy Association, Spring 1994, p. 3-69.
61. MYDANS, S. Scientists developing super rice to feed Asia. New York Times, April 6, 1997. p. 9.
62. MYERS, N. and KENT, J. Environmental exodus—An emergent crisis in the global arena. Washington, D.C., Climate Institute, June 1995, p. 14-160.
63. NELSON, T. Closing the nutrient loop. World Watch 9(6): 10-17. November-December 1996.
64. PEARCE, F. Crop gurus sow some seeds of hope. New Scientist, November 9, 1996. p. 6.
65. PEARCE, F. Crying out for food. New Scientist, November 9, 1996. p. 14-15.
66. PEARCE, F. To feed the world, talk to the farmers. New Scientist, November 23, 1996. p. 6-7.
67. PHILDHRRA JOURNAL. Of empty bowls and promises. Phildhrra Journal 1(1): 22-26. 1996.
68. PIMENTEL, D., HOUSER, J., PREISS, E., WHITE, O., FANG, H., MESNICK, L., BARSKY, T., TARICHE, S., SCHRECK, J., and ALPERT, S. Water resources: Agriculture, the environment and society. BioScience 47(2): 97-105. February 1997.
* 69. PONTING, C. A green history of the world. New York, Penguin Books, 1991. 430 p.
70. POPULAR COALITION FOR ACTION (PCA). Conference on hunger and poverty: An overview. Brussels, PCA, November 1995. p. 2-24.
71. POPULATION ACTION INTERNATIONAL (PAI). Catching the limits: Population and the decline of fisheries. [Wall chart] Washington, D.C., PAI, 1995.
72. POPULATION REFERENCE BUREAU (PRB). World Population Data Sheet 1997. [Wall Chart]. Washington, D. C., PRB, 1997.
73. POSTEL, S. Dividing the waters: Food security, ecosystem health, and the new politics of scarcity. Washington, D.C., Wo watch Institute, September 1996. p. 5-64.
74. POTTS, M. Too many people pose global risk. Forum Applied Research and Public Policy 12(2): 6-15. Summer 199
75. PRESIDENT'S COUNCIL ON SUSTAINABLE DEVELOME (PCSD). Population and consumption: Task force report. Wa ington, D.C., PCSD, 1996. 96 p.
76. REPETTO, R. The second India revisted: Population grov poverty, and environment over two decades. In: Tata Ene Research Institute (TERI) and World Resources Institute (W Proceedings of the Conference on Population, Environment Development, Washington, D.C., March 13-14, 1996. p. 2-31
77. REYES, L.S. Philippines—Lucrative fisheries disappeari Food Summit Watch, November 12, 1996. p. 4.
78. ROBEY, B., PIOTROW, P.T., and SALTER, C. Family plann lessons and challenges: Making programs work. Population ports, Series J, No. 40. Baltimore, Johns Hopkins School of Pu Health, Population Information Program, August 1994. 28 p.
79. ROBEY, B., ROSS, J., and BHUSHAN, I. Meeting unı need—New strategies. Population Reports, Series J, No. 43. E timore, Johns Hopkins School of Public Health, Population In mation Program, September 1996. 36 p.
* 80. ROBEY, B., RUTSTEIN, S.O., MORRIS, L., and BLACKBUR R. The reproductive revolution: New survey findings. Populat Reports, Series M, No. 11. Baltimore, Johns Hopkins School Public Health, Population Information Program, December 19 44 p.
81. ROCA, Z. Urbanization and rural women: Impact of rural urban migration. Rome, United Nations Food and Agricult Organization, November 1993. p. 1-10.
82. ROSEGRANT, M.W. From falling prices to security. Solag Courrier de la Planete (European Commission), April 1996. 10-11.
* 83. SAGOFF, M. Do we consume too much? Atlantic Month June 1997. p. 80-96.
84. SCHMIDT, K. Whatever happened to the gene revolutio New Scientist, January 7, 1995. p. 21-25.
85. SCOMMEGNA, P. UN Food Summit tries to focus wo attention on hunger. Population Today 24(11): 1-2. Novemb 1996.
86. SEN, A. The economics of life and death. Scientific America May 1993. p. 40-47.
87. SEYMOUR, J. Hungry for a new revolution. New Scienti March 30, 1996. p. 34-41.
88. SIMON, J.L. The ultimate resource. Princeton, New Jerse Princeton University Press, 1981. 415 p.
89. SOUTHGATE, D. and BASTERRECHEA, M. Populati growth, public policy and resource degradation: The case Guatemala. Ambio 21(7): 460-464. November 1992.
90. STOREY, J.D., ILKHAMOV, A., and SAKSVIG, B. Perceptio of family planning and reproductive health issues: Focus grou discussions in Kazakhstan, Turkmenistan, Kyrgyzstan, and Uzbe istan. Baltimore, Johns Hopkins Center for Communication Pr grams, August 1997. (Field Report No. 10)
91. TYLER, P. Nature and economic boom devouring China farmland. New York Times, March 27, 1994. p. 1 and 8.
92. UNITED NATIONS CHILDREN'S FUND (UNICEF). The pr gress of nations 1997. New York, UN, 1997. 68 p.
* 93. UNITED NATIONS DEVELOPMENT PROGRAMME (UNDF Urban agriculture—Food, jobs and sustainable cities. New Yo UNDP, 1996. p. 3-205.
94. UNITED NATIONS DEVELOPMENT PROGRAMME (UNDF Sustainable human development and agriculture. New Yor UNDP, 1994. p. 1-78.
95. UNITED NATIONS. DIVISION FOR SUSTAINABLE DEVELO MENT (UNDSD). Earth summit +5, backgrounder. New Yor UNDSD, 1997. p. 1-6.
96. UNITED NATIONS (UN). DEPARTMENT FOR ECONOMI AND SOCIAL INFORMATION AND POLICY ANALYSIS. Popula tion and development: 1. Programme of Action adopted at th International Conference on Population and Development, Cair 5-11 September 1994. Geneva, UN, 1995. 107 p.
* 97. UNITED NATIONS (UN). DEPARTMENT FOR POLICY COOF DINATION AND SUSTAINABLE DEVELOPMENT. Critica trends—Global change and sustainable development. New Yor UN, 1997. p. 1-76.
* 98. UNITED NATIONS. FOOD AND AGRICULTURE ORGAN ZATION (FAO). Dimensions of need: An atlas of food and agricu ture. Rome, FAO, 1995. p. 16-98.
* 99. UNITED NATIONS. FOOD AND AGRICULTURE ORGAN ZATION (FAO). Food for all. Rome, FAO, 1996. 64 p.
100. UNITED NATIONS. FOOD AND AGRICULTURE ORGAN ZATION (FAO). Food requirements and population growth Rome, FAO, 1996. p. 1-15.
101. UNITED NATIONS. FOOD AND AGRICULTURE ORGAN ZATION (FAO). Harvesting nature's diversity. Rome, FAO, Octo ber 1993. p. 7-25.
102. UNITED NATIONS. FOOD AND AGRICULTURE ORGAN ZATION (FAO). Initiatives to protect agrobiological diversity. AC March 1994. p. 1.
103. UNITED NATIONS. FOOD AND AGRICULTURE ORGAN ZATION (FAO). Land, food and people. Rome, FAO, 1984. p 1-77.
104. UNITED NATIONS. FOOD AND AGRICULTURE ORGAN ZATION (FAO). Review of the state of world fishery resources Marine fisheries. Rome, FAO, 1995. p. 1-56.
105. UNITED NATIONS. FOOD AND AGRICULTURE ORGAN ZATION (FAO). Safeguarding the diversity of plant genetic re sources. In: World Agriculture 1993. Rome, FAO, 1993. p. 11-13

106. UNITED NATIONS. FOOD AND AGRICULTURE ORGANI-ZATION (FAO). The special programme for food security. Rome, FAO, 1996. 12 p.

107. UNITED NATIONS. FOOD AND AGRICULTURE ORGANI-ZATION (FAO). Women in agricultural development—Women, food systems and agriculture. Rome, FAO, 1990. p. 15-44.

108. UNITED NATIONS. FOOD AND AGRICULTURE ORGANI-ZATION (FAO). World Food Day 1996: Fighting hunger and malnutrition. Rome, FAO, 1996. 16 p.

109. UNITED NATIONS. FOOD AND AGRICULTURE ORGANI-ZATION (FAO). World Food Summit: Rome declaration on world food security and World Food Summit plan of action. Rome, FAO, 1996. 43 p.

110. UNITED NATIONS. FOOD AND AGRICULTURE ORGANI-ZATION (FAO). World Food Summit: Vol 1. Technical Background Documents 1-5. Rome, FAO, 1996. 200 p.

111. UNITED NATIONS. FOOD AND AGRICULTURE ORGANI-ZATION (FAO). World Food Summit: Vol. 2. Technical Background Documents 6-11. Rome, FAO, 1996. 200 p.

112. UNITED NATIONS. FOOD AND AGRICULTURE ORGANI-ZATION (FAO). World Food Summit: Vol. 3. Technical Background Documents 12-15. Rome, FAO, 1996. 102 p.

113. UNITED NATIONS. FOOD AND AGRICULTURE ORGANI-ZATION. COMMITTEE ON WORLD FOOD SECURITY (CWFS). FAO/NGO consultation on the World Food Summit (19-21 September 1996): Key points of the consultation. New York, CWFS, 1996. 6 p. (Mimeo).

114. UNITED NATIONS. FOOD AND AGRICULTURE ORGANI-ZATION. FAO Production Yearbook 1995. Rome, FAO, 1996.

115. UNITED NATIONS DEVELOPMENT FUND FOR WOMEN (UNIFEM). UNIFEM in Beijing and beyond. New York, UNIFEM, 1995. p. 26-29.

116. UNITED NATIONS POPULATION FUND (UNFPA). Advocating change: Population, empowerment, development. New York, UNFPA, 1995. p. 1-16.

• 117. UNITED NATIONS POPULATION FUND (UNFPA). Food for the future: Women, population and food security. New York, UNFPA, 1996. p. 1-16.

118. UNITED NATIONS POPULATION FUND (UNFPA). India: PRSD background document. New Delhi, UNFPA, 1996. 128 p. (Mimeo)

• 119. UNITED NATIONS POPULATION FUND (UNFPA). Population and sustainable development—Five years after Rio. New York, UNFPA, 1997. p. 1-36.

120. UNITED NATIONS POPULATION FUND (UNFPA). Population issues briefing kit, 1996. New York, UNFPA, 1996. p. 2-24.

121. UNITED NATIONS POPULATION FUND (UNFPA). The state of world population 1996. New York, UNFPA, 1996. p. 5-66.

122. UNITED STATES (US). BUREAU OF THE CENSUS. World population profile: 1994. Washington, D.C., US Government Printing Office, 1994. (Report WP/94) 139 p.

123. VALENTE, T.W. Network models of the diffusion of innovations. Cresskill, New Jersey, Hampton Press, 1995.

• 124. VITOUSEK, P.M., MOONEY, H.A., LUBCHENCO, J., and MELILLO, J.M. Human domination of earth's ecosystems. Science 277: 494-499. July 25, 1997.

125. WESTOFF, C.F. and BANKOLE, A. The potential demographic significance of unmet need. International Family Planning Perspectives 22(1): 16-20. March 1996.

126. WIRTH, T.E. Statement of The Honorable Timothy E. Wirth, Under Secretary of State for Global Affairs, before the Committee on International Relations United States House of Representatives, July 24, 1997. 1997. 5 p. (Unpublished)

127. WORLD BANK (WB). Biodiversity and agricultural intensification. Washington, D.C., WB, 1996. p. 1-129.

128. WORLD BANK (WB). Food security for the world. Washington, D.C., WB, 1996. 12 p.

129. WORLD BANK (WB). From scarcity to security—Averting a water crisis in the Middle East and North Africa. Washington, D.C., WB, December 1995. 32 p.

• 130. WORLD BANK (WB). Global food supply prospects. Washington, D.C., WB, 1996. 23 p.

131. WORLD BANK (WB). Rural Development—Putting the pieces in place. Washington, D.C., WB, 1996. 29 p.

132. WORLD FOOD PROGRAMME (WFP). Tackling hunger in a world full of food: Tasks ahead for food aid. Rome, WFP, 1996. p. 7-24.

• 133. WORLD HEALTH ORGANIZATION (WHO). Health and environment in sustainable development—Five years after the earth summit. Geneva, WHO, 1997. p. 1-202.

134. WORLD RESOURCES INSTITUTE. and UNITED NATIONS ENVIRONMENT PROGRAMME. and UNITED NATIONS DEVELOPMENT PROGRAMME. and WORLD BANK. World resources 1996-97. New York, Oxford University Press, 1996. 379 p.

135. ZAKHAROVA, N. The role of rural women in food security. New York, United Nations Division for the Advancement of Women, October 1995. p. 1-6 (Mimeo)

136. ZAMORA, O. The real roots of security. Our Planet 8(4): 25-26. 1996.

### ADDENDUM

137. PINSTRUP-ANDERSEN, P., PANDYA-LORCH, R., and ROSEGRANT, M.W. The world food situation: Recent developments, emerging issues, and long-term prospects. Washington, D.C., Consultation Group on International Agricultural Research, October 27, 1997. 53 p. (Mimeo)

ISSN 0887-0241

[Editor's Note: Some notes apply to articles that are not included in this three-part essay. See *Population Reports*, December 1997.]

# *It's not called a famine, but thousands starve*

## **Sudan:** A vicious civil war and years of drought combine to push a people accustomed to adversity over the edge.

By GILBERT A. LEWTHWAITE
**SUN FOREIGN STAFF**

AKUEM, Sudan—Ajok Luah Luah, 25, a young mother of upright bearing but dwindling strength, is the anguished face of famine-threatened Sudan today.

For three days, she has eaten nothing but wild leaves, walking by night, sheltering under the shade trees by day, all the time cradling her 14-month-old baby in her arms as she flees from civil war.

Her little daughter is sick, coughing and perspiring with fever; her hair is copper-tinted, the tell-tale sign of malnutrition.

Ajok still suckles the baby at breasts that may soon be as arid as the terrain across which she trudges in her soiled cream and purple garb, a figure of wretchedness.

She is just one of tens, if not hundreds, of thousands facing starvation in this benighted place.

"Time has basically run out," says Diane de Guzman, field program manager for southern Sudan with Britain's Save the Children Fund.

From *The Baltimore Sun*, May 17, 1998, pp. 1A, 26A. © 1998 by The Baltimore Sun. Reprinted by permission.

Fifteen years of civil war and two years of drought have overwhelmed the centuries-old coping mechanisms of a people who know how to counter adversity but now hover daily between life and death.

"We knew that by this year, if nothing complicated their coping mechanisms, there could still be a disaster," says David Kugunda, of UNICEF. "Unfortunately, something happened, and that something was war."

The war between the Muslim-led government forces of the north and the secessionist Christians and animists—believers in traditional spirits—of the south intensified earlier this year.

It is a seemingly endless conflict in which arms are more plentiful than food, with the government said to be supplied by China, Iraq, Iran and Malaysia and the rebels getting arms through Uganda and Eritrea. Neither side seems able to win.

At peace talks this month in Nairobi, Kenya, the rebels obtained the promise of a referendum on independence for the south but rejected the government's offer of a ceasefire, suspecting that the government forces wanted time to recover from losing battles.

The rebels are poised to take garrison towns in Bahr el Ghazal.

Displaced by the ebb and flow of the conflict, which has left their villages razed, their homes and crops burned, people and livestock seized, the refugees have been deprived of all means of self-sufficiency.

The Islamic government's reaction to the food crisis has been confused. In February, when the rebels were on the offensive, it banned all relief flights.

"The government has been using food as a weapon of war," says one aid program manager, asking not to be named.

Then, this month, the government finally agreed that five C-130 Hercules and three Buffalo cargo planes could have unfettered access to the hunger area for the month of May.

Khartoum authorizes flights on a month-by-month basis.

There is however, suspicion now that Khartoum's belated acquiescence is cruelly timed.

"I'm afraid Khartoum may have almost set us up here to fail," says de Guzman: "Now it is just too late, and they are going to say, 'We gave you the planes, and people are still dying. You guys failed.' That's what really worries me."

And as if the conflict itself were not enough, help from international aid donors has been slow in coming.

The major donor countries played down the first warning signals from October's annual assessment by the World Food Program. Only after the fighting displaced 100,000 refugees around the city of Wau in January did they respond to an emergency appeal with $28 million worth of aid.

The United States has provided 48 percent of the aid, supplying 8,500 tons of food worth $2.4 million. With transport included, the U.S. contribution has cost $13.3 million.

The original estimate by the World Food Program was that 30 percent of the 1.5 million people in the region might be victims of the seasonal "hunger gap," facing a calorie deficit of 15 percent to 20 percent.

Now the calculation is that 40 percent of the population lacks up to 40 percent of the normal diet.

## Could have acted earlier

"It didn't have to reach this level," says Jason Matus, food economic officer with the WFP. "We could have responded earlier with less if we had had the [airlift] capacity and the access."

Barbara Barton, WFP spokeswoman in Nairobi, says, "Many of the people are now starting to move in search of food."

In Gogrial County, where aid agencies are expected to feed 250,000, they now have an additional 100,000 hungry war refugees.

East Aweil County, where the local population of 203,000 is unable to feed itself, is expected to become the haven for as many as 300,000 fugitives from the fighting in West Aweil.

People have been reduced to eating the seed they were saving to plant for the late August harvest.

They frequently also eat the aid seed, although it is chemically treated and makes them sick. To counter this, aid agencies are trying to distribute food and seed simultaneously, hoping to get the seed in the ground before it is consumed.

But much of the land still lies fallow, baking ever harder under the relentless equatorial sun.

"There's not enough land being cultivated out there," says de Guzman. "I don't see how we can possibly have a harvest that can resolve this situation. It may just stave it off a little bit."

Another problem: The international seed is neither suited to the weather here nor resistant to local pests. Agriculturists estimate that less than half the available land will be cultivated, and the germination rate on that land will be less than 40 percent.

## Specter of continued drought

Most ominous of all, the rains that should have started in mid-April have yet to fall, raising the specter of a third annual drought to deprive the earth of new life.

This has not been officially declared a famine, when people, deprived of all the means of survival, die like flies—the babies first, then the frail, followed by those whose ebbing strength is finally overcome.

Technically, it is being called "a hunger gap," or "a food deficit." But the distinction is hard to see.

"There is nothing, no food," says Nyal Chan Nyal, elderly chief of the village of Akon. "I tell my people they have to be patient."

But how many more days can Nji-bol Deng, already a skeletal figure, sit in the blazing heat loosening the earth with a hand-broom of dried grass in search of tiny brownish-red akaudo seeds, a form of wild rice.

This day, she has been here since sunrise, her pot-bellied daughter, Ayen Akol, 5, at her feet.

She fled from the fighting around her home at Agalit in August last year and came here to join her mother-in-law, who had nothing to offer but the barest of shelter.

She sits with her legs straight out, her back erect, methodically removing the seed from the dirt, first winnowing it from one basket to another, then rubbing it through her hands.

In six hours of painstaking separation, she has produced about a pound of seed, insufficient for herself, two children and her mother-in-law. She must scrape on to live another day.

Awien Dut's diet today will be the kernels of the tamarind fruit, their hard shells roasted off in the small fire of dried grass she is tending. Already the 36-year-old and her six children have nibbled the fruit off the nuts.

"Look at me," she says, kneeling up to show her skinny frame. "The hunger shows in my body." Not since February has she eaten anything but wild fruits, roots and seeds, she says.

It is a diet that would be suitable as supplemental food. Eaten exclusively, it produces stomach problems and diarrhea, particularly among children. But for weeks, this has been the staple food of thousands of Sudanese.

In the jargon of official aid papers, it is termed "famine wild food"—the last chance of survival without outside help.

## Suffering of children

"The worst thing is the kids," says Buzz Sharp, head of the World Food Program's food economics of-fice in Lokichokio, Kenya, the jumping-off place for most aid agencies.

He has seen 800 children—130 of them severely malnourished—at a feeding station run by the Belgium branch of Medecins Sans Frontieres (Doctors Without Borders) in the village of Ajiep.

"If they were anywhere else, they would be in hospital having 12 feeds a day," he says. "That is not going to happen. If a lot of them live, it will be a miracle."

Medecins Sans Frontieres is caring for 3,000 children, 25 percent of them severely malnourished—defined as at least a third under normal body weight.

"That is a lot for children," says Dr. Els Mathieu, MSF's medical coordinator for southern Sudan. "It is getting closer and closer to famine. Now people are starving.

"We have also adults dying. I think now you can say it will become a famine."

The rainy season, if and when it starts, will bring the onset of mosquito-borne malaria. It will also make delivery of aid, by road and air, more difficult.

To reach the worst-hit areas takes a three-hour flight over largely uninhabited terrain to land on a stretch of red earth, cleared in the bush and little longer than a football field, in Bahr el Ghazal.

Akuem is in East Aweil County, a normally self-sufficient region that today is almost totally dependent on outside help. A campaign by government forces in neighboring West Aweil has started an exodus.

"It is an organized war," says Aleu Akechak Jok, commissioner of West Aweil, who arrived here with the bulk of his people last weekend.

"This place is far from the enemy. It is the nearest airstrip, and it is beside a river," he added, explaining his decision to lead the way here. "Anybody from outside who wants to help us will find it easier here."

Ajok Luah Luah, her daughter still in her arms, says she ran away from the village of Nyamlell, in West Aweil, because most of the people were killed.

"I had to escape with my child," she says. "The houses were burning. I decided to walk at night for cover. I was hiding and walking. For three days, I didn't stop. Now I need medicine for my child—and water."

Four babies died of thirst on the 80-mile trek, according to Simon Woh, representative of the rebels' Sudanese Relief and Rehabilitation Association.

Now hundreds of families squat under shade trees, waiting for help. They can do little, except scratch for wild roots or pick leaves, to fend for themselves.

## Food from the sky

Alerted to the local crisis, the World Food Program arranges two immediate 32-ton food drops. The white bags of sorghum and lentils separate from their wooden pallets and cascade down like huge snowflakes as a C-130 sharply tips up its nose 700 feet over the drop zone.

A few bags burst on impact. The hundreds squatting around the area watch and wait. They have been told that the bags will be shared under a system established among the aid agencies, local chiefs and women leaders.

Men with sticks patrol the perimeter, threatening to strike anyone who advances.

The bags are collected and neatly stacked.

Then chaos breaks out. The women run to the cleared drop zone. They fall to their knees, scrambling to get as much food spilled from the burst bags as their bowls will hold. The dust flies as they push and shove, scrape and grab for a few tiny grains.

"To see a Mum on her knees with a baby on one breast and another on her hand, groveling around in the dust, just shows the level of desperation of these people," says Sharp.

Not far from the drop zone, Boll Akok has slaughtered a cow in the ope of making some money to buy perhaps 60 pounds of grain, enough to give him food and seed, but no one has any cash—or grain to barter—and the meat is turning black in the heat of the sun.

For a Dinka to kill a cow is equivalent to a Westerner selling off the family silver. Cows here are the symbols of wealth, used for dowries, in ceremonies, but rarely slaughtered for meat.

"You cannot kill a cow if you are not dying," says Luka Lual Lual, 60, a farmer and entrepreneur reputed to be the richest man in Akon, whose herd of 500 cattle has been reduced to 200 since he was forced to flee the fighting last year.

"But if you are dying, you have no option," he says.

Thus, the growing hunger, ironically, has brought a surplus of beef.

In Akon today, auctioneer Mawien Deng has 20 head of cattle tied to stakes beneath a towering tamarind tree, where normally he might have two or three.

One of those waiting to be put on the block is the small white heifer brought here by Deng Deng, 38, a typically tall, thin Dinka, who has led the animal three hours from his riverside tukul—the traditional round, thatched home in these parts—at Akerkaui.

"I would not sell it if I wasn't hungry," says the father of four. "I am feeling ashamed, but because of the children what can I do?"

A year ago he had four cows. Now he is left with one milk cow. When he left home early in the morning, his wife, Acol Madut, 23, reassured him: "You take it to the market, and if there is a good price, then that is for the survival of our children."

Perhaps Deng's animal will end up on Benjamin Aguang's butcher stall, less than 50 yards away from the auction. Meat prices, he says, have come down by a third or more in a few months, just as grain prices have shot up.

"To save their lives, that's why they are killing the cows," he says.

"It is the worst time. They are starving. They are suffering."

# Thunder in the Distance

## A University of California study on poverty estimates that two million California children are hungry. What happens when that hunger turns to anger, and those children grow up?

## Al Martinez

*Al Martinez is an award-winning columnist for the* Los Angeles Times *and the author of several books, including a collection of essays published under the title "Ashes in the Rain."*

The year was 1936. I was in the second grade and we were living in a shack on a hillside in East Oakland. It was Thanksgiving. I remember the feelings of festivity in the air, and the good smells that seemed to emanate from the kitchens of others. It didn't come from ours. We were poor, and lived like we were poor. Our shack had no gas and no electricity. It hovered precariously over a steep slope, partially propped up by a single board wedged against a tree. We cooked on a wood stove and lighted the house with kerosene lanterns.

It was the time of the Great Depression, and my angry old stepfather had been out of work for God knows how long, and it gnawed at his soul like a hound of heaven. I remember we were on "relief" and were given occasional handouts of food and clothing by abrupt and harried people at long tables in cold and cavernous buildings.

I hated the grayness of the buildings, the attitudes of the workers and the terrible oppressiveness of those who stood in lines that wound out the door, waiting their turn for food and clothing. Even at age seven, I disliked being there. I could feel the resentment of a relief worker who jammed new shoes on my feet to see if they fit, handling me as though I were less than human, a job he hated that had to be done.

I suppose, in a way, I could have taken all that had it not been for Thanksgiving. I mentioned the smells and the warmth of other households in the neighborhood. No one

was rich on Burr Street, but they had somehow managed to put together a holiday dinner. In our house, it was bread and a homemade meatless soup. Even in our terrible poverty, I had somehow expected there would be a Thanksgiving, but there wasn't. The shock of the meager dinner remains etched on my memory. And I think of all the children, in this Golden Age and this Golden State, who are today what I was back then: hungry, angry and terribly sad.

I was reminded of it recently by a report from the University of California, Berkeley, that said there are five million hungry people in California, and two million of them are children—enough to create a city more than twice the size of San Francisco. They comprise about 25 percent of all the children in the state up to age 18, a figure that, according to the U.S. Census Bureau, almost doubled in the decade of the 1980s. More children have entered poverty in the past five years than in the previous 20.

We don't always recognize them as poor by their outward appearance. They go to school, play outside and then disappear. Some go to houses, some to trailers and some to the cars or trucks or vans they call home. What awaits them are the kinds of meals that awaited me back then, or possibly less. They're what John Steinbeck called the children of fury, pushing at the thin line between hunger and anger.

We are coming full circle in my lifetime from an era of intense privation, through war and full bellies, to a period in which children wonder once more what became of Thanksgiving. The poor, the unseen people, have always been with us, and no doubt always will be, but their ranks, like armies of despair, are steadily growing. The number of Californians living below poverty level rose from 11 percent in 1980 to

From *California Journal*, July 1995, pp. 22-25. © 1995 by Information for Public Affairs, Inc. Reprinted by permission.

18.2 percent in 1993. What makes their existence more painful than ever is a widening gap between the haves and have-nots, bringing into sharper contrast those who sign multimillion dollar contracts for hitting balls and sinking baskets and those with no place to go and nothing to eat.

Social scientist Michael Harrington, acknowledging the invisibility of the poor, observed that "They are not simply neglected and forgotten as in the old rhetoric of reform; what is much worse, they are not seen." And yet, evidence of their existence surfaces occasionally with such poignancy that we can't deny their pain.

I wrote once in my column for the *Los Angeles Times* of my search for a homeless family I had heard of living in a small cluster of trees near a freeway off-ramp. There are about 80,000 homeless people living in Los Angeles County, and I, like most everyone else, had tended to ignore their existence. They were like passing traffic, or leaves carried on a stray breeze, sensed briefly and gone quickly. I wanted to correct my own dispassion by writing about a family I'd been told lived in an encampment at the northern terminus of the Long Beach Freeway. So I went looking.

Neighbors told me they'd been there but had been chased off by the police. I searched the abandoned encamp-

ment and found the debris of their existence: a barbecue grill, a paper cup, a few cans, a ragged shirt . . . and a note. It was written in black crayon on a piece of lined notebook paper by a child who might have been seven or eight years old. On one side was a picture of a house in rough outline, without doors or windows, standing bleakly alone. On the other, printed with determined care, were the words, "I love you mom."

I looked at that note for a long time, drawn into it by the terrible sadness of its circumstances. I could picture a little girl, the age of my own granddaughters, sitting in that vacant lot, carefully printing the words, and just as meticulously drawing a picture of a home that might have existed in a small corner of her memory. It was a house without her in it, a place beyond the horizons of her reach, cold and distant and empty.

When I think of that child, and of all the children in California whose dreams are trampled by poverty, I wince at the dogged efforts of those who would deny them assistance in order to drive them away. The passage of Proposition 187 and attacks on welfare, affirmative action and free food programs burn with acrimony bordering on hatred toward the kinds of people who need help the most. Frustrated by

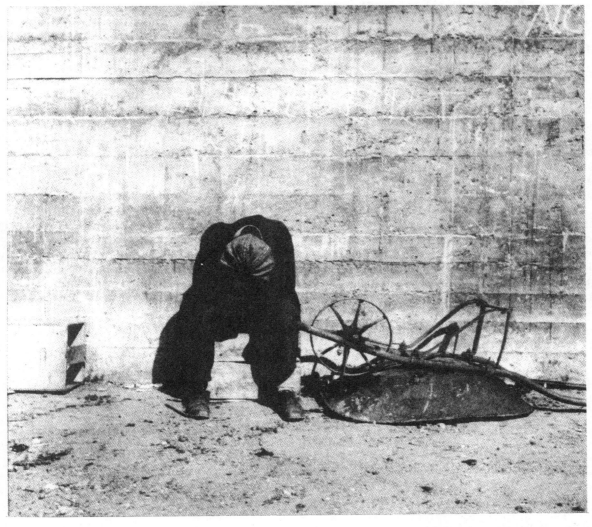

**Man Beside Wheelbarrow**

Dorothea Lange, San Francisco, 1934,
Courtesy of the Oakland Museum

growing tax burdens and crushing unemployment, we look around for someone to blame and place it on the shoulders of the poor, whether they are immigrants, the mentally ill we dumped into the streets when we stopped "warehousing" them, or those who forever wander in search of existence.

**P**overty isn't always a choice we make by reasons of indolence or the absence of skill. Sometimes it is thrust upon its victims when wars end, government contracts dry up and huge industries move away. We've seen the aerospace plants shut down and General Motors move and a recession-rooted downsizing of businesses from Yreka to San Diego. It all happened for reasons so complex that only a small percentage of the population even begins to understand them. We didn't deliberately add to the problem of poverty, and if you sat down with the guy next door you'd find he hates the idea of people being out of work and kids going hungry.

But poverty in the abstract is something else, and politicians can easily transform the homeless into bums and welfare recipients into leeches as they play upon the fears of a vast middle class to enhance their own positions on the political spectrum. We're going broke, they say, because bums refuse to work; we're going broke because Mexicans are taking our jobs; we're going broke because illegals are burdening our social systems and driving our taxes upward.

They find ready listeners, because many Californians stand a paycheck away from poverty themselves. The same University of California report that found five million Californians hungry found another 8.4 million at risk of being hungry. They're the working poor, to whom a layoff can mean disaster. I saw it happen when the General Motors plant shut down in Van Nuys and 26,000 employees were suddenly out of work. Unexpected illness can similarly wipe out a lifetime of building. I've seen that happen too among those who least expected it.

One of them was Liz McVey.

She was a successful woman in her mid-40s, a restaurateur and the owner of two private detective agencies. A graduate of Bryn Mawr, she was raised in a gray stone mansion in a wealthy section of Chester, Pennsylvania, and numbered the DuPonts among her schoolmates. She came to California in the mid-1950s as an Air Force comptroller, then, intrigued by detective work, earned a private investigator's license. By 1970, she owned two agencies. Such was the success of the agencies that within 10 years she had opened a pair of restaurants. Then the roof fell in.

Business setbacks were followed by a bad fall, followed by a series of illness that kept her hospitalized for seven months. Without medical insurance, her savings disappeared. Lacking the ability to function, her businesses failed. If it is true we are all fate's children, she was selected for punishment beyond reason.

Once out of the hospital, she remained on medication for asthma and diabetes. When I saw her, she was still on oxygen and bedbound. She had no money for food or rent and was about to be evicted from the small Hollywood apartment she occupied alone. "I always wondered why homeless people couldn't just pull themselves up by the bootstraps," she said to me. "I guess I'll find out."

As it turned out, McVey was helped by friends and ultimately gained enough public assistance to get her back on her feet. But this was a university graduate who finally could figure out how to work her way through a maze of bureaucracies to get the help she needed to keep her off the streets. This was a woman with friends.

The five million people in California who live below the poverty level lack the mental resources McVey had. There are damned few university graduates among them, and no friends to extend helping hands. We are their friends. We are their resources. If the California Dream, already blurred, is not to end up as a nightmare, we've got to stop ignoring the armies of despair that occupy our state, and, even more urgently, stop attempting to deprive them of the little they receive from us.

I keep coming back to that Thanksgiving almost 60 years ago and the feelings of hopelessness and despair that poverty created; they are an indelible part of my soul. And I keep coming back to the children of poverty, because by the year 2000 they will be one-third of all the children in California. I grew up in an age relatively free of an inclination toward street violence and found avenues for my rage that were socially acceptable. But this is a different world, a different state, a place that bristles with new armaments and new hatreds, and I can't help but wonder how the anger in the bellies of the children, the sad and hungry kids in the shadows, will react when they're grown up enough to let us know how they feel. I hear thunder in the distance, and wonder when the storm will arrive.

UNICEF Report Says Malnutrition Kills Millions Each Year

# Hunger Plagues Children

**The report says half the children in South Asia and a third of the children in sub-Saharan Africa suffer from malnutrition.**

*By Joseph Schuman*
**The Associated Press**

PARIS, Dec. 16—Malnutrition kills between 6 million and 7 million children every year, and leaves millions more stunted both physically and intellectually, UNICEF said today. Hunger—which is now more lethal than any disease since the bubonic plague—isn't confined to the developing world, said the organization's annual "State of the World's Children" report.

## U.S. Does Not Fare Well

An estimated 13 million children in the United States, or one in four children under 12, do not get enough food, the report said.

"It tends to be worse at the end of the month, when people's paychecks run out," said Carol Bellamy, executive director of the United Nations Children's Fund. Bellamy added that one-sixth of U.S. children are born into poverty—a higher proportion than in any other industrialized nation.

In developing nations, malnutrition is even more endemic. Half the children in South Asia suffer from it, as well as a third of children in sub-Saharan Africa. "Those malnourished children who do survive often don't grow well," Bellamy said. "They have more frequent and severe bouts of illness. They are at high risk and have very bad intellectual development." The report paints a devastating picture of children left without access to enough food, vitamins and minerals they need to develop.

## Some of the Report's Findings

Anemia in infancy and early childhood, brought on by a lack of iron, can lower a child's IQ by about nine points. It also contributes to more than 20 percent of all postpartum deaths of mothers in Africa and Asia.

• A lack of iodine in the diets of pregnant mothers can cause "profound mental retardation" in their children.

• Vitamin A deficiency, affecting about 100 million young children worldwide, can cause blindness and impair immune systems. It reduces resistance to diarrhea, which kills 2.2 million children a year.

• By stunting growth, malnutrition leaves a child open to countless other risks in adulthood. A study in Guatemala, for example, tied malnutrition to the deaths of women during childbirth, with shorter women at greater risk.

## The News Was Not All Bad

The percentage of malnourished children in Latin America has shrunk by half since 1970, from 20 percent to 10 percent, even though those countries have seen income levels rise only slightly in the past 27 years, Bellamy said.

And to fight iodine deficiency, more than 60 percent of the world's salt has been iodized, up from 12 percent five years ago.

"That's the best way for anyone to get the small amount of iodine they need," Bellamy said. She said such small changes are the most effective ways governments can fight malnutrition.

From http://www.abcnews.com, December 16, 1997. © 1997 by Associated Press. All rights reserved. Reprinted with permission.

# Glossary

**Absorption** The process by which digestive products pass from the gastrointestinal tract into the blood.

**Acid/base balance** The relationship between acidity and alkalinity in the body fluids.

**Amino acids** The structural units that make up proteins.

**Amylase** An enzyme that breaks down starches; a component of saliva.

**Amylopectin** A component of starch, consisting of many glucose units joined in branching patterns.

**Amylose** A component of starch, consisting of many glucose units joined in a straight chain, without branching.

**Anabolism** The synthesis of new materials for cellular growth, maintenance, or repair in the body.

**Anemia** A deficiency of oxygen-carrying material in the blood.

**Anorexia nervosa** A disorder in which a person refuses food and loses weight to the point of emaciation and even death.

**Antioxidant** A substance that prevents or delays the breakdown of other substances by oxygen; often added to food to retard deterioration and rancidity.

**Arachidonic acid** An essential polyunsaturated fatty acid.

**Arteriosclerosis** Condition characterized by a thickening and hardening of the walls of the arteries and a resultant loss of elasticity.

**Ascorbic acid** Vitamin C.

**Atherosclerosis** A type of arteriosclerosis in which lipids, especially cholesterol, accumulate in the arteries and obstruct blood flow.

**Avidin** A substance in raw egg white that acts as an antagonist of biotin, one of the B vitamins.

**Basal metabolic rate (BMR)** The rate at which the body uses energy for maintaining involuntary functions such as cellular activity, respiration, and heartbeat when at rest.

**Basic four** The food plan outlining the milk, meat, fruits and vegetables, and breads and cereals needed in the daily diet to provide the necessary nutrients.

**Beriberi** A disease resulting from inadequate thiamin in the diet.

**Beta-carotene** Yellow pigment that is converted to vitamin A in the body.

**Biotin** One of the B vitamins.

**Bomb calorimeter** An instrument that oxidizes food samples to measure their energy content.

**Buffer** A substance that can neutralize both acids and bases to minimize change in the pH of a solution.

**Calorie** The energy required to raise the temperature of one gram of water one degree Celsius.

**Carbohydrate** An organic compound composed of carbon, hydrogen, and oxygen in a ratio of 1:2:1.

**Carcinogen** A cancer-causing substance.

**Catabolism** The breakdown of complex substances into simpler ones.

**Celiac disease** A syndrome resulting from intestinal sensitivity to gluten, a protein substance of wheat flour especially and of other grains.

**Cellulose** An indigestible polysaccharide made of many glucose molecules.

**Cheilosis** Cracks at the corners of the mouth, due primarily to a deficiency of riboflavin in the diet.

**Cholesterol** A fat-like substance found only in animal products; important in many body functions but also implicated in heart disease.

**Choline** A substance that prevents the development of a fatty liver; frequently considered one of the B-complex vitamins.

**Chylomicron** A very small emulsified lipoprotein that transports fat in the blood.

**Cobalamin** One of the B vitamins (B$_{12}$).

**Coenzyme** A component of an enzyme system that facilitates the working of the enzyme.

**Collagen** Principal protein of connective tissue.

**Colostrum** The yellowish fluid that precedes breast milk, produced in the first few days of lactation.

**Cretinism** The physical and mental retardation of a child resulting from severe iodine or thyroid deficiency in the mother during pregnancy.

**Dehydration** Excessive loss of water from the body.

**Dextrin** Any of various small soluble polysaccharides found in the leaves of starch-forming plants and in the human alimentary canal as a product of starch digestion.

**Diabetes (diabetes mellitus)** A metabolic disorder characterized by excess blood sugar and urine sugar.

**Digestion** The breakdown of ingested foods into particles of a size and chemical composition that can be absorbed by the body.

**Diglyceride** A lipid containing glycerol and two fatty acids.

**Disaccharide** A sugar made up of two chemically combined monosaccharides, or simple sugars.

**Diuretics** Substances that stimulate urination.

**Diverticulosis** A condition in which the wall of the large intestine weakens and balloons out, forming pouches where fecal matter can be entrapped.

**Edema** The presence of an abnormally high amount of fluid in the tissues.

**Emulsifier** A substance that promotes the mixing of foods, such as oil and water in a salad dressing.

**Enrichment** The addition of nutrients to foods, often to restore what has been lost in processing.

**Enzyme** A protein that speeds up chemical reactions in the cell.

**Epidemiology** The study of the factors that contribute to the occurrence of a disease in a population.

**Essential amino acid** Any of the nine amino acids that the human body cannot manufacture and that must be supplied by the diet as they are necessary for growth and maintenance.

**Essential fatty acid** A fatty acid that the human body cannot manufacture and that must be supplied by the diet, as it is necessary for growth and maintenance.

**Fat** An organic compound whose molecules contain glycerol and fatty acids; fat insulates the body, protects organs, carries fat-soluble vitamins, is a constituent of cell membranes, and makes food taste good.

**Fatty acid** A simple lipid—containing only carbon, hydrogen, and oxygen—that is a constituent of fat.

**Ferritin** A substance in which iron, in combination with protein, is stored in the liver, spleen, and bone marrow.

**Fiber** Indigestible carbohydrate found primarily in plant foods; high fiber intake is useful in regulating bowel movements, and may lower the incidence of certain types of cancer and other diseases.

**Flavoprotein** Protein containing riboflavin.

**Folic acid (folacin)** One of the B vitamins.

**Fortification** The addition of nutrients to foods to enhance their nutritional values.

**Fructose** A six-carbon monosaccharide found in many fruits as well as honey and plant saps; one of two monosaccharides forming sucrose, or table sugar.

**Galactose** A six-carbon monosaccharide, one of the two that make up lactose, or milk sugar.

**Gallstones** An abnormal formation of gravel or stones, composed of cholesterol and bile salts and sometimes bile pigments, in the gallbladder; they result when substances that normally dissolve in bile precipitate out.

**Gastritis** Inflammation of the stomach.

**Glucagon** A hormone produced by the pancreas that works to increase blood glucose concentration.

**Glucose** A six-carbon monosaccharide found in sucrose, honey, and many fruits and vegetables; the major carbohydrate found in the body.

**Glucose tolerance factor (GTF)** A hormone-like substance containing chromium, niacin, and protein that helps the body to use glucose.

**Glyceride** A simple lipid composed of fatty acids and glycerol.

**Glycogen** The storage form of carbohydrates in the body; composed of glucose molecules.

**Goiter** Enlargement of the thyroid gland as a result of iodine deficiency.

**Goitrogens** Substances that induce goiter, often by interfering with the body's utilization of iodine.

**Heme** A complex iron–containing compound that is a component of hemoglobin.

**Hemicellulose** Any of various indigestible plant polysaccharides.

**Hemochromatosis** A disorder of iron metabolism.

**Hemoglobin** The iron-containing protein in red blood cells that carries oxygen to the tissues.

**High-density lipoprotein (HDL)** A lipoprotein that acts as a cholesterol carrier in the blood; referred to as "good" cholesterol because relatively high levels of it appear to protect against atherosclerosis.

**Hormones** Compounds secreted by the endocrine glands that influence the functioning of various organs.

**Humectants** Substances added to foods to help them maintain moistness.

**Hydrogenation** The chemical process by which hydrogen is added to unsaturated fatty acids, which saturates them and converts them from a liquid to a solid form.

**Hydrolyze** To split a chemical compound into smaller molecules by adding water.

**Hydroxyapatite** The hard mineral portion (the major constituent) of bone, composed of calcium and phosphate.

**Hypercalcemia** A high level of calcium in the blood.

**Hyperglycemia** A high level of "sugar" (glucose) in the blood.

**Hypocalcemia** A low level of calcium in the blood.

**Hypoglycemia** A low level of "sugar" (glucose) in the blood.

**Incomplete protein** A protein lacking or deficient in one or more of the essential amino acids.

**Inorganic** Describes a substance not containing carbon.

**Insensible loss** Fluid loss, through the skin and from the lungs, that an individual is unaware of.

**Insulin** A hormone produced by the pancreas that regulates the body's use of glucose.

**Intrinsic factor** A protein produced by the stomach that makes absorption of B12 possible; lack of this protein results in pernicious anemia.

**Joule** A unit of energy preferred by some professionals instead of the heat energy measurements of the calorie system for calculating food energy; sometimes referred to as "kilojoule."

**Keratinization** Formation of a protein called keratin, which, in vitamin A deficiency, occurs instead of mucus formation; leads to a drying and hardening of epithelial tissue.

**Ketogenic** Describes substances that can be converted to ketone bodies during metabolism, such as fatty acids and some amino acids.

**Ketone bodies** The three chemicals—acetone, acetoacetic acid, and betahydroxybutyrie—that are normally involved in lipid metabolism and accumulate in blood and urine in abnormal amounts in conditions of impaired metabolism (such as diabetes).

**Ketosis** A condition resulting when fats are the major source of energy and are incompletely oxidized, causing ketone bodies to build up in the bloodstream.

**Kilocalorie** One thousand calories, or the energy required to raise the temperature of one kilogram of water one degree Celsius; the preferred unit of measurement for food energy.

**Kilojoule** *See* Joule.

**Kwashiorkor** A form of malnutrition resulting from a diet severely deficient in protein but high in carbohydrates.

**Lactase** A digestive enzyme produced by the small intestine that breaks down lactose.

**Lactation** Milk production/secretion.

**Lacto-ovo-vegetarian** A person who does not eat meat, poultry, or fish but does eat milk products and eggs.

**Lactose** A disaccharide composed of glucose and galactose and found in milk.

**Lactose intolerance** The inability to digest lactose due to a lack of the enzyme lactase in the intestine.

**Lacto-vegetarian** A person who does not eat meat, poultry, fish, or eggs but does drink milk and eat milk products.

**Laxatives** Food or drugs that stimulate bowel movements.

**Lignins** Certain forms of indigestible carbohydrate in plant foods.

**Linoleic acid** An essential polyunsaturated fatty acid.

**Lipase** An enzyme that digests fats.

**Lipid** Any of various substances in the body or in food that are insoluble in water; a fat or fat-like substance.

**Lipoprotein** Compound composed of a lipid (fat) and a protein that transports both in the bloodstream.

**Low-density lipoprotein (LDL)** A lipoprotein that acts as a cholesterol carrier in the blood; referred to as "bad" cholesterol because relatively high levels of it appear to enhance atherosclerosis.

**Macrocytic anemia** A form of anemia characterized by the presence of abnormally large blood cells.

**Macroelements (also macronutrient elements)** Those elements present in the body in amounts exceeding 0.005 percent of body weight and required in the diet in amounts exceeding 100 mg/day; include sodium, potassium, calcium, and phosphorus.

**Malnutrition** A poor state of health resulting from a lack, excess, or imbalance of the nutrients needed by the body.

**Maltose** A disaccharide whose units are each composed of two glucose molecules, produced by the digestion of starch.

**Marasmus** Condition resulting from a deficiency of calories and nearly all essential nutrients.

**Melanin** A dark pigment in the skin, hair, and eyes.

**Metabolism** The sum of all chemical reactions that take place within the body.

**Microelements (also micronutrient elements; trace elements)** Those elements present in the body in amounts under 0.005 percent of body weight and required in the diet in amounts under 100 mg/day.

**Monoglyceride** A lipid containing glycerol and only one fatty acid.

**Monosaccharide** A single sugar molecule, the simplest form of carbohydrate; examples are glucose, fructose, and galactose.

**Monosodium glutamate (MSG)** An amino acid used in flavoring foods, which causes allergic reactions in some people.

**Monounsaturated fatty acid** A fatty acid containing one double bond.

**Mutagen** A mutation-causing agent.

**Negative nitrogen balance** Nitrogen output exceeds nitrogen intake.

**Niacin (nicotinic acid)** One of the B vitamins.

**Nitrogen equilibrium (zero nitrogen balance)** Nitrogen output equals nitrogen intake.

**Nonessential amino acid** Any of the 13 amino acids that the body can manufacture in adequate amounts, but which are nonetheless required in the diet in an amount relative to the amount of essential amino acids.

**Nutrients** Nourishing substances in food that can be digested, absorbed, and metabolized by the body; needed for growth, maintenance, and reproduction.

**Nutrition** (1) The sum of the processes by which an organism obtains, assimilates, and utilizes food. (2) The scientific study of these processes.

**Obesity** Condition of being 15 to 20 percent above one's ideal body weight.

**Oleic acid** A monounsaturated fatty acid.

**Organic foods** Those foods, especially fruits and vegetables, grown without the use of pesticides, synthetic fertilizers, etc.

**Osmosis** Passage of a solvent through a semipermeable membrane from an area of higher concentration to an area of lower concentration until the concentration is equal on both sides of the membrane.

**Osteomalacia** Condition in which a loss of bone mineral leads to a softening of the bones; adult counterpart of rickets.

**Osteoporosis** Disorder in which the bones degenerate due to a loss of bone mineral, producing porosity and fragility; normally found in older women.

**Overweight** Body weight exceeding an accepted norm by 10 or 15 percent.

**Ovo-vegetarian** A person who does not eat meat, poultry, fish, milk, or milk products but does eat eggs.

**Oxidation** The process by which a substrate takes up oxygen or loses hydrogen; the loss of electrons.

**Palmitic acid** A saturated fatty acid.

**Pantothenic acid** One of the B vitamins.

**Pellagra** Niacin deficiency syndrome, characterized by dementia, diarrhea, and dermatitis.

**Pepsin** A protein-digesting enzyme produced by the stomach.

**Peptic ulcer** An open sore or erosion in the lining of the digestive tract, especially in the stomach and duodenum.

**Peptide** A compound composed of amino acids that are joined together.

**Peristalsis** Motions of the digestive tract that propel food through the tract.

**Pernicious anemia** One form of anemia caused by an inability to absorb vitamin B12, owing to the absense of intrinsic factor.

**pH** A measure of the acidity of a solution, based on a scale from 0 to 14: a pH of 7 is neutral; greater than 7 is alkaline; less than 7 is acidic.

**Phenylketonuria (PKU)** A genetic disease in which phenylalanine, an essential amino acid, is not properly metabolized, thus accumulating in the blood and causing early brain damage.

**Phospholipid** A fat containing phosphorus, glycerol, two fatty acids, and any of several other chemical substances.

**Polypeptide** A molecular chain of amino acids.

**Polysaccharide** A carbohydrate containing many monosaccharide subunits.

**Polyunsaturated fatty acids** A fatty acid in which two or more carbon atoms have formed double bonds, with each holding only one hydrogen atom.

**Positive nitrogen balance** Condition in which nitrogen intake exceeds nitrogen output in the body.

**Protein** Any of the organic compounds composed of amino acids and containing nitrogen; found in the cells of all living organisms.

**Provitamins** Precursors of vitamins that can be converted to vitamins in the body (e.g., beta-carotene, from which the body can make vitamin A).

**Pyridoxine** One of the B vitamins (B6).

**Pull date** Date after which food should no longer be sold but still may be edible for several days.

**Recommended Daily Allowances (RDAs)** Standards for daily intake of specific nutrients established by the Food and Nutrition Board of the National Academy of Sciences; they are the levels thought to be adequate to maintain the good health of most people.

**Rhodopsin** The visual pigment in the retinal rods of the eyes which allows one to see at night; its formation requires vitamin A.

**Riboflavin** One of the B vitamins (B2).

**Ribosome** The cellular structure in which protein synthesis occurs.

**Rickets** The vitamin D deficiency disease in children characterized by bone softening and deformities.

**Saliva** Fluid produced in the mouth that helps food digestion.

**Salmonella** A bacterium that can cause food poisoning.

**Saturated fatty acid** A fatty acid in which carbon is joined with four other atoms; i.e., all carbon atoms are bound to the maximum possible number of hydrogen atoms.

**Scurvy** A disease characterized by bleeding gums, pain in joints, lethargy, and other problems; caused by a deficiency of vitamin C (ascorbic acid).

**Standard of identity** A list of specifications for the manufacture of certain foods that stipulates their required contents.

**Starch** A polysaccharide composed of glucose molecules; the major form in which energy is stored in plants.

**Stearic acid** A saturated fatty acid.

**Sucrose** A disaccharide composed of glucose and fructose, often called "table sugar."

**Sulfites** Agents used as preservatives in foods to eliminate bacteria, preserve freshness, prevent browning, and increase storage life; can cause acute asthma attacks, and even death, in people who are sensitive to them.

**Teratogen** An agent with the potential of causing birth defects.

**Thiamin** One of the B vitamins (B1).

**Thyroxine** Hormone containing iodine that is secreted by the thyroid gland.

**Toxemia** A complication of pregnancy characterized by high blood pressure, edema, vomiting, presence of protein in the urine, and other symptoms.

**Transferrin** A protein compound, the form in which iron is transported in the blood.

**Triglyceride** A lipid containing glycerol and three fatty acids.

**Trypsin** A digestive enzyme, produced in the pancreas, that breaks down protein.

**Underweight** Body weight below an accepted norm by more than 10 percent.

**United States Recommended Daily Allowance (USRDA)** The highest level of recommended intakes for population groups (except pregnant and lactating women); derived from the RDAs and used in food labeling.

**Urea** The main nitrogenous component of urine, resulting from the breakdown of amino acids.

**Uremia** A disease in which urea accumulates in the blood.

**Vegan** A person who eats nothing derived from an animal; the strictest type of vegetarian.

**Vitamin** Organic substance required by the body in small amounts to perform numerous functions.

**Vitamin B complex** All known water-soluble vitamins except C; includes thiamin (B1), riboflavin (B2), pyridoxine (B6), niacin, folic acid, cobalamin (B12), pantothenic acid, and biotin.

**Xerophthalmia** A disease of the eye resulting from vitamin A deficiency.

# AE Article Review Form

We encourage you to photocopy and use this page as a tool to assess how the articles in **Annual Editions** expand on the information in your textbook. By reflecting on the articles you will gain enhanced text information. You can also access this useful form on a product's book support Web site at **http://www.dushkin.com/ online/.**

NAME: _____ DATE: _____

TITLE AND NUMBER OF ARTICLE: _____

BRIEFLY STATE THE MAIN IDEA OF THIS ARTICLE: _____

LIST THREE IMPORTANT FACTS THAT THE AUTHOR USES TO SUPPORT THE MAIN IDEA:




WHAT INFORMATION OR IDEAS DISCUSSED IN THIS ARTICLE ARE ALSO DISCUSSED IN YOUR TEXTBOOK OR OTHER READINGS THAT YOU HAVE DONE? LIST THE TEXTBOOK CHAPTERS AND PAGE NUMBERS:




LIST ANY EXAMPLES OF BIAS OR FAULTY REASONING THAT YOU FOUND IN THE ARTICLE:




LIST ANY NEW TERMS/CONCEPTS THAT WERE DISCUSSED IN THE ARTICLE, AND WRITE A SHORT DEFINITION

ANNUAL EDITIONS revisions depend on two major opinion sources: one is our Advisory Board, listed in the front of this volume, which works with us in scanning the thousands of articles published in the public press each year; the other is you—the person actually using the book. Please help us and the users of the next edition by completing the prepaid article rating form on this page and returning it to us. Thank you for your help!

## ANNUAL EDITIONS: Nutrition 99/00

### ARTICLE RATING FORM

Here is an opportunity for you to have direct input into the next revision of this volume. We would like you to rate each of the 65 articles listed below, using the following scale:

1. **Excellent: should definitely be retained**
2. **Above average: should probably be retained**
3. **Below average: should probably be deleted**
4. **Poor: should definitely be deleted**

Your ratings will play a vital part in the next revision. So please mail this prepaid form to us just as soon as you complete it. Thanks for your help!

**RATING**

**ARTICLE**

1. "What We Eat in America" Survey
2. Are Reduced-Fat Foods Keeping Americans Healthier?
3. Low-Calorie Sweeteners: Adding Reduced-Calorie Delights to a Healthful Diet
4. Are Fruits and Vegetables Less Nutritious Today?
5. The Freshness Fallacy
6. The Truth about Organic 'Certification'
7. Clearing up Common Misconceptions about Vegetarianism
8. Doing the DRIs
9. An FDA Guide to Dietary Supplements
10. Fruits and Vegetables: Nature's Best Protection
11. Are You Getting Enough Fat?
12. Trans Fat: Another Artery Clogger?
13. A 'Bran-New' Look at Dietary Fiber
14. Food for Thought about Dietary Supplements
15. Vitamin Supplements
16. Vitamin E Supplements: To E or Not to E?
17. Do You Need More Minerals?
18. Making the Most of Calcium: Factors Affecting Calcium Metabolism
19. How Important Is Salt Restriction?
20. Fighting Cancer with Food
21. Most Frequently Asked Questions . . . about Diet and Cancer
22. Heart Association Dietary Guidelines
23. Answering Nine of Your Cholesterol Questions
24. Evidence Mounts for Heart Disease Marker
25. New Blood Pressure Guidelines Emphasize Nutrition
26. Smarten Up: Certain Foods Help Maintain Brain Power as You Age
27. When Eating Goes Awry: An Update on Eating Disorders
28. Food Allergy Myths and Realities
29. Physical Activity and Nutrition
30. Alcohol and Health: Straight Talk on the Medical Headlines
31. Guidelines Call More Americans Overweight
32. Body Mass Index and Mortality

**RATING**

**ARTICLE**

33. Obesity and the Brain
34. What It Takes to Take Off Weight (and Keep It Off)
35. The Skinny on Weight Loss
36. Several Small Meals Keep Off Body Fat Better than One or Two Large Ones
37. Winnowing Weight-Loss Programs to Find a Match for You
38. "Natural" Therapeutics for Weight Loss: Garden of Slender Delights or Dangerous Alchemy?
39. The History of Dieting and Its Effectiveness
40. Congress Asked to Take Eating Disorders Seriously
41. Binge Eating
42. Dysfunctional Eating: A New Concept
43. Foodborne Illness: Role of Home Food Handling Practices
44. New Risks in Ground Beef Revealed
45. Why You Need a Kitchen Thermometer
46. For Safety's Sake: Scrub Your Produce
47. Mad Cows and Americans
48. Irradiation: A Safe Measure for Safer Food
49. Codex: Protecting Consumers' Health and Facilitating International Trade
50. Twenty-Five Ways to Spot Quacks and Vitamin Pushers
51. How Quackery Sells
52. Yet Another Study—Should You Pay Attention?
53. How to Spot a "Quacky" Web Site
54. Alternative Medicine—The Risks of Untested and Unregulated Remedies
55. The 'Dietary Supplement' Mess
56. Minding Your Memory with Ginkgo?
57. Ephedrine's Deadly Edge
58. Hard Facts on Colloidal Minerals
59. Can Nutrition Cure ADHD?
60. Don't Buy Phony 'Ergogenic Aids'
61. The Unethical Behavior of Pharmacists
62. Winning the Food Race
63. It's Not Called a Famine, but Thousands Starve
64. Thunder in the Distance
65. Hunger Plagues Children

(Continued on next page)

**We Want Your Advice**

NO POSTA
NECESSA
IF MAILE
IN THE
UNITED STA

## BUSINESS REPLY MAIL
FIRST-CLASS MAIL  PERMIT NO. 84  GUILFORD CT

POSTAGE WILL BE PAID BY ADDRESSEE

**Dushkin/McGraw-Hill
Sluice Dock
Guilford, CT 06437-9989**

---

## ABOUT YOU

Name                                                          Date

Are you a teacher? ☐  A student? ☐
Your school's name

Department

Address                                      City                         State      Zip

School telephone #

## YOUR COMMENTS ARE IMPORTANT TO US !

Please fill in the following information:
For which course did you use this book?

Did you use a text with this *ANNUAL EDITION*? ☐ yes ☐ no
What was the title of the text?

What are your general reactions to the *Annual Editions* concept?

Have you read any particular articles recently that you think should be included in the next edition?

Are there any articles you feel should be replaced in the next edition? Why?

Are there any World Wide Web sites you feel should be included in the next edition? Please annotate.

May we contact you for editorial input? ☐ yes ☐ no
May we quote your comments? ☐ yes ☐ no